IMMUNITY AGAINST ANIMAL PARASITES

IMMUNITY AGAINST ANIMAL PARASITES

By JAMES T. CULBERTSON

ASSISTANT PROFESSOR OF BACTERIOLOGY
COLLEGE OF PHYSICIANS AND SURGEONS
COLUMBIA UNIVERSITY

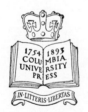

NEW YORK : MORNINGSIDE HEIGHTS

COLUMBIA UNIVERSITY PRESS

1941

PREFACE

IN PRESENTING this volume the author hopes to supply a text
which will be of value to those just beginning the study of immunity to the parasitic forms, by acquainting them with the fundamental principles of the subject as now understood. He wishes also
to aid those who are more experienced, through orienting and col-
lating the voluminous and heterogeneous recent literature dealing
with immunity in parasitic infection. He has therefore treated the
available material in the manner which he deems will prove most
useful to the beginning student, the trained investigator, and the
practicing physician or veterinarian. Personal concepts and the-
ories, both of the author and of others, are held to a minimum—in
fact they are wholly avoided unless supported by experimental
data. Some arbitrary preferences in viewpoint are acknowledged,
but these are few and generally of such limited significance as to
have but little influence on the utility of the book as a whole.

The reader is assumed to be well trained in the two subjects:
parasitology and immunology. Hence no elementary delineation is
given either of parasite life history or of general principles of immunity. To have done so would have required a much larger volume than this and the restatement of much that is already available
in many excellent textbooks in the separate fields of parasitology
and immunology.

The author desires to express his indebtedness to the many investigators, including his students and others with whom he has
collaborated, whose researches form the basis of this book, and he
hopes that without exception he has stated their results accurately
and with correct interpretation. He wishes also to acknowledge the
inspiration which has come to him from certain men long prominent in the field with whom he has had occasional contact. Most

especially among these are Professor W. H. Taliaferro, of the University of Chicago, Professor W. W. Cort, of The Johns Hopkins University, and Professor J. E. Ackert, of Kansas State College of Agriculture and Applied Science, who both personally and through their many students have contributed so largely to the subject. Mention should also be made of Dr. N. H. Fairley and Professor R. T. Leiper, of the London School of Hygiene and Tropical Medicine, Professor R. Matheson, of Cornell University, and Professor H. W. Stunkard, of New York University, under all of whom the author was privileged briefly to study.

Special thanks must go to the John Simon Guggenheim Memorial Foundation, which supported some of the author's own studies which are referred to in the text. The author is also indebted specifically to Professor W. H. Taliaferro for Figure 2 and Chart III, to Dr. M. P. Sarles for Figure 1, to Drs. L. T. Coggeshall and H. W. Kumm for Chart II, and to Dr. H. M. Miller, Jr., for Figure 3, which have been included. Finally, grateful acknowledgment is made to the author's wife, Louise Barber Culbertson, who encouraged him to undertake the writing of this volume, to Professors A. R. Dochez and C. W. Jungeblut, of the Department of Bacteriology of Columbia University, who read parts of the manuscript, and to Mr. Lee Morrison and Miss Ida M. Lynn, of the Columbia University Press, who carefully edited the manuscript.

JAMES T. CULBERTSON

Columbia University
July 2, 1941

CONTENTS

CONTENTS

Part Three

APPLIED IMMUNOLOGY

ILLUSTRATIONS

CHARTS AND TABLES

CHARTS

TABLES

IMMUNITY AGAINST
ANIMAL PARASITES

Chapter I

INTRODUCTION

THE PRESENCE of a parasite in a host is the resultant of many forces. Through some of these the parasite seeks to establish itself upon, or even to overwhelm, the host. Through others the host seeks to eradicate the parasite or at least to check its ravages. In order to survive together, both the parasite and the host must make many mutual adjustments. Each must protect itself from the other, and each must carry on its essential life processes in spite of the presence of the other.

The various modes of resistance which a host offers to invasion represent forces which the parasite must be able to contend with before it can hope for prolonged residence in that host. The capacity of a host to resist a given parasite is sometimes the natural endowment of that host species and completely protects the host throughout its life against that parasite. Usually, this natural resistance is, not a specific quality, but one exerted equally and with similar effect upon a variety of parasites. Such natural resistance is not always enjoyed from birth, but it sometimes is developed to certain parasites only after the host has grown older—possibly even after it has reached maturity. Young individuals, then, are often readily susceptible to parasites which cannot infect older hosts. As these susceptible young individuals reach the resistant age, they frequently expel such of the parasites as they then harbor.

To some parasites, on the other hand, the host never becomes naturally resistant and remains susceptible to infection on initial exposure so long as it lives. As a result of a first exposure, however, forces distinct from those responsible for natural resistance are set in motion by the host which generally enable it to check the progress of the parasite and sometimes cause the parasite to leave the host. Usually these forces are less powerful than those which account for natural resistance, but they are at the same time more specific in action upon the parasites. Furthermore, a host in which such specific forces have once been stimulated is likely to remain immune to that parasite, since it is able thereafter to call forth the same forces again when invasion by the same parasite threatens.

It is exclusively with these matters of natural resistance and acquired immunity against the animal parasites that this book will deal. In many respects the fundamental principles which apply in the case of the parasites apply equally with respect to bacteria, spirochetes, filterable viruses, and other infectious agents. Similar variation among different host species is observed in susceptibility to all these forms. Furthermore, after infection the same humoral and cellular defense forces are called into play by the host, whether the infecting agent is an animal parasite or of different nature, and these same defense forces protect the host against subsequent reinfection with all. Moreover, vaccination with the antigens of a parasite or the administration of an immune serum will often protect normal animals from the parasites, as is true also in other infections. Finally, the existence of a parasitic infection can sometimes be proved by demonstrating antibodies in the blood serum or by performing skin tests, these methods of diagnosis having the same relative specificity with parasitic diseases which they have in infections with other agents. As complete information becomes available, it appears more and more probable that no fundamental differences exist in the character of the immune responses to the parasites and to other agents of disease. Indeed, the essentially gross similarities which have just been pointed out and which will be amplified in the succeeding pages of this book suggest the identity of the governing principles.

HISTORY OF IMMUNITY AGAINST PARASITIC INFECTION

The first clear demonstration of an acquired immunity to animal parasites was reported in 1893 by Theobald Smith and F. L. Kilbourne,[1] who showed that recovery from one attack of Texas fever conferred immunity to cattle against subsequent attacks of the same disease. In 1899 the rat was shown to acquire immunity by

[1] T. Smith and F. L. Kilbourne, Bur. Animal Industry (U. S. Dept. Agri.), *Bull.* No. 1, pp. 1–301 (1893).

recovery from an initial infection with its natural blood parasite *Trypanosoma lewisi*.[2] These two observations represent practically all that was known of the specific immunity to animal parasites at the dawn of the twentieth century. In the years since, however, nearly all the significant parasites of man and of domesticated animals have been studied from the immunological point of view, and a large store of knowledge has been accumulated.

The history of immunity to parasitic infections during the first three decades of the twentieth century is chiefly concerned with the development of tests for the diagnosis of the various infections of man and of domesticated animals. Eminent success has been attained in some diseases, particularly with the somatic helminthiases. A complement fixation test for echinococcus disease was developed as early as 1906,[3] and a precipitin test was reported the next year.[4] A delayed type of skin test was devised for the same infection in 1911,[5] and an immediate type in 1921.[6] For schistosomiasis a fixation test was reported in 1910,[7] a skin test in 1927,[8] and a precipitin test in 1928.[9] Precipitin[10] and skin tests[11] for trichiniasis were described in 1928, and a complement fixation test the following year.[12] Skin tests were reported for ascariasis in 1924,[13] for strongyloidiasis[14] in 1925, and for filariasis[15] in 1930:

Somewhat less was done with immunological tests in the diagnosis of protozoan diseases, although in a few instances fair success was reported. Agglutination and precipitation tests for human leishmaniasis[16] were developed by 1913, and a complement fixa-

[2] L. Rabinowitsch and W. Kempner, *Ztschr. f. Hyg. u. Infektionskr.*, 30: 251 (1899).

[3] G. Ghedini, *Gazz. d. osp.*, 27: 1616 (1906).

[4] C. Fleig and M. Lisbonne, *Compt. rend. Soc. de biol.*, 62: 1198 (1907).

[5] T. Casoni, *Folia clin., chim., et micr.*, 4: 5 (1911–12).

[6] T. B. Magath, *M. Clin. North America*, 5: 549 (1921).

[7] M. Yoshimoto, *Ztschr. f. Immunitätsforsch. u. exper. Therap.*, 5: 438 (1910).

[8] N. H. Fairley and F. E. Williams, *M. J. Australia*, 2: 811 (1927).

[9] S. Miyaji and B. Imai, *Centralbl. f. Bakt.*, 106: 237 (1928) ; W. H. Taliaferro, W. A. Hoffman, and D. H. Cook, *J. Prevent. Med.*, 2: 395 (1928).

[10] G. W. Bachman, *J. Prevent. Med.*, 2: 35 (1928).

[11] *Ibid.*, pp. 169, 513 (1928).

[12] G. W. Bachman and P. E. Menendez, *J. Prevent. Med.*, 3: 471 (1929).

[13] B. H. Ransom, W. T. Harrison, and J. F. Couch, *J. Agric. Res.*, 28: 577 (1924).

[14] F. Fülleborn, *Klin. Wchnschr.*, 4: 1709 (1925).

[15] W. H. Taliaferro and W. A. Hoffman, *J. Prevent. Med.*, 4: 261 (1930).

[16] G. di Cristina, *Pathologica*, 3: 399 (1911) ; G. Caronia, *Ztschr. f. Immunitätsforsch. u. exper. Therap.*, 20: 174 (1913).

tion test for animal trypanosomiasis [17] in the same year. A precipitin test for amoebiasis of the cat [18] was described in 1924, and a
fixation test of much greater utility for the human disease [19] in
1927. A fixation test for rabbit coccidiosis [20] was devised in 1930.
Positive fixation tests were reported in human malaria as early as
1913,[21] and a precipitin test was described for the same disease in
1928.[22]

Compared with the tremendous volume of practical work on the
diagnosis of infection, other contributions on immunity to animal
parasites in the first thirty years of the twentieth century appear
rather small. Nevertheless, many different aspects of the subject
were investigated, some with notable success. For example, it
was clearly shown that at least a partial immunity to reinfection
was acquired through recovery from various parasitic diseases.
This was fairly well established experimentally in cutaneous
leishmaniasis of man by 1910,[23] in infections with the pathogenic
trypanosomes in animals by 1911,[24] and in a number of the animal
piroplasmoses by 1912.[25] In 1912 birds were shown to acquire an
immunity to bird malaria.[26] Even before this man was suspected
likewise to develop immunity to the human malarias,[27] although
convincing evidence for it was not forthcoming till much later.[28]
In 1925 it was shown that fowls build up an immunity to coccidiosis.[29]

The acquisition of immunity to certain helminths was also
clearly proved. In 1916 horses and calves were shown to acquire
immunity to *Schistosoma japonicum*.[30] An acquired immunity was

[17] J. Mohler, A. Eichhorn, and J. Buck, *J. Agric. Res.*, 1: 99 (1913).
[18] E. H. Wagener, *Univ. California Publ., Zoology*, 26: 15 (1924).
[19] C. F. Craig, *Am. J. Trop. Med.*, 7: 225 (1927).
[20] G. W. Bachman, *Am. J. Hyg.*, 12: 624 (1930).
[21] A. Gasbarrini, *Ztschr. f. Immunitätsforsch. u. exper. Therap.*, 20: 178 (1913).
[22] W. H. Taliaferro and L. G. Taliaferro, *J. Prevent. Med.*, 2: 147 (1928).
[23] C. Nicolle and L. Manceaux, *Ann. Inst. Past.*, 24: 673 (1910).
[24] A. Laveran, *Compt. rend. Acad. de Sc.*, 152: 63 (1911).
[25] K. Wölfel, *Ztschr. f. Infektionskr.*, 12: 247 (1912); A. Theiler, *Ztschr. f. Infektionskr.*, 11: 193 (1912).
[26] J. Moldovan, *Centralbl. f. Bakt.*, 66: 105 (1912).
[27] R. Koch, *Ztschr. f. Hyg. u. Infektionskr.*, 32: 1 (1899).
[28] J. E. Nicole and J. P. Steel, *J. Trop. Med.*, 28: 428 (1925).
[29] J. R. Beach and J. C. Corl, *Poult. Sci.*, 4: 92 (1925).
[30] A. Fujinami, *China M. J.*, 31: 81 (1916). Reviewed by R. G. Mills.

demonstrated in trichiniasis of rats in 1921,[31] in strongyloidiasis of dogs and cats in 1928,[32] and in *Haemonchus* infection of sheep in the same year.[33] Convincing evidence of acquired immunity in rats to somatic cestodes was presented in 1930.[34] Relatively little evidence for the acquisition of immunity to arthropods, however, was obtained up to 1930. Nevertheless, the guinea pig was shown in 1923 to acquire an immunity to somatic myiasis.[35]

Various special antibodies of the normal and of the immune serum were discovered. The normal serum of man and of some apes was shown as early as 1902 to be destructive for certain trypanosomes pathogenic for animals.[36] A similar property was described in the serum of sheep effective upon *Trypanosoma duttoni* of the mouse.[37] A highly specialized type of antibody called an ablastin, which is acquired by certain rodents to their natural trypanosomes and which inhibits the reproduction of these parasites in the infected animal, was described in 1924.[38] Beginnings were also made in the classification of parasites by immunological methods, particularly the trypanosomes,[39] leishmanias,[40] and the coccidia,[41] among protozoans, and the ascarids [42] among the helminths. The significance of the age of the host in natural resistance was recognized, particularly in infections with some of the nematodes.[43] The influence of such factors as the vitamins and other elements of the diet upon natural resistance to the helminths was also suggested.[44]

The study of immunity in the parasitic infections took its first

[31] R. Ducas, *L'immunité dans la trichinose*, Thèse, Paris, Jouve et Cie., 1921, p. 47.
[32] J. H. Sandground, *Am. J. Hyg.*, 8: 507 (1928).
[33] N. R. Stoll, *J. Parasitol.*, 15: 147 (1928).
[34] H. M. Miller, Jr., *Proc. Soc. Exper. Biol. & Med.*, 27: 926 (1930).
[35] D. B. Blacklock and M. G. Thompson, *Ann. Trop. Med.*, 17: 443 (1923).
[36] A. Laveran, *Compt. rend. Acad. d. sc.*, 134: 735 (1902).
[37] A. Thiroux, *Compt. rend. Acad. d. sc.*, 149: 534 (1909).
[38] W. H. Taliaferro, *J. Exper. Med.*, 39: 171 (1924).
[39] A. Laveran and F. Mesnil, *Compt. rend. Acad. d. sc.*, 140: 831 (1905).
[40] H. Noguchi, *Proc. Internat. Conf. Health Prob. in Trop. America,* United Fruit Company, Boston, 1924, p. 455.
[41] E. E. Tyzzer, *Am. J. Hyg.*, 10: 269 (1929).
[42] B. Schwartz, *J. Parasitol.*, 6: 115 (1920) ; L. Hektoen, *J. Infect. Dis.*, 39: 342 (1926).
[43] A. Looss, *Records of Egypt. Gov't. Med. School,* Cairo, 4: 163 (1911) ; C. A. Herrick, *Am. J. Hyg.*, 6: 153 (1925).
[44] J. E. Ackert, M. L. Fisher, and N. B. Zimmerman, *J. Parasitol.*, 13: 219 (1927).

form and direction with the publication of W. H. Taliaferro's valued book, *The Immunology of Parasitic Infections,*[45] in 1929. No history of the subject would be complete without specific reference to this volume. It is the most important source book available in the field, for nearly all the significant papers which appeared before its publication are there referred to, and many of them are fully analyzed. Furthermore, it is responsible more than any other book for the vast number of studies done in the years since it appeared, for it pointed the way to new workers by indicating where additional investigation was needed. The present volume has adopted Taliaferro's book, in a manner, as its point of departure. Only very few of the many references here cited antedate 1929. For most of the literature preceding that year the reader must refer to the Taliaferro monograph. An effort has been made, however, in the present book to cite all the significant studies of the twelve years since 1929. It is hoped and believed that these citations will prove useful to the audience for which this book is designed.

[45] W. H. Taliaferro, *The Immunology of Parasitic Infections,* New York, Century, 1929.

Part One

NATURAL RESISTANCE AND ACQUIRED IMMUNITY

Chapter II

NATURAL RESISTANCE

ALL ANIMALS are more or less constantly exposed to natural infection by a wide variety of parasites. The limits of exposure and potential infection of an animal are largely contingent upon its geographical distribution and the character and variety of the activities in which it is engaged. The kinds of food it utilizes, its habits in procuring food, its capacity to swim or to burrow through earth, and its associations with other animals all govern what types of parasite a given host will have.

A parasite can be expected to develop in any host which supplies an adequate physiological environment, provided the parasite is equipped to contact that host.[1] Favorable physiological conditions are usually provided best by the natural host or its near relatives. Often, however, even in certain remotely related host species no physiologically antagonistic conditions are met, and the parasite may grow well if it enters such forms. The absence of antagonistic factors in the host explains many of the sporadic cases of infection with unnatural parasites occasionally seen in man and animals. Such sporadic infections are rare, however, since commonly animals are utterly intolerant of the parasites of physiologically distantly related hosts.[2]

No species of animal is susceptible to all parasites, and no parasite is able to infect all hosts. In fact, only a limited number of parasite species can regularly establish themselves in a given host, and most parasites infect comparatively few closely related hosts. In some extreme cases only a single species of host is susceptible to infection by a given parasite.

Natural resistance must not, however, be confused with mere

[1] E. R. Becker, *Am. J. Trop. Med.*, 13: 505 (1933).
[2] W. T. M. Cameron, *Canad. J. Research*, 15: 77 (1937).

absence of infection. A given animal may simply never have been exposed to infection with a given parasite, even though it is readily susceptible when exposed. The sporadic infections often reported with strange forms also illustrate this point—the hosts in these cases having experienced a chance contact with the parasite. Before true natural resistance can be claimed for a host against any parasite, therefore, such resistance must first be experimentally demonstrated by exposure to infection.

HOST-PARASITE RELATIONSHIPS

The ideal relationship between a host and parasite is one which favors both, or in which each is at least permitted to experience approximately optimal development. Certainly, for satisfactory adjustment the parasite must be able to continue as much of its life cycle as necessary in the host, although in doing so it must not cause such extensive damage that the host suffers significantly. If the host dies from effects of the parasite, then the parasite itself is endangered, for it is confronted with the usually perilous task of finding a new host if its own life is to continue. In such a case the host-parasite relationship is not in perfect balance, but rather is tilted strongly in the parasite's favor. Not infrequently, however, the host has the better of the relationship and either prevents entirely a parasite from becoming established within itself or else soon after its establishment checks its development or even destroys it.

WELL-ADJUSTED RELATIONSHIPS

In general, parasites which can establish themselves with the least damage to the host have the best chance for prolonged residence in it, for against these the host's capacity for affecting the parasite either by natural powers or by specific immune response is meager or sluggish and generally ineffectual. The best adjustment with their hosts is found, therefore, in the case of the numerous parasites limited to the alimentary canal, for these, in contrast to any of the somatic parasites, do essentially no damage whatsoever. Persons may harbor tapeworms such as *Taenia saginata* or flukes such as *Fasciolopsis buski* for many years with no physical effects so long as the diet is sufficient for both the individual and his parasite. Likewise, the intestinal flagellates as a group, as well as the nonpathogenic amoebae, may persist in the intestines for years without the host's even being aware of his infection, because these forms are essentially commensals.

POORLY ADJUSTED RELATIONSHIPS

Maladjustment between a parasite and its hosts sometimes results directly in the death of one or the other. For example, when *Trypanosoma equiperdum* of the horse is inoculated to rats, the rats die within four or five days; but if inoculated to man, no infection whatsoever occurs. The parasite in each of these cases is poorly adjusted to the host, and its survival is unlikely or impossible. In the horse, in contrast, a chronic type of infection characteristically develops, which lasts for months. In this interval, opportunity is provided for infection of new hosts, and the parasite is thus enabled to perpetuate itself.

Another frequent outcome of poor adjustment is imperfect development of the parasite, the parasite perhaps failing to attain maturity or to complete its life cycle. The human amoeba *Endamoeba histolytica*, for example, after transfer to the dog or cat, fails to develop the cyst stage, essential for the natural transmission of the parasite to other animals. Likewise, the hookworms of man and the dog, respectively, if given to the alternate host species will never or only seldom attain their full maturity as intestinal parasites. The infective stage of the dog hookworm may migrate for years in the human skin, unable to develop beyond the stage which first penetrated the skin. In these instances, the host-parasite relationship may slightly favor the parasite at first, permitting it to invade the host, but soon swings over to favor the host and prevents subsequent development of the parasite.

Usually, poorly adjusted parasites are those which have only recently—in an evolutionary sense—been acquired by a host. Such recent acquisitions are often seriously pathogenic. Gradually, however, the parasite loses some of its virulence for the host or the host by selection or otherwise becomes more tolerant of the parasite until finally the two get along together comparatively well. An example of such gradual adjustment is seen in the two species of trypanosomes which infect man in Africa. *Trypanosoma gambiense* has invaded man for so long a period that man is now considered its natural host, whereas *Trypanosoma rhodesiense* has been only recently acquired by man. In fact, *Trypanosoma rhodesiense* may more properly be deemed merely a sporadic human form and a natural parasite of antelopes or cattle. The difference in time of acquisition of the parasites is reflected by the relative pathogenicity of these organisms for man. The Gambian trypanosome is decidedly the less virulent form, producing in man a slowly developing, lingering type of disease which, although eventually fatal in untreated cases, is mild in character when compared with the rapidly fatal infection with the Rhodesian parasite. As time passes, *Trypanosoma rhodesiense* also may become better adjusted to human beings. One might even suspect that ages hence both these trypanosomes will eventually lose their extraordinary pathogenicity for man, even though they retain their capacity to propagate themselves in his blood and tissues. In certain game animals of Africa the infections are even now milder than in man, thus suggesting a longer residence in and a more complete adjustment to these animals.

Examples of extreme maladjustment between host and parasite do not occur, of course, in natural infections, but only in experimentally induced or sporadic infections. If parasites were forced to depend on abnormal hosts to sustain their development, they would, in many cases, be unable to propagate themselves at all and would soon become extinct.

HOST RESTRICTION AMONG PARASITES

Some species of parasites are narrowly limited as to the hosts in which they can establish themselves; others have broader choice. Certain forms which require a different host for each successive stage in their complete development have a broad choice at one stage of growth and a narrow choice at another. For all parasites, however, there are definite limits to the range of possible hosts, however wide the range may be. Accordingly, the host-parasite relationship must always be considered specific in character.

In the following paragraphs the principal human parasites and a few strictly animal forms are grouped according to their range of hosts. Especial attention is paid to relationships among the hosts.

For example, a parasite is considered to have a broader host range if it infects only the dog among carnivores and the rat among rodents than if it infects exclusively animals in one of these orders. Even when several animals in one order are susceptible—for example, rat, mouse, guinea pig, and rabbit among rodents—the actual range of the host is considered narrow, since these several hosts are very closely related.

PARASITES WHICH INFECT FEW HOSTS

Protozoa.—The narrowest host range is presented by the protozoan parasites of the class Sporozoa and by a few species of the class Mastigophora. Essentially all the sporozoans, whether of the blood or of the intestinal tract, have an extraordinarily limited host range. The four species of blood sporozoa causing human malaria, for example, infect none but primate animals and among these only one or two species besides man himself. *Plasmodium vivax* will sometimes infect chimpanzees, and *Plasmodium falciparum* will persist and multiply for some time in the howler monkey; [3] but other animals, including such divers forms as horses, dogs, guinea pigs, hedgehogs, bats, birds, and cold-blooded species, are refractory to all the human malaria organisms. If malaria-infected blood be put into common laboratory rodents, the parasites are quickly destroyed, for blood transferred back to a nonimmune person within a few hours is no longer infective for him.[4]

Similarly, the malarias of animals have a narrow choice of hosts. Monkey malarias infect only monkeys, except for one species, *Plasmodium knowlesi,* which infects man as well.[5] Bird malarias, although never found in mammals or in cold-blooded forms, seem to have a comparatively broad host range among birds. *Plasmodium cathemerium,* for example, is infective not only for canaries but also for the duck and the common fowl,[6] as well as for several sparrows and the wood thrush.

The intestinal sporozoans, the coccidia, have a similarly restricted host range, the restriction equaling that of the blood spo-

[3] W. H. Taliaferro and P. R. Cannon, *Am. J. Hyg.,* 19: 335 (1934).

[4] J. Segál, *Ann. de parasitol.,* 8: 590 (1930).

[5] D. F. Milam and L. T. Coggeshall, *Am. J. Trop. Med.,* 18: 331 (1938).

[6] R. D. Manwell, *Am. J. Trop. Med.,* 13: 97 (1933); F. Wolfson, *Am. J. Hyg.,* 28: 317 (1938).

Table 1

HOST RANGE OF REPRESENTATIVE PROTOZOAN AND HELMINTH PARASITES

Mammalian orders representatives of which can be infected are indicated by a plus sign (+).

Parasite Group	Parasite Name	ZOOLOGIC ORDERS TO WHICH SUSCEPTIBLE HOSTS BELONG									Hosts in Other Orders or Classes
		Marsupialia	*Insectivora*	*Chiroptera*	*Carnivora*	*Rodentia*	*Edentata*	*Primates*	*Artiodactyla*	*Perissodactyla*	
Protozoa Rhizopoda	Endamoeba histolytica				+	+		+			
Mastigophora	Trichomonas hominis				+	+		+			Fowl
	Giardia lamblia							+			
	Leishmania donovani			+	+	+		+			
	Trypanosoma talpae		+								
	Trypanosoma vespertilionis			+							
	Trypanosoma pestanai				+						
	Trypanosoma lewisi					+					Bandicoot ?
	Trypanosoma legeri						+				
	Trypanosoma cruzi	+		+	+	+	+	+			
	Trypanosoma brucei	+	+	+	+	+	+	+	+	+	Some birds
	Trypanosoma rhodesiense	+	+	±	+	+	+	+	+	+	Some birds
	Trypanosoma gambiense				+	+		+	+		Fowl, infected with difficulty
	Trypanosoma congolense				+	±			+	+	
	Trypanosoma vivax								+	+	
	Trypanosoma evansi				+	+		+	+	+	Elephant
	Trypanosoma equiperdum				+	+		+	+	+	
	Trypanosoma hippicum				+	+			+	+	
Sporozoa	Plasmodium vivax							+			
	Plasmodium malariae							+			
	Plasmodium falciparum							+			
	Plasmodium ovale							+			
	Plasmodium knowlesi							+			
	Eimeria stiedae					+					
	Isospora hominis							+			
Ciliata	Balantidium coli				+			+	+		
Helminths Trematoda	Schistosoma hematobium					+		+			
	Schistosoma mansoni					+		+			
	Schistosoma japonicum				+	+		+	+	+	
	Schistosoma bovis							+	+	+	
	Schistosoma spindale					+		+?	+	+	
	Fasciola hepatica	+			+	+		+	+	+	Elephant
	Fasciolopsis buski				+			+	+		
	Echinostoma ilocanum				+	+		+			
	Dicrocoelium dendriticum				+	+		+	+	+	
	Heterophyes heterophyes				+			+			
	Metagonimus yokogawai				+	+		+	+		Pelican
	Clonorchis sinensis				+	+		+	+		
	Paragonimus westermanni				+	+		+	+		

Parasite Group	Parasite Name	Marsupialia	Insectivora	Chiroptera	Carnivora	Rodentia	Edentata	Primates	Artiodactyla	Perissodactyla	Hosts in Other Orders or Classes
	ZOOLOGIC ORDERS TO WHICH SUSCEPTIBLE HOSTS BELONG										
Cestoda	Diphyllobothrium latum										
	Plerocercoid										Fish
	Adult				+			+	+		
	Diphyllobothrium mansoni										
	Plerocercoid				+			+			Birds, snakes, frogs
	Adult				+						
	Dipylidium caninum										
	Adult				+			+			
	Raillietina madagascariensis										
	Adult					+		+			
	Hymenolepis nana										
	Adult					+		+			
	Hymenolepis diminuta										
	Adult				+?	+		+			
	Taenia solium										
	Cysticercus							+	+		
	Adult							+			
	Taenia saginata										
	Cysticercus								+		
	Adult							+			
	Multiceps multiceps										
	Coenurus							+	+	+	
	Adult				+						
	Multiceps serialis										
	Coenurus					+		+			
	Adult				+						
	Echinococcus granulosus										
	Hydatid	+			+	+		+	+	+	Elephant
	Adult				+						
Nematoda	Trichinella spiralis				+	+		+	+		Certain birds
	Trichocephalus dispar							+	+		
	Capillaria hepatica				+	+		+	+		
	Strongyloides stercoralis				+?			+			
	Ancylostoma duodenale				+?			+	+?		
	Ancylostoma caninum				+						
	Necator americanus				+?	+		+	+?	+	Pangolin
	Enterobius vermicularis							+			
	Ascaris lumbricoides							+	+		
	Wuchereria bancrofti							+			
	Loa loa							+			
	Onchocerca volvulus							+			
	Dracunculus medinensis				+			+	+	+	
Acanthocephala	Moniliformis moniliformis				+	+		+			
	Gigantorhynchus gigas				+			+	+		

rozoa. The human coccidian *Isospora hominis,* for example, has never been established in any species besides man, and man resists infection with all the known species of animal coccidia. The somewhat closely related cat and dog coccidians, *Isospora felis* and *Isospora rivolta,* will infect both these animals, as well as several other carnivores, but no other mammals.[7] Coccidia of the genus *Eimeria* almost all infect only a single host: *Eimeria perforans* infects only the rabbit; *Eimeria caviae* only the guinea pig; and so forth. Even the avian coccidia of this genus are largely infective only for a single host. Those from such closely related birds as turkey, quail, pheasant, and chicken generally infect only the host from which each is naturally derived.[8]

In the protozoan class Mastigophora several trypanosomes and certain intestinal species have a sharply restricted host range. The trypanosomes are nonpathogenic forms belonging to the *lewisi* group. The type species, *Trypanosoma lewisi,* infects wild rats naturally and can be introduced to albino rats and to guinea pigs experimentally. All other laboratory animals besides rats and guinea pigs are, however, resistant. Related trypanosomes, such as *Trypanosoma duttoni* of mice, *Trypanosoma vespertilionis* of bats, and *Trypanosoma legeri* of anteaters, all are specific for the hosts mentioned and are not known to invade others.

The intestinal flagellates of the genus *Giardia* also are highly specific forms. *Giardia lamblia* of man, for example, infects no animal besides man, with the possible exception of the monkey. Humans are not susceptible to infection with the corresponding forms found in rodents and other lower animals.

Helminths.—The best examples of helminths with a sharply restricted host range are found in the classes Cestoda and Nematoda. Among the cestodes, the beef tapeworm, *Taenia saginata,* presents the most limited host range. Its adult form is found only in the human intestine, and its larval or cysticercus stage only in the tissues of cattle. *Taenia solium,* the human pork tapeworm, has only slightly broader choice. The adult of this form resides exclusively in the human intestine, but the larval form occurs in the somatic tissues of both the human and the pig. In general cestodes

[7] J. Andrews, *Am. J. Hyg.,* 28: 317 (1926).
[8] E. E. Tyzzer, *Am. J. Hyg.,* 10: 269 (1929).

of the family Taeniidae are restricted in choice of host for the adult stage much more than for the larva. Even the adult of *Echinococcus granulosus* infects only the dog and two or three of its closest relatives (for example, the wolf and the fox), but the larva infects a broad range of mammals. Cestodes outside the family Taeniidae generally have less restriction in choice of host even for their adult stage.

The nematodes having the most restricted host selection are the pinworms, the various species of *Strongyloides,* and the filarids. Man is the only host of the human pinworm, *Enterobius vermicularis,* and of the filarids *Wuchereria bancrofti, Loa loa, Acanthocheilonema perstans,* and *Mansonella ozzardi.* He is, furthermore, entirely resistant to the related forms found in many animals, since these species generally exhibit just as great restriction in host range as does the corresponding species from man. *Strongyloides stercoralis* occurs almost exclusively in man, although possibly sometimes in the dog, the fox, and the cat also. The lack of susceptible animals for these various human nematodes has seriously handicapped the experimental study of the infections they cause.

PARASITES WHICH INFECT MANY HOSTS

Protozoa.—The pathogenic amoeba, certain intestinal flagellates, the leishmanias, and the pathogenic trypanosomes all have a comparatively broad potential host range. *Endamoeba histolytica* infects man, several species of monkey,[9] the dog,[10] the cat,[11] and the rat.[12] The *Macacus rhesus* is considered a natural host for the parasite. The complete life cycle of the parasite goes on in this monkey quite as in man, with comparable lesions in the large intestine.[13] Extraordinarily serious infections with *Endamoeba histolytica* are the rule among dogs and cats, with extensive ulceration and death as the final outcome. Cysts are not often developed in

[9] R. Hegner, C. M. Johnson, and R. M. Stabler, *Am. J. Hyg.,* 15: 394 (1932); H. E. Meleney and W. W. Frye, *Am. J. Pub. Health,* 27: 505 (1937).

[10] T. Simïc, *Ann. de parasitol.,* 13: 345 (1935); O. Wagner, *Arch. f. Schiffs-u. Tropen-Hyg.,* 39: 1 (1935).

[11] T. Simïc, *Ann. de parasitol.,* 13: 345 (1935); O. Wagner, *Arch. f. Schiffs-u. Tropen-Hyg.,* 39: 1 (1935).

[12] H. Tsuchiya, *Am. J. Trop. Med.,* 19: 151 (1939).

[13] C. Dobell, *Parasitology,* 23: 1 (1931).

these animals. On the other hand, tissue invasion is not known to occur in the rat, and cysts have seldom been observed, yet it is often suspected that this animal has importance in the natural transmission of the parasite among human beings.

Of all the intestinal flagellates the trichomonads have the broadest choice of hosts. *Trichomonas hominis* can certainly infect at least the rat, the mouse, the kitten, and the chick, besides man.[14] The rat appears important as a disseminator of the human trichomonad, since experimental infections persist in this animal for more than a year and spread naturally from rat to rat.[15] Some observers consider that trichomonads found in the mouth, the intestine, and the vagina of man have the same organ preference after transfer to the rat or the kitten, although this point of view requires further substantiation.[16] Another intestinal flagellate, *Chilomastix mesnili,* can infect both man and the chick.[17]

Leishmania donovani infects several kinds of animal, including particularly the monkey, the dog, the cat, and the Chinese hamster, as well as white rats and mice, voles, Chinese house mice, and house rats.[18]

The trypanosome with the broadest choice of hosts is *Trypanosoma brucei.* This form can infect representatives of essentially all orders of mammal. Only man and the baboon, among primate mammals, resist it. Sometimes even fowls and other birds will harbor the parasite for considerable periods after inoculation, although the parasite does not propagate itself well in avian hosts. The human trypanosomes also infect a wide variety of hosts. *Trypanosoma rhodesiense* has about the same host range as *Trypanosoma brucei* and, like it, causes infections of great severity. *Trypanosoma gambiense* develops in many carnivores, rodents, and even-toed ungulates, as well as in many primates. The South American form, *Trypanosoma cruzi,* infects such species as armadillos, opossums, dogs, cats, bats, and primates, as well as the usual laboratory rodents.

The balantidias are more or less intermediate as far as host

[14] R. Hegner, *Am. J. Hyg.,* 9: 529 (1929).
[15] R. Hegner and L. Eskridge, *Am. J. Hyg.,* 21: 135 (1935) ; 26: 124 (1937).
[16] A. E. Bonestell, *J. Parasitol.,* 22: 511 (1936).
[17] R. Hegner, *J. Parasitol.,* 23: 1 (1937) ; G. H. Ball, *Am. J. Hyg.,* 16: 85 (1932).
[18] C. W. Young, M. Hertig, and L. Pao-Yung, *Am. J. Hyg.,* 10: 183 (1929).

range is concerned. They do not have such extraordinary restriction as the sporozoans, yet are more restricted than the other protozoans mentioned in the present section. *Balantidia* from man, monkey, and pig will infect the alternate hosts, and those from the chimpanzee and the pig can be established fairly well in the rat and the guinea pig.[19] Colonic lesions have not, however, been demonstrated in such experimentally infected rodents,[20] although they have been described in man, the pig, and the monkey. Also, encystment does not occur in the rodent intestine, although cysts are produced in the natural hosts.[21]

Helminths.—The trematodes as a class have a comparatively broad choice of hosts. For example, *Fasciola hepatica* can establish itself in such forms as kangaroo, dog, rabbit, sheep, cow, horse, and elephant. *Metagonimus yokogawai* infects certain primates, carnivores, rodents, and ruminants, as well as pelicans, although its close relative *Heterophyes heterophyes* is more restricted, invading only certain primates and carnivores. The schistosomes have rather broad infectivity. *Schistosoma japonicum* has been found naturally in such hosts as man, cat, and cow and is readily infective experimentally in laboratory monkeys and rodents, as well as horses. Similarly, other significant trematodes generally can invade many varieties of host.

The cestodes of families other than the Taeniidae usually infect several varieties of animal. *Hymenolepis nana* and *Hymenolepis diminuta,* for example, occur in both man and certain rodents, and *Dipylidium caninum* occurs in man and dogs. *Diphyllobothrium latum* has an even broader choice of hosts, since it occurs in practically all fish-eating mammals, including man, dog, cat, fox, mink, bear, and pig.

Among nematode parasites, *Trichinella spiralis* has the broadest choice of host. This parasite regularly infects not only man and other primates but also nearly all other mammals, including carnivores, rodents, and ungulates. It will also infect the

[19] F. O. Atchley, *J. Parasitol.,* 21: 183 (1935); A. Gabaldon, *J. Parasitol.,* 21: 386 (1935); E. C. Nelson, *Am. J. Hyg.,* 22: 26 (1935); E. Schumaker, *Science,* 70: 385 (1929); *Am. J. Hyg.,* 12: 341 (1930).

[20] F. O. Atchley, *J. Parasitol.,* 21: 183 (1935).

[21] F. O. Atchley, *J. Parasitol.,* 21: 183 (1935); E. Schumaker, *Am. J. Hyg.,* 12: 341 (1930).

young of a number of species of birds, although avian hosts are probably not of importance in the natural transmission of the parasite.[22] The New World hookworm, *Necator americanus,* likewise will develop not only in man but also, at least occasionally, in dog, rat, pig, horse, and pangolin. Similarly, the guinea worm, *Dracunculus medinensis,* infects man, several carnivores, and possibly a number of ungulates. Such a broad range of hosts is, however, exceptional among the nematode parasites, restriction being distinctly greater as a rule than among trematodes and cestodes.

FACTORS INFLUENCING NATURAL RESISTANCE

The factors influencing natural resistance and more or less explaining it are quite numerous, and no one of them applies to all examples. Certain fundamental factors, such as the genetic constitution of the host and perhaps also of the parasite, undoubtedly play a profound role in natural resistance. But other more superficial and decidedly more variable characteristics of the individual also are significant, such as age, diet, intercurrent infection, and debility or stimulation from other causes.[23] The influence of these several factors, as well as others, upon natural resistance will be briefly discussed.

GENETIC CONSTITUTION OF THE HOST

The difference in natural resistance against a given parasite manifested by two different races or breeds within a single species of host is best explained through the genetic constitution of the individuals. The best example of a racial difference in resistance among human parasitic infections is found in malaria. From studies carried on chiefly in induced malaria therapy of neurosyphilis it is clear that the Negro race has greater resistance to malaria than has the white race. Negroes sometimes resist absolutely all attempts to infect them with *Plasmodium vivax,* and when they do contract the infection, they suffer only comparatively mild cases after prolonged incubation periods. Even young

---

[22] K. Matoff, *Tierärztl. Rundschau,* 42: 401 (1936) ; *Ztschr. f. Infektionskr.,* 54: 116 (1938).

[23] A. C. Chandler, *J. Parasitol.,* 18: 135 (1932).

Negro children resist this parasite.[24] White persons, on the other hand, are uniformly susceptible to *Plasmodium vivax*. According to one report, all but 16 of 103 white persons contracted malaria after the first experimental inoculation by infected mosquito, and 11 of 12 of those escaping the first time promptly contracted the disease on second inoculation.[25] Failure to infect Caucasians with *Plasmodium vivax* can generally be referred to premunition in the host or to the administration of parasites of degraded virulence.[26]

Generally Negroes can be infected with *Plasmodium falciparum* adequately for the purposes of malaria-induced therapy, but they suffer milder infections than do white persons.[27] They seldom experience the important sequel of prolonged *falciparum* infection, blackwater fever. Negroes also suffer milder infections than do white persons with *Plasmodium knowlesi,* the monkey parasite sometimes used in the therapy of neurosyphilis of man.[28]

Some evidence for racial differences in resistance is also seen among the helminthiases. Negroes in the United States seem less susceptible to *Hymenolepis nana* than are whites.[29] The hookworm larvae penetrate the skin of Negroes less readily than that of white persons.[30] The Javanese and the bushmen in Paramaribo are reported to resist clinical effects of filariasis more successfully than do Creoles with equal filarial infection.[31] Among animals, Cheviot sheep are more tolerant of infection with *Haemonchus contortus* than are lowland breeds of sheep,[32] and heavier breeds of chickens (Rhode Island Reds, Plymouth Rocks) are more resistant to *Ascaridia lineata* than are lighter breeds (Leghorns, Buff Orpingtons, Minorcas).[33] Even within a given breed (Mi-

---

[24] M. F. Boyd, *South. M. J.*, 27: 155 (1934); M. F. Boyd and W. K. Stratman-Thomas, *Am. J. Hyg.*, 18: 485 (1933).

[25] M. F. Boyd, *South. M. J.*, 27: 155 (1934).

[26] M. F. Boyd and W. K. Stratman-Thomas, *Am. J. Hyg.*, 19: 541 (1934).

[27] M. F. Boyd and S. F. Kitchen, *Am. J. Trop. Med.*, 17: 213 (1937).

[28] D. F. Milam and L. T. Coggeshall, *Am. J. Trop. Med.*, 18: 331 (1938); D. F. Milam and E. Kusch, *South. M. J.*, 31: 947 (1938).

[29] G. F. Otto, *J. Parasitol.*, 21: 443 (1935).

[30] W. G. Smillie and D. L. Augustine, *J. A. M. A.*, 85: 1958 (1925).

[31] L. Elsbach, *Geneesk. Tijdschr. v. Nederl.-Indië*, 73: 647 (1933).

[32] W. T. M. Cameron, *Proc. Int. Vet. Congr., N.Y.*, 3: 44 (1935).

[33] J. E. Ackert, *Tr. Dynamics of Develop.*, 10: 413 (1935).

norca) heavier strains of fowl are more resistant to *Ascaridia* than lighter ones.

The significance of the genetic constitution in natural resistance has been well shown experimentally in chickens infected with *Ascaridia lineata*. In the second of two successive years a flock of Minorca chickens became much more susceptible to this parasite. The difference was finally attributed to a change in the genetic constitution of the flock, resulting from the introduction of new cockerels at the end of the first year. The birds in the second year's flock were significantly lighter in weight, and their susceptibility to the nematode increased as their weight fell.[34]

The blood group.—No connection is known between any human blood group and natural resistance to parasitic infection. One large study, involving two thousand Tamile, concluded that malaria was contracted equally by persons of all blood groups.[35] When possible in malaria-induced therapy, inoculation should be made from a donor of the same blood group as the patient so that the parasites will not be injured by the agglutination of the injected erythrocytes.[36]

AGE

The age of the host influences significantly its natural resistance. Very young animals can be easily infected with many parasites which older animals resist perfectly. These forms are usually eradicated naturally as the host matures. The phenomenon of age resistance is, however, so large a subject and one of such importance that a complete chapter will be given to its consideration. The subject will not be discussed further here, therefore, but will be presented in detail in Chapter III.

SEX AND REPRODUCTION

Given equal exposure to infection, male and female persons or animals are generally about equal in their natural resistance to most parasitic infections. In amoebiasis and in kala azar, however, a disproportionate number of cases are found among males,

---

[34] J. E. Ackert and J. H. Wilmoth, *J. Parasitol.*, 20: 323 (1934).
[35] R. Green, *Tr. Roy. Soc. Trop. Med. and Hyg.*, 23: 161 (1929).
[36] G. Hopf, *München. med. Wchnschr.*, 75: 1755 (1928).

which is not attributable to greater exposure. Usually under the strain incident to some phase of reproduction, both males and females are less resistant than normally to both protozoan and helminth infection.[37] A latent infection with malignant malaria, for example, often flares up during pregnancy, labor, or after parturition.[38] Likewise, the natural resistance of sheep to *Haemonchus contortus* is reduced in rams during the breeding season and in ewes during reproduction and especially during lactation.[39] Furthermore, female partridges are more susceptible to *Syngamus trachea* than are males,[40] at least during the period of egg laying.[41] On the other hand, female guinea pigs are relatively resistant to *Trypanosoma equiperdum* during pregnancy,[42] and mice assume enhanced resistance to *Hymenolepis fraterna* for some days after parturition.[43]

Attempts to influence the resistance of rats to trichomonads by the administration of sex hormones or other such products have not been very successful.[44] On the other hand, their resistance to *Trypanosoma lewisi* is reported to be reduced by bilateral gonadectomy.[45] Female rats have greater natural resistance to cysticercosis than males.[46] Ovariectomy or the administration of the male hormone reduces the resistance of the female rat. The analogous treatment enhances resistance in the male.

INTERCURRENT INFECTION

It would seem possible that if an animal were already infected with one disease agent at the time he was exposed to a second, the chance for infection with the second would be greater because of some depressing effect the initial infection might have

[37] G. A. W. Wickramasuriya, *Malaria and ancylostomiasis in the pregnant woman*, London, Humphrey Milford, 1937.
[38] D. S. Karve, *Kenya and East African M. J.*, 6: 43 (1929); P. Daleas, *Bull. Soc. méd.-chir. de l'Indochine*, 13: 432 (1935).
[39] N. R. Stoll, *J. Am. Vet. M. A.*, 96: 305 (1940).
[40] P. A. Clapham, *J. Helminthol.*, 17: 192 (1935).
[41] S. C. Whitlock, *J. Parasitol.*, 23: 426 (1937).
[42] H. A. Poindexter, *Am. J. Trop. Med.*, 13: 555 (1933).
[43] A. V. Hunninen, *Am. J. Hyg.*, 22: 414 (1935).
[44] R. Hegner and L. Eskridge, *J. Parasitol.*, 22: 410 (1936).
[45] D. Perla and J. Marmorston-Gottesman, *J. Exper. Med.*, 52: 601 (1930).
[46] D. H. Campbell, *Science*, 89: 415 (1939); D. H. Campbell and L. R. Melcher, *J. Infect. Dis.*, 66: 184 (1940).

upon the natural powers of resistance of the host. On the other hand, the possibility certainly remains that the powers of resistance of the host would have been set in motion by the initial infection so that the second agent would encounter a resistance of higher level and be unable to establish itself at all in the host. A third possibility also exists—namely, that each infection runs its course independently of an earlier or concurrent one. Of the many studies involving parasites carried out on the problem, from either the clinical or the experimental point of view, a majority have suggested that the natural resistance is altered in one way or the other—either enhanced or depressed—by an intercurrent infection. The finding of a disproportionally large number of human infections with two or more species of amoebae or with amoebae and intestinal flagellates, for example, has been suggested as evidence that infection with one of these forms predisposes to infection with the other.[47] Monkeys, likewise, appear more susceptible to experimental *Leishmania donovani* infection if already infected with malaria.[48] On the other hand, if mice be simultaneously infected with spirochetes and pathogenic trypanosomes they live longer than if given the trypanosome alone,[49] the development of the trypanosome not infrequently being completely inhibited.[50] A similar observation is made in malaria: when *Plasmodium vivax* and *Plasmodium falciparum* are injected simultaneously into white persons, *Plasmodium falciparum* assumes the greater prominence first, but this more malignant infection declines as *Plasmodium vivax* increases, since the *vivax* parasite is the dominant one.[51] When *Plasmodium vivax* and *Plasmodium malariae* are given simultaneously, a similar circumstance is observed, *Plasmodium malariae* often being completely inhibited by *Plasmodium vivax*.[52] Similarly, one spe-

[47] D. C. Boughton and E. E. Byrd, *Am. J. Hyg.*, 27: 88 (1938).

[48] L. E. Napier, R. O. A. Smith, and K. V. Krishnan, *Indian J. M. Research*, 21: 553 (1934).

[49] J. G. Thomson and P. De Muro, *J. Trop. Med.*, 35: 33 (1932).

[50] K.-D. Gno, *Zentralbl. f. Bakt.*, 139: 113 (1937); J. Stroder, *Ztschr. f. Immunitätsforsch. u. exper. Therap.*, 89: 161 (1936); F. Tanzer, *Arch. ital. di sc. med. colon.*, 11: 91 (1930).

[51] M. F. Boyd and S. F. Kitchen, *Am. J. Trop. Med.*, 17: 855 (1937).

[52] B. Mayne and M. D. Young, *Pub. Health Rep.*, 53: 1289 (1939).

cies of trypanosome often depresses another inoculated at the same time.[53] Repeated malaria infection in infants is said to protect them against trypanosomiasis in endemic areas.[54] No mutual influence, on the other hand, can be noted between malaria and typhoid fever;[55] but malaria superimposed on tuberculosis is said to depress tuberculin sensitivity[56] and to lead to extension of the tuberculous lesions[57] or even to relapse in those about to recover.[58]

Very few studies have been carried out on the effect of intercurrent infection upon the helminthiases. Mice are known to suffer internal autoreinfection with *Hymenolepis fraterna* if they are suffering from paratyphoid infection.[59] On the other hand, in turkeys with blackhead the nematode *Heterakis gallinae* is retarded in development and reduced in number compared with healthy birds.[60] Birds with leukaemia harbor a more intense infection with *Heterakis gallinae*,[61] although those with tuberculosis appear peculiarly resistant to this nematode.[62] Infection with other helminths appears to be one of the most significant predisposing factors to infection with *Heterakis gallinae*.

From what has been said, it is obvious that the effect of intercurrent infection upon the natural resistance of a host to any parasite is as yet poorly understood. Usually resistance is altered by the intercurrent infection, but in some cases it is increased and in others decreased, without a very definite trend being discernible. Nevertheless the most significant effects have seemed to result when the two agents concerned are closely related—for example, two species of human malaria parasite.

[53] C. Schilling, *J. Trop. Med.*, 23: 334 (1930); H. Tseng, *Zentralbl. f. Bakt.*, 134: 153 (1935).

[54] R. E. Barrett, *Tr. Roy. Soc. Trop. Med. and Hyg.*, 25: 191 (1931).

[55] G. Giglioli, *Riv. di malariol.*, 12: 708 (1933).

[56] H. Ishioka, *J. M. A. Formosa*, 36: 1502 (1937); B. Boggian, *Riv. di patol. e clin. d. tuberc.*, 8: 513 (1934).

[57] S. Collari, *Riv. di malariol.*, 11: 308 (1932); B. Boggian, *Riv. di patol. e clin. d. tuberc.*, 8: 513 (1934).

[58] A. Manai, *Riv. di malariol.*, 13: 443 (1934).

[59] A. V. Hunninen, *J. Parasitol.*, 22: 84 (1936).

[60] Baker, *Scientific Agric.*, 13: 356 (1933).

[61] P. A. Clapham, *J. Helminthol.*, 16: 53 (1938).

[62] D. O. Morgan and J. E. Wilson, *J. Helminthol.*, 16: 165 (1938), and 17: 177 (1939).

DIET

The character of the diet influences very profoundly certain parasitic infections. The most conspicuous effects are seen upon those parasites which reside in the alimentary canal or the tissues lining it, yet some evidence for an influence of the diet upon somatic infections also is available.

Protozoan infections.—A generally balanced and ample diet favors the resistance of man to amoebiasis, since infected individuals suffer less often from clinical symptoms when the diet is good.[63] Experimental infections with amoebae in dogs usually improve if the animals are placed on a diet of raw liver, the parasite often thereafter being wholly eradicated.[64] A high-protein diet, favoring proteolytic bacteria, decreases the intensity of natural infections with *Endamoeba muris* in mice.[65] The intestinal flagellates of rats also are adversely affected by a high protein diet,[66] although little clinical evidence is yet available that the nature of the diet affects the presence of these parasites in man.[67] Rats are not freed of their intestinal flagellates by starvation,[68] and certain bile salts,[69] as well as liver [70] (which acts so favorably on experimental amoebic infections in dogs), actually favor the increase of these flagellates in the rat. The intestinal ciliate, *Balantidium coli,* becomes established in the gut of rats only if hosts are on a high carbohydrate diet [71] and is reduced in number or eliminated after infected animals are transferred to a diet high in protein.[72]

The animal coccidioses are particularly susceptible to control

---

[63] F. D. Alexander and H. E. Meleney, *Am. J. Hyg.,* 22: 704 (1935).

[64] E. C. Faust and E. S. Kagy, *Am. J. Trop. Med.,* 14: 235 (1934).

[65] H. L. Ratcliffe, *J. Parasitol.,* 16: 75 (1929).

[66] R. Hegner, *Am. J. Trop. Med.,* 13: 535 (1933); R. Hegner and L. Eskridge, *J. Parasitol.,* 21: 313 (1935); H. L. Ratcliffe, *Am. J. Hyg.,* 11: 159 (1930); H. L. Ratcliffe, *Am. J. Hyg.,* 8: 910 (1928); H. Tsuchiya, *Am. J. Hyg.,* 15: 232 (1932).

[67] J. Andrews and J. W. Landsberg, *Am. J. Hyg.,* 24: 416 (1937); C. D. De Langen, *Acta leidensia scholae med. trop.,* 2: 137 (1927); R. Hegner and L. Eskridge, *Am. J. Hyg.,* 21: 121 (1935).

[68] R. Hegner and L. Eskridge, *J. Parasitol.,* 23: 225 (1937).

[69] R. Hegner and L. Eskridge, *Am. J. Hyg.,* 26: 186 (1937).

[70] R. Hegner and L. Eskridge, *Am. J. Hyg.,* 26: 127 (1937).

[71] R. Hegner, *J. Parasitol.,* 23: 1 (1937); E. C. Nelson, *Am. J. Hyg.,* 18: 185 (1933); E. Schumaker, *Am. J. Hyg.,* 13: 576 (1931).

[72] E. Schumaker, *Am. J. Hyg.,* 12: 341 (1930).

through the diet.[73] Large amounts of vitamin G favor more intense coccidiosis in the experimentally infected rat, and the strict limitation of this vitamin is, therefore, recommended for controlling the infection in this animal.[74] Vitamin B_1 exerts a restraining influence upon the rat coccidian.[75] In fowl coccidiosis, dried skim milk or buttermilk plus wheat middlings added to the diet increases the severity of the disease.[76] The addition of sulphur to the ration, on the other hand, decreases the infection among fowls,[77] although this element is often toxic to the hosts.[78] Vitamins A and D have slight or no effect on the course of coccidial infection.[79]

In humoral protozoan infections, the effect of diet is less obvious. A generally poor diet is not found to affect resistance in trypanosomiasis,[80] and vitamin A specifically has no effect in experimental *Trypanosoma brucei* disease of rats.[81] Vitamin C, however, occasionally aborts *Trypanosoma brucei* infections of guinea pigs, although no such action is seen in mice which harbor the same parasite.[82] Pigeons can be rendered susceptible to *Trypanosoma brucei* by starvation or by a deficiency of vitamin B.[83] The addition of copper and iron or both to the diet of rats elevates their resistance to *Trypanosoma lewisi*.[84] The severity of infections with the pathogenic trypanosomes can be to some extent controlled by regulating the blood sugar: parenteral injections of glucose elevate the blood sugar and lead to earlier death,[85] whereas insulin administration prolongs the life of the infected host.[86] The diet plays only a minor role in malaria, al-

[73] E. R. Becker, *Science,* 86: 403 (1937).
[74] E. R. Becker and N. F. Morehouse, *J. Parasitol.,* 22: 60 (1936) ; *Proc. Soc. Exper. Biol. & Med.,* 33: 487 (1936).
[75] E. R. Becker, *Proc. Soc. Exper. Biol. & Med.,* 42: 597 (1939).
[76] E. R. Becker and P. C. Waters, *Iowa State Coll. J. Sci.,* 12: 405 (1938).
[77] C. A. Herrick and C. E. Holmes, *Vet. Med.,* 31: 390 (1936).
[78] C. E. Holmes, H. J. Deobald, and C. A. Herrick, *Poult. Sci.,* 17: 136 (1938).
[79] E. R. Becker and N. F. Morehouse, *J. Parasitol.,* 22: 60 (1936) ; *Proc. Soc. Exper. Biol. & Med.,* 33: 487 (1936).
[80] M. H. French and H. E. Hornby, Tangan. Terr., *Ann. Rep., Dept. Vet. Sci. and Animal Husb.,* Part V (1934).
[81] J. Fine, *J. Hyg.,* 34: 154 (1934).   [82] D. Perla, *Am. J. Hyg.,* 26: 374 (1937).
[83] G. Sollazzo, *Ztschr. f. Immunitätsforsch. u. exper. Therap.,* 60: 239 (1929).
[84] D. Perla, *J. Exper. Med.,* 60: 541 (1934).
[85] H. A. Poindexter, *Am. J. Trop. Med.,* 13: 555 (1933).
[86] H. A. Poindexter, *J. Parasitol.,* 21: 292 (1935).

though relapse in benign tertian infections is said to occur more often if the diet is rich in sugar.[87] Canaries are found to suffer only a lower-grade infection with *Plasmodium cathemerium* if treated with insulin so as to maintain a low blood sugar.[88]

Helminth infections.—The quality of the diet is important also in a number of helminth diseases, particularly in experimental hookworm infection of dogs. Animals on a poor diet manifest definitely less resistance to hookworm disease than those on a good diet.[89] The natural resistance of older animals can be broken down by providing these animals with a poor ration,[90] although their resistance is regained when a good ration is resumed.[91] The heaviest human infections with hookworm also occur in those on a poor diet.[92] Essentially similar conditions are observed also in human ascariasis,[93] in rats with *Nippostrongylus muris,*[94] and in lambs with *Haemonchus contortus,*[95] although the dietary effects must often be extreme before resistance is significantly altered. On a white bread and water diet rats become less resistant to the cestode *Hymenolepis fraterna,* although the worms fail to reach maturity in animals on such a diet.[96] The starvation of fowls for twenty to forty-eight hours upsets the metabolism of *Raillietina cesticillus* which they harbor, long chains of proglottids of the parasite commonly being broken off and eliminated.[97]

The significance of vitamin A in resistance against helminth infections has been studied almost to the exclusion of other accessory factors. A deficiency of vitamin A is found by some to increase the susceptibility of pigs to *Ascaris lumbricoides,* although most studies conclude that this vitamin has no effect in this in-

---

[87] W. Bird, *Indian J. M. Research,* 16: 109 (1928).

[88] R. Hegner, *J. Parasitol.,* 23: 1 (1937).

[89] W. W. Cort and G. F. Otto, *Rev. Gastroenterol.,* 7: 2 (1940); W. W. Cort, *J. Parasitol.,* 19: 142 (1932); A. O. Foster and W. W. Cort, *Science,* 73: 681 (1931); *Am. J. Hyg.,* 16: 241 (1932); *Am. J. Hyg.,* 21: 302 (1935); G. F. Otto and J. W. Landsberg, *Am. J. Hyg.,* 31: 37 (1940, sec. D).

[90] A. O. Foster and W. W. Cort, *Am. J. Hyg.,* 21: 302 (1935).

[91] A. O. Foster and W. W. Cort, *Science,* 73: 681 (1931).

[92] A. O. Foster and W. W. Cort, *Am. J. Hyg.,* 16: 241 (1932).

[93] C. F. Ahmann and L. M. Bristol, *South. M. J.,* 26: 959 (1933).

[94] D. A. Porter, *Am. J. Hyg.,* 22: 467 (1935).

[95] A. H. H. Fraser and D. Robertson, *Emp. J. Exp. Agric.,* 1: 17 (1933).

[96] D. A. Shorb, *Am. J. Hyg.,* 18: 74 (1933).

[97] W. M. Reid, *J. Parasitol. (Suppl.),* 26: 16 (1940).

fection.[98] More marked results from vitamin A deficiency have
been reported in dogs infected with *Toxocara canis,* older dogs being susceptible to the parasite only when they are on such a diet.
The greater susceptibility of dogs on an A-deficient diet is trace-
able to a deficiency in intestinal juice, this juice providing normally a chemical barrier which prevents young larval worms in
the intestine from penetrating tissues of the gut wall.[99] Likewise,
the resistance of fowls to *Ascaridia lineata* is less when on an
A-deficient diet, more and larger worms developing in such animals, probably because of diminished peristalsis and the consequent prolonged presence of the food in the intestine.[100] Resistance of rats to *Nippostrongylus muris* [101] and to *Trichinella
spiralis* [102] is less if the diet is low in vitamin A, no specific resistance then being acquired against a second infection with
Trichinella spiralis.[103] The effect of a vitamin-E deficiency in the
diet seems to be in an opposite direction in trichiniasis, rats on
such a diet suffering less severe infections.[104]

The presence or absence of certain chemicals in the ration also
affects resistance. Chicks on a diet lacking manganese become
more susceptible to the tapeworm *Raillietina cesticillus,*[105] and
cats and dogs on a diet low in minerals are more susceptible to
nonspecific strains of hookworms.[106] The addition of iron alone
to a poor diet is of little use in raising resistance to hookworm
disease, but a more substantial effect is attained by a general improvement in the ration.[107] Parathormone is found helpful by
some in accelerating the calcification of trichina cysts,[108] although
others cannot confirm this result.[109]

[98] E. de Boer, *Tijdschr. v. Diergeneesk.,* 62: 965 (1935); P. Clapham, *J. Helminthol.,* 12: 165 (1934).

[99] W. H. Wright, *J. Parasitol.,* 21: 433 (1935).

[100] J. E. Ackert, M. F. McIlvaine, and N. Z. Crawford, *Am. J. Hyg.,* 13: 320
(1931).

[101] L. A. Spindler, *J. Parasitol.,* 20: 72 (1933).

[102] O. R. McCoy, *Am. J. Hyg.,* 20: 169 (1934).   [103] *Ibid.*

[104] H. Zaiman, *J. Parasitol. (Suppl.),* 26: 44 (1940).

[105] P. D. Harwood and G. W. Luttermoser, *Proc. Helminthol. Soc. Washington,*
5: 60 (1938).

[106] A. O. Foster and W. W. Cort, *Am. J. Hyg.,* 16: 582 (1932).

[107] G. F. Otto and J. W. Landsberg, *Am. J. Hyg.,* 31: 37 (1940, sec. D).

[108] W. W. Wantland, *Proc. Soc. Exper. Biol. & Med.,* 32: 438 (1934).

[109] T. v. Brand, G. F. Otto, and E. Abrams, *Am. J. Hyg.,* 27: 461 (1938).

SIGNIFICANCE OF SPECIFIC ORGANS AND TISSUES

The relationship of certain organs and tissues to natural resistance has been investigated with great care, although with by no means uniform results. The usual manner of determining the part each organ plays is by comparing the resistance of animals from which that organ has been functionally eliminated—either through extirpation or otherwise—with that of normal animals. The parasites used in most studies on the significance of specific organs and tissues are the somatic protozoans, especially the leishmanias, trypanosomes, and malarial organisms.

Effect of the reticulo-endothelial system and the spleen.—The reticulo-endothelial system is believed to have more to do with the resistance of an animal than any other organ or tissue. Conditions which limit the function of this system of tissues seem to interfere seriously with the resistance which an animal can manifest against any parasite. If the reticulo-endothelial system is blockaded by an injection of a solution of India ink or other material which can lodge in its cells, antibody production is usually depressed and resistance is proportionately reduced. A much greater effect is obtained if reticulo-endothelial blockade is combined with splenectomy, the spleen representing the largest single mass of reticulo-endothelial tissue which can be surgically extirpated. According to reports of many experimenters, removal of the spleen alone suffices to lower resistance drastically.

Unfortunately, the many experimental investigations upon the role of the reticulo-endothelial system and spleen have led to confusing results. In trypanosomiasis, for example, reticulo-endothelial blockade by India ink often decreases resistance,[110] although sometimes no effect whatsoever can be observed.[111] Likewise, splenectomy is believed by some to increase the severity or duration of a subsequently induced infection,[112] and the

[110] T. H. Amako, *Zentralbl. f. Bakt.* 116: 280 (1930); N. v. Jancsó and H. v. Jancsó, *Ann. Trop. Med.,* 28: 419 (1934).

[111] W. Pookels, *Arb. a. d. Staatsinst. f. exper. Therap.,* No. 29: 12 (1934); M. Zolog and O. Comsia, *Compt. rend. Soc. de biol.,* 122: 1138 (1936).

[112] D. Perla and J. Marmorston-Gottesmann, *J. Exper. Med.,* 52: 601 (1930); P. Regendanz, *Ztschr. f. Immunitätsforsch. u. exper. Therap.,* 76: 437 (1932); I. J. Kligler, *Ann. Trop. Med.,* 23: 315 (1929); H. Galliard, *Bull. Soc. path. exot.,* 26: 609 (1933); W. H. Taliaferro and Y. Pavlinova, *J. Parasitol.,* 22: 29 (1936).

implantation of splenic tissue to splenectomized animals occasionally restores this resistance.[113] Others note, however, little or no such alteration in resistance.[114] Even combined reticulo-endothelial blockade and splenectomy does not always successfully depress resistance, although generally it is effective in doing so.[115] Exposure to X ray is said to be without effect in experimental trypanosomiasis.[116]

In experimental kala azar, hamsters become more susceptible after treatment with benzol or after splenectomy, both these procedures depressing reticulo-endothelial function.[117] No difference has been found, on the other hand, between the resistance of splenectomized and normal mice to *Leishmania donovani*.[118] Splenectomy is often resorted to with apparently some success as a means of therapy in human visceral leishmaniasis.[119]

The results of studies with malaria are much more in agreement as to the importance of the spleen in natural resistance than are those with the flagellate parasites. Human infections with clinically cured malaria very frequently relapse after splenectomy.[120] Monkeys also are more susceptible to the monkey malarias after splenectomy,[121] and often the monkeys succumb to species of parasites which are well tolerated by the normal monkey.[122] Not infrequently operated monkeys relapse after clinical cure.[123]

Other organs.—The removal of the adrenal glands [124] or of the hypophysis [125] results in the death of rats after infection with

[113] W. Pookels, *Arb. a. d. Staatsinst. f. exper. Therap.*, No. 29: 12 (1934).

[114] F. D. Wood, *Am. J. Trop. Med.*, 14: 497 (1934); W. H. Taliaferro, P. R. Cannon, and S. Goodloe, *Am. J. Hyg.*, 14: 1 (1931); J. Schwetz, *Bull. Soc. path. exot.*, 27: 62, and 253 (1934); P. Regendanz, *Zentralbl. f. Bakt.*, 116: 256 (1930).

[115] N. v. Jancsó and H. v. Jancsó, *Ann. Trop. Med.*, 28: 419 (1934).

[116] I. J. Kligler and R. Comaroff, *Am. J. Hyg.*, 22: 11 (1935).

[117] C. W. Wang and H.-L. Chung, *Proc. Soc. Exper. Biol. & Med.*, 44: 35 (1940).

[118] K. V. Krishnan, *Indian M. Research Mem., Suppl. Ser. to Indian J. M. Research*, Mem. No. 25: 109 (1932).

[119] P. Timpano, *Policlinico*, 37: 1710 (1930).

[120] E. Benhamou, *Bull. Soc. path. exot.*, 25: 685 (1932).

[121] J. A. Sinton, *Records of Malaria Survey of India*, 5: 501 (1935); K. V. Krishnan, R. O. A. Smith, and C. Lal, *Indian J. M. Research*, 21: 639 (1934).

[122] K. V. Krishnan, R. O. A. Smith, and C. Lal, *Indian J. M. Research*, 21: 343 (1933); B. Malamos, *Arch. f. Schiffs- u. Tropen-Hyg.*, 38: 326 (1934).

[123] *Ibid.*, p. 639 (1934).

[124] D. Perla and J. Marmorston-Gottesman, *J. Exper. Med.*, 52: 601 (1930).

[125] J. T. Culbertson and N. Molomut, *Proc. Soc. Exper. Biol. & Med.*, 39: 28 (1938).

Trypanosoma lewisi, death usually occurring in about five days. The parasite counts are not raised above the usual level in the operated animals, and death appears to be related more to changes in the chemical balance of the blood than to an alteration in the resistance mechanism itself. Thymectomy, on the other hand, enhances resistance to *Trypanosoma lewisi,* both the severity and duration of an infection being less in operated rats. Bilateral gonadectomy depresses the resistance of rats to this parasite, although unilateral nephrectomy has no effect.[126] The infection of chicks with caecal flagellates can be rendered impossible by caecectomy, the parasites evidently being unable to survive in other parts of the food canal.[127]

ADDITIONAL FACTORS: HEMORRHAGE; ALCOHOL

A number of other factors significantly influence resistance. For example, repeated hemorrhage lowers resistance against the intestinal nematodes.[128] The administration of alcohol to mice for one or two weeks prior to infection with *Trypanosoma gambiense* is said to lead to earlier death of the animals.[129] The abuse of alcohol is said to predispose humans to amoebic infection. When alcohol is given simultaneously with infective cysts of *Trichinella spiralis,* however, the severity of ensuing infections is sharply reduced, presumably because the alcohol prevents the excystation of the parasites.[130]

SPECIAL DEFENSIVE AND INVASIVE FACTORS

Natural resistance is often explained through the possession of special means of defense by the host or of special means of invasion by the parasite. Many of these mechanisms are without the scope of this text and will not be mentioned. Others, however, do have an immunological basis and will, therefore, be described briefly.

[126] J. Marmorston-Gottesman, D. Perla, and J. Vorzimer, *J. Exper. Med.,* 52: 587 (1930) ; D. Perla and J. Marmorston-Gottesman, *J. Exper. Med.,* 52: 601 (1930).
[127] F. L. Richardson, *Am. J. Hyg.,* 30: 69 (1939, sec. C).
[128] W. W. Cort, *J. Parasitol.,* 19: 142 (1932) ; D. A. Porter and J. E. Ackert, *Am. J. Hyg.,* 17: 252 (1933) ; A. O. Foster, *Am. J. Hyg.,* 24: 109 (1936).
[129] L. B. Levinson, *Zentralbl. f. Bakt.,* 114: 488 (1929).
[130] J. B. McNaught and G. N. Pierce, *Am. J. Clin. Path.,* 9: 52 (1939).

DEFENSIVE MECHANISMS OF THE HOST

The natural defensive mechanisms of the host usually depend basically on the action of its cells or, somewhat more obviously, on the secretions of these cells, especially as found in the blood plasma or serum and in the digestive juices. Infection with amoebae, for example, seems to depend upon the absence of free hydrochloric acid from the stomach of the host,[131] and coccidial infection occurs only in animals whose digestive juice contains components causing excystation of the parasite.[132] Conversely, infection with the adult of *Echinococcus granulosus* is possible only in those few animals whose intestinal juice does not digest the scolices of the larval stage of this cestode.[133]

The normal serum of certain animals also contains antagonistic substances for a number of parasites. Human serum, for example, as well as that of a few other primates, will lyse either in vitro or in the animal body any of the numerous pathogenic trypanosomes of animals, despite its inactivity upon the human pathogens.[134] These parasites from animals cannot infect man, perhaps because of this action of human serum. Essentially similar phenomena are seen when the normal serum of a wide range of animals is added in vitro to certain species of cercariae.[135] These parasites are killed and lysed by the serum even when this is added in considerable dilution. A similar effect is produced when fish trematodes are exposed to the mucus of certain resistant fish.[136] All these studies suggest that susceptibility or resistance is related to components of the serum or the body secretions of the host.

The action of the body cells themselves also is a definite factor in natural resistance, although their activity in the normal animal is often difficult to demonstrate. Their function is much more easily seen when specific antibody is also present in the serum. Nevertheless, in experimental malaria of monkeys, for example,

[131] H. Tsuchiya, *Am. J. Trop. Med.*, 19: 151 (1939).

[132] J. M. Andrews, *J. Parasitol.*, 13: 183 (1927).

[133] D. A. Berberian, *J. Helminthol.*, 14: 21 (1936).

[134] J. T. Culbertson, *Arch. Path.*, 20: 767 (1935).

[135] J. T. Culbertson and S. B. Talbot, *Science*, 82: 525 (1935); J. T. Culbertson, *J. Parasitol.*, 22: 11 (1936); M. A. Tubangui and V. A. Masilungan, *Philippine J. Sc.*, 60: 393 (1936).

[136] R. F. Nigrelli, *J. Parasitol.*, 21: 438 (1935).

the macrophages of the normal animal can, even in the beginning, phagocytize the infected red cells, although at a rate too slow to keep the infection in check.[137] After the crisis or after antibody is supplied passively these cells immediately manifest enhanced phagocytizing potentialities, and the infection is soon controlled. Likewise, a cellular infiltration is noted about migrating nematode larvae in the somatic tissues of normal animals, although much less in both amount and effect than in immunized animals.[138]

INVASIVE MECHANISMS OF THE PARASITE

Trematode cercariae that invade tissue are equipped with glands which assist the organism to penetrate the tissue. These glands secrete a ferment which digests the tissue through which the cercariae must pass. This ferment can also be demonstrated in vitro after extraction from the bodies of the cercariae, and extracts containing it readily digest tissue from susceptible animals.[139] The action of this lysin is more or less analogous with that of the cytolysin believed to be formed by *Endamoeba histolytica*. Cercariae devoid of glands for producing this ferment are not tissue invaders. The lysin of the amoebae just mentioned is considered to enable that protozoan to make its way beneath the intestinal epithelium.

Certain of the other helminth parasites, particularly nematodes, are believed to produce antienzymes which not only protect the worm from digestion by the ferments of the host but also inhibit the action of the host's digestive juices upon ingested food. The extreme emaciation and generally poor condition of animals which have heavy infections with these parasites is believed to result from the action of the antienzymes produced by the parasites.[140]

[137] W. H. Taliaferro and P. R. Cannon, *J. Infect. Dis.*, 52: 72 (1936).

[138] W. H. Taliaferro and M. P. Sarles, *J. Infect. Dis.*, 64: 157 (1939).

[139] D. J. Davis, *J. Parasitol.*, 22: 108 (1936); G. W. Hunter, III, and W. S. Hunter, *J. Parasitol.*, 23: 572 (1937).

[140] J. Stewart, *3rd Rep., Univ. Cambridge, Inst. Animal Pathol.*, 77 (1932–33).

Chapter III

AGE RESISTANCE

YOUNG ANIMALS often suffer intense or even fatal infections with parasites which either fail entirely to establish themselves in older hosts or else produce only mild infections. This follows because these animals become naturally resistant to the parasite as they grow older, without experiencing an infection with it. The refractory state of normal older animals which belong to species whose young are susceptible is commonly termed "age resistance." The young animals appear either to lack the defensive mechanisms which enable the older hosts to resist the parasite or else to provide a more favorable milieu in which the parasite may develop. Often such parasites as the young host has acquired are expelled when the host attains the resistant age.

EXAMPLES OF AGE RESISTANCE

Age resistance occurs with respect to both protozoan and helminth parasites. Examples will first be given of each of these groups, and then explanations of the phenomenon of age resistance will be suggested.

PROTOZOA

Age resistance has been demonstrated to protozoans of such diverse groups as amoebae, intestinal flagellates, trypanosomes, coccidia, and malaria organisms. *Endamoeba histolytica* has its greatest incidence in young adults; persons over thirty-five years old seldom harbor the parasite. Among inmates of institutions, however, where perhaps greater opportunity for infection obtains than in the population at large, the incidence of infection often remains high even among the aged.[1] Young dogs and cats suffer

---

[1] D. H. Wenrich and J. H. Arnett, *J. Parasitol.*, 23: 318 (1937).

more severe experimental infections with *Endamoeba histolytica* than do older animals.[2]

Age resistance has been demonstrated only to *Giardia lamblia* [3] among the intestinal flagellates. No resistance is developed with age to either natural or experimental infection with the trichomonads.[4]

Only a few examples of age resistance to trypanosomes have been reported. The phenomenon has been repeatedly shown with respect to *Trypanosoma cruzi*, both in man and in animals.[5] A definite age resistance is also manifested to *Trypanosoma lewisi*, the natural trypanosome of rats.[6] An inverse age resistance occurs to the effects of *Trypanosoma equiperdum* infection in rats, although the parasite is lethal to all age groups.[7] The more frequent relapse in young rats after treatment of *Trypanosoma brucei* infection with arsenicals and antimonials may be the reflection of an age resistance by the animals to this parasite.[8]

Chicks of all ages are susceptible to the pathogenic coccidian *Eimeria tenella*, but those over three months old are considerably more resistant than are younger birds.[9] An inverse age resistance has been reported in chicks to *Eimeria necatrix*, young birds suffering less from this infection than older ones.[10]

Children experience more frequent and more intense infection with *Plasmodium vivax* malaria than do adults.[11] The age group most frequently infected is that between five and nine years.[12]

[2] O. Wagner, *Arch. f. Schiffs- u. Tropen-Hyg.*, 39: 1 (1935).

[3] K. M. Lynch, *Am. J. Trop. Med.*, 8: 345 (1928); T. B. Magath and P. W. Brown, *Am. J. Trop. Med.*, 10: 113 (1930).

[4] K. M. Lynch, *Am. J. Trop. Med.*, 8: 345 (1928); R. Hegner, *Am. J. Hyg.*, 9: 529 (1929).

[5] S. Niimi, *Jap. J. Exper. Med.*, 13: 543 (1935); P. Regendanz, *Zentralbl. f. Bakt.*, 116: 256 (1930); M. H. Kolodny, *Am. J. Hyg.*, 29: 13, 155 (1939, sec. C).

[6] B. Borghi, Soc. internaz di microbiol., *Boll. d. sez ital.*, 4: 69 (1932); C. A. Herrick and S. X. Cross, *J. Parasitol*, 22: 126 (1936); C. J. Duca, *Am. J. Hyg.*, 29: 25 (1939, sec. C).

[7] H. A. Poindexter, *Am. J. Hyg.*, 29: 111 (1939, sec. C).

[8] H. Neumann, *Ztschr. f. Immunitätsforsch. u. exper. Therap.*, 74: 177 (1932).

[9] C. A. Herrick, G. L. Ott, and C. E. Holmes, *J. Parasitol.*, 22: 264 (1936).

[10] E. E. Tyzzer, H. Theiler, and E. E. Jones, *Am. J. Hyg.*, 15: 319 (1932).

[11] I. Balteanu and I. Alexa, *Arch. roumaines de path. expér. et de microbiol.*, 8: 491 (1935); M. Ciuca, L. Ballif, and M. Vieru, *Arch. roumaines de path. expér. et de microbiol.*, 3: 209 (1930); P. S. Djaparidse, *Arch. f. Schiffs- u. Tropen-Hyg.*, 36: 476 (1932); W. C. Earle, *Puerto Rico J. Pub. Health & Trop. Med.*, 15: 3 (1939); L. H. Henderson, *Tr. Roy. Soc. Trop. Med. & Hyg.*, 28: 157 (1934); F. Pistoni, *Arch. ital. di sc. med. colon.*, 18: 138 (1937).

[12] W. C. Earle, *Puerto Rico J. Pub. Health & Trop. Med.*, 15: 3 (1939).

Age resistance to *Plasmodium falciparum* has also been described,[13] although some authorities find the percentage of carriers increases with age.[14]

HELMINTHS

There is as yet but little data available upon age resistance to trematodes. The maximum incidence of human schistosomiasis occurs in persons between ten and fifteen years of age.[15] The disease rarely affects those over thirty years old.[16] Other human trematode infections have as yet been too little studied for generalization. Herring gulls seem to acquire resistance with age to the cloacal trematode *Parorchis acanthus*,[17] and frogs resist *Diplostomum flexicaudum* following their metamorphosis from tadpoles.[18] Certain marine fish show an inverse age resistance to a monogenetic trematode *Epibdella melleni*.[19]

Age resistance has been demonstrated with cestodes of the genera *Diphyllobothrium, Hymenolepis,* and *Raillietina. Hymenolepis nana* has its greatest incidence in persons from five to fourteen years of age.[20] Rats and mice five to seven months old are much more resistant to the rodent form *Hymenolepis fraterna* than are animals two months of age.[21] Chicks more than two months old resist *Raillietina cesticillus* better than do those below this age.[22] Gulls naturally eliminate certain *Diphyllobothrium* tapeworms when they reach an age at which a constant high body temperature is established and when complete feathering has taken place.[23]

Among the many nematode parasites, age resistance has been demonstrated with respect to *Trichinella spiralis,* the ascarids,

[13] B. Wilson, *Acta Conventus Tertii de Tropicis Atque Malariae Morbis,* Part 2: 346 (1939).

[14] P. S. Djaparidse, *Arch. f. Schiffs- u. Tropen-Hyg.,* 36: 476 (1932) ; M. Rankov, *Arch. f. Schiffs- u. Tropen-Hyg.,* 40: 277 (1936).

[15] P. K. Dixon, *Tr. Roy. Soc. Trop. Med. & Hyg.,* 27: 505 (1934) ; G. W. St. C. Ramsay, *West African M. J.,* 8: 2 (1935).

[16] A. C. Fisher, *Tr. Roy. Soc. Trop. Med. & Hyg.,* 28: 277 (1934).

[17] R. M. Cable, *J. Parasitol.,* 23: 559 (1937).

[18] D. J. Davis, *J. Parasitol.,* 22: 329 (1936).

[19] R. F. Nigrelli and C. M. Breder, Jr., *J. Parasitol.,* 20: 259 (1934).

[20] G. F. Otto, *J. Parasitol.,* 21: 443 (1935).

[21] D. A. Shorb, *Am. J. Hyg.,* 18: 74 (1933) ; A. V. Hunninen, *Am. J. Hyg.,* 22: 414 (1935).

[22] J. E. Ackert and W. M. Reid, *J. Parasitol.,* 23: 558 (1937).

[23] L. J. Thomas, *Anat. Rec. (Suppl.),* 78: 104 (1940).

and the hookworms, as well as the related forms of each. Young dogs are more susceptible to both the muscle and the gut stages of *Trichinella spiralis* than are older dogs. The resistance of the old animals appears to result from the failure of ingested larvae to mature in the intestine.[24] An age resistance to *Trichinella spiralis* is also seen in pigeons, muscle being invaded only in the young birds despite the fact that the ingested larvae develop to adults in pigeons of all ages.[25] Rats develop an age resistance to the related nematode *Capillaria hepatica.*[26]

Ascariasis is primarily an infection of children, the peak incidence occurring among those about five years of age.[27] Age resistance has also been demonstrated to such animal ascarids as *Toxocara canis* of dogs,[28] *Ascaridia lineata,*[29] *Ascaridia galli,*[30] and perhaps *Heterakis gallinae*[31] of chickens, and *Ascaris lumbricoides* of pigs.[32]

Hookworm infection is most severe in children below fifteen years of age.[33] From experimental studies it is clear that dogs as well as cats acquire resistance with age to *Ancylostoma caninum*[34] and that a marked age resistance is manifested to *Nippostrongylus muris* by rats[35] and mice.[36] Lambs gradually become naturally resistant to *Dictyocaulus filaria.*[37] Chicks over ten weeks old resist *Syngamus trachea,*[38] although even yearling fowls sometimes are susceptible.[39] Equines over fifteen years old

[24] K. Matoff, *Tierärztl. Rundschau,* 43: 399 (1937).
[25] K. Matoff, *Tierärztl. Rundschau,* 42: 401 (1936).
[26] G. Luttermoser, *Am. J. Hyg.,* 27: 321 (1938).
[27] G. F. Otto and W. W. Cort, *Am. J. Hyg.,* 19: 657 (1934); W. W. Cort and G. F. Otto, *South. M. J.,* 26: 273 (1933).
[28] E. H. Hinman and D. D. Baker, *J. Trop. Med.,* 39: 101 (1936).
[29] J. E. Ackert, D. A. Porter, and T. D. Beach, *J. Parasitol.,* 21: 205 (1935).
[30] D. O. Morgan and J. E. Wilson, *J. Helminthol.,* 16: 165 (1938).
[31] P. A. Clapham, *J. Helminthol.,* 12: 71 (1934).
[32] D. O. Morgan, *J. Helminthol.,* 9: 121 (1931).
[33] F. C. Caldwell and E. L. Caldwell, *J. Parasitol.,* 17: 209 (1931).
[34] C. A. Herrick, *Am. J. Hyg.,* 8: 125 (1928); J. A. Scott, *Am. J. Hyg.,* 8: 158 (1928); M. P. Sarles, *Am. J. Hyg.,* 10: 453 (1929); A. O. Foster, *Am. J. Hyg.,* 22: 65 (1935).
[35] C. M. Africa, *J. Parasitol.,* 18: 1 (1931); A. C. Chandler, *Am. J. Hyg.,* 16: 750 (1932).
[36] D. A. Porter, *Am. J. Hyg.,* 22: 444 (1935).
[37] G. Kauzal, *Australian Vet. Jour.,* 10: 100 (1934).
[38] P. A. Clapham, *Proc. Roy. Soc. London,* s. B, 115: 18 (1934).
[39] D. O. Morgan, *J. Helminthol.,* 9: 117 (1931); R. H. Waite, Maryland State Coll. Agric., *Bull.* 234, p. 103.

have smaller numbers of strongylid worms than those below this age.[40]

An age resistance to *Strongyloides ratti* is manifested by rats eight months old or more. A smaller percentage of the larvae administered reach the adult stage in the intestine of the older rats, and these persist for a briefer time than do those which develop to adults in the intestines of the young rats.[41]

EXPLANATIONS OF AGE RESISTANCE

Several possible explanations for age resistance present themselves. One of these considers age resistance merely an extension of natural resistance and is based primarily upon the fact that a parasite never infects animals which do not provide a favorable physiological medium in which it may live. Many animals, when young, have not attained their complete physiological differentiation, and during such time are susceptible to a given parasite. As the animals grow older and their tissues and fluids take on mature characteristics, they may become physiologically unsuited to the parasite. Infection with that parasite cannot thereafter occur, and such forms as it picked up earlier may be expelled. Age resistance, according to this view, would be least expected in natural host-parasite relationships. In fact the hypothesis has been offered that age resistance is manifested by hosts chiefly against unnatural, newly acquired, or otherwise imperfectly adjusted parasites.[42]

According to another view, the greater susceptibility of young animals to many parasites is a reflection of their poorer capacity to manifest a specific immune response after infection. The capacity of the specific antibody-forming mechanism of young animals is known often to be poor compared with that of adults.[43] In such young animals a parasite will be able to establish itself and perhaps cause an intense infection, whereas, in animals able to respond with specific antagonistic antibodies, the infection may be largely inhibited and quickly eliminated. This mechanism has been shown to obtain in the experimental infections of rats with

[40] A. O. Foster, *Am. J. Hyg.*, 25: 66 (1937).
[41] A. J. Sheldon, *Am. J. Hyg.*, 26: 355 (1937) ; H. J. Lawlor, *J. Parasitol. (Suppl.)*, 25: 30 (1939).
[42] J. H. Sandground, *Parasitology*, 21: 227 (1929).
[43] L. Baumgartner, *Yale J. Biol. and Med.*, 6: 403 (1934).

Trypanosoma lewisi and with *Trypanosoma cruzi*. Nursling rats
are usually killed by either parasite, and they invariably suffer
intense infections. Old rats, in contrast, seldom die from either

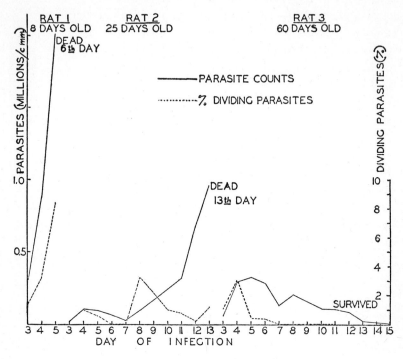

CHART I

ANTIBODY PRODUCTION AGAINST *TRYPANOSOMA LEWISI*
BY RATS OF DIFFERENT AGE GROUPS

As the ablastin (reproduction-inhibiting) antibody increases in amount in
the blood, the percentage of trypanosomes seen in division decreases. The
antibody is produced only poorly, if at all, in very young rats (for example,
No. 1, eight days old) and these animals generally succumb. It is produced
well by older rats (for example, No. 3, sixty days old), and these animals
generally survive. The capacity to produce the antibody in adequate amount
is acquired at about twenty-five days of age (for example, No. 2). Animals
of this age sometimes survive, but they often succumb after a prolonged
infection, as in the case of the example given.

infection and in the case of *Trypanosoma cruzi* they experience
infections of exceedingly low intensity. The greater susceptibility
of young rats to each of these forms results from their poorer

capacity to form specific antibody rapidly and thus to prevent the infection from overwhelming them.[44] An essentially similar explanation has been offered for the age resistance of rats to the nematode *Strongyloides ratti*.[45]

Still other mechanisms have been presented to explain specific examples of age resistance. The inverse age resistance of chicks to *Eimeria necatrix* may be the result of the extraordinarily high natural rate of growth of the affected tissue—namely, the intestinal epithelium—of the young birds.[46] The resistance of mature frogs, compared with tadpoles, to *Diplostomum flexicaudum* has been explained by the inability of the parasite to penetrate the tougher skin of the old frog.[47] The greater resistance of older chicks to *Ascaridia lineata* and *Ascaridia galli* is probably due to their secretion of protective mucus from the proportionately more numerous goblet cells in their duodenal epithelium.[48] The age resistance of dogs to *Ancylostoma caninum* may be related to the natural age curve of the hemoglobin level of the host,[49] but certainly in part it depends upon the function of the body defense cells in checking the progress of larval forms migrating through the skin or other tissue.[50]

OTHER FACTORS INFLUENCING AGE RESISTANCE

A number of other factors besides those mentioned in the previous section influence age resistance. Among these are the diet, the environmental temperature, and the hormone balance. If animals of species which normally become resistant with age are kept on a diet deficient in essential elements, they will fail to become resistant as they mature. This has been shown especially well in such nematode infections of dogs as hookworm disease

[44] J. T. Culbertson and R. M. Wotton, *Am. J. Hyg.*, 30: 101 (1939, sec. C) ; J. T. Culbertson and W. R. Kessler, *Am. J. Hyg.*, 29: 33 (1939, sec. C) ; M. H. Kolodny, *Am. J. Hyg.*, 31: 7 (1940, sec. C).

[45] H. J. Lawlor, *J. Parasitol. (Suppl.)*, 25: 30 (1939).

[46] E. E. Tyzzer, H. Theiler, and E. E. Jones, *Am. J. Hyg.*, 15: 319 (1932).

[47] D. J. Davis, *J. Parasitol.*, 22: 329 (1936).

[48] J. E. Ackert and S. A. Edgar, *J. Parasitol.*, 24: 13 (1938); J. E. Ackert, S. A. Edgar, and L. P. Frick, *Tr. Am. Micro. Soc.*, 58: 81 (1939) ; J. E. Ackert and S. A. Edgar, *J. Parasitol. (Suppl.)*, 26: 14 (1940) ; J. E. Ackert and L. P. Frick, *J. Parasitol. (Suppl.)*, 26: 14 (1940).

[49] A. O. Foster, *Am. J. Hyg.*, 24: 109 (1936).

[50] M. P. Sarles, *Am. J. Hyg.*, 10: 683 (1929) ; 10: 693 (1929).

and ascariasis.[51] The natural resistance of older rats to trypanosomes (*Trypanosoma cruzi*) can be partially overcome by keep-
ing the animals in a low temperature environment.[52]

One might suspect that hormones would exert almost a governing role in age resistance and that by prematurely aging young
animals through supplying the hormones of sex organs or other
body tissues a precocious resistance could be developed. Some of
the attempts to produce resistance experimentally by supplying
these hormones have resulted in success. For example, it has been
reported that young rats can be rendered significantly resistant
to *Trypanosoma lewisi* by implanting the pituitary gland from
adult nonimmune rats intramuscularly or by injecting oestrin
cutaneously to the young.[53] The majority of such efforts, however, have failed to influence age resistance. Their failures are
difficult to explain, but may result from the fact that most
hormone-containing extracts yet available have a comparatively
limited sphere of influence rather than a complete or general effect
upon the body as a whole. When hormone preparations are available which are capable of artificially aging the entire organism
simultaneously, the experimental development of age resistance
may be regularly possible of achievement.

[51] A. O. Foster and W. W. Cort, *Am. J. Hyg.*, 21: 302 (1935); W. H. Wright,
J. Parasitol., 21: 43 (1935).
[52] M. H. Kolodny, *Am. J. Hyg.*, 32: 21 (1940, sec. C).
[53] C. A. Herrick and S. X. Cross, *J. Parasitol.*, 22: 126 (1936).

Chapter IV

SPECIFICALLY ACQUIRED
IMMUNITY

MANY ANIMALS can be infected with a given parasite on first exposure to it, but as a direct result of this initial exposure they may acquire a specific immunity which prevents a subsequent infection with the same parasite. In the present chapter the different manners in which animals may acquire immunity are described, and examples of each are cited.

Specific immunity may be acquired actively or passively. In actively acquired immunity, the immune animal himself has responded to a prior infection with a parasite or to vaccination with the parasite antigens by producing specific substances antagonistic for that parasite. In passively acquired immunity, these antagonistic substances are produced by one animal, but introduced by transfer of its serum to another animal in which they act. The antagonistic substances are identical as to specificity of action, whether acquired actively or passively. Actively acquired immunity often endures for long periods, and may continue for life; whereas passively acquired immunity is usually of distinctly brief duration, since the antagonistic substances seldom persist in an animal to which they have been transferred for more than four to six weeks. The longer persistence of the actively acquired immune state results because the production of antagonistic substances usually continues for a considerable period once it is initiated. An actively immunized animal can, furthermore, resume the production of the specific antagonistic substances at some later time, if an occasion requiring them arises.

IMMUNITY ACQUIRED BY INFECTION

Specific immunity is acquired after infection with either protozoans or helminths. Examples are known in nearly all types of protozoan diseases—amoebiasis, trichomoniasis, leishmaniasis, trypanosomiasis, coccidiosis, and malaria. Immunity is also acquired after such somatic helminth infections as cysticercosis, trichiniasis, ascariasis, hookworm disease, and strongyloidiasis.

Protozoa.—Man apparently resists a superimposed infection with *Endamoeba histolytica,* although the conclusive demonstration of such an acquired resistance has not been reported. Kittens, however, are believed to acquire some immunity after repeated experimental reinfection with this parasite.[1] Cattle which have recovered from infection with *Trichomonas foetus* are not susceptible to reinfection.[2] Man resists the leishmanias of oriental sore after recovering from an initial lesion.[3] Specific immunity is developed likewise by monkeys as well as by sheep and goats against *Trypanosoma gambiense,*[4] by cattle against *Trypanosoma congolense* [5] and *Trypanosoma brucei,*[6] by rats to *Trypanosoma lewisi,* by mice to *Trypanosoma duttoni,* by cotton rats to *Trypanosoma sigmodoni,*[7] and by various rodents to *Trypanosoma cruzi.*[8] Among the coccidioses, immunity against reinfection is acquired by rabbits to *Eimeria perforans,*[9] by rats to *Eimeria mayairii,*[10] by cats to *Isospora felis* and *Isospora rivolta,*[11] and by chicks to *Eimeria tenella* and *Eimeria necatrix,*[12] to state but

[1] O. Wagner, *Arch. f. Schiffs- u. Tropen-Hyg.,* 39: 1 (1935).

[2] J. Andrews, *Am. J. Hyg.,* 27: 149 (1935).

[3] A. P. Lawrow and P. A. Dubowskoj, *Arch. f. Schiffs- u. Tropen-Hyg.,* 41: 374 (1937); E. I. Marzinowsky, *Bull. Soc. path. exot.,* 21: 638 (1928).

[4] P. Le Gac, *Bull. Soc. path. exot.,* 24: 372 (1931); L. Van Hoof, *Bull. Soc. path. exot.,* 27: 167 (1934); H. L. Duke, *Parasitology,* 20: 427 (1928).

[5] R. Van Saceghem, *Bull. Soc. path. exot.,* 31: 296 (1938).

[6] C. Schilling, *J. Trop. Med.,* 37: 70 (1934).

[7] J. T. Culbertson, *J. Parasitol.,* 27: 45 (1941).

[8] W. A. Collier, *Ztschr. f. Hyg. u. Infektionskr.,* 112: 88 (1931); F. D. Wood, *Am. J. Trop. Med.,* 14: 497 (1934); J. T. Culbertson and M. H. Kolodny, *J. Parasitol.,* 24: 83 (1938).

[9] G. W. Bachman, *Am. J. Hyg.,* 12: 641 (1930).

[10] E. R. Becker and P. R. Hall, *Am. J. Hyg.,* 18: 220 (1933).

[11] J. M. Andrews, *Am. J. Hyg.,* 6: 784 (1926).

[12] E. E. Tyzzer, H. Theiler, and E. E. Jones, *Am. J. Hyg.,* 15: 319 (1932).

a few examples. Among the malaria organisms, immunity to re-infection is acquired by man to *Plasmodium vivax* [13] or *Plasmodium knowlesi*,[14] by Malayan monkeys to *Plasmodium knowlesi*,[15] by Panamanian monkeys to *Plasmodium brasilianum*,[16] and by birds to, among others, *Plasmodium cathemerium, Plasmodium circumflexum, Plasmodium rouxi,* and *Plasmodium elongatum.*[17]

Helminths.—Few examples are available to illustrate acquired immunity to the trematodiases. Certain marine fish resist reinfection with monogenetic trematodes.[18] The *Macacus* monkey, as well as horses and cattle, resist superimposed infection with schistosomes,[19] but experimental evidence for the acquisition of such resistance by man is as yet unavailable.

Among the cestodiases, infections with larval forms provide the best immunity to reinfection. This has been demonstrated with cysticerci of *Taenia serrata* in rabbits,[20] *Taenia crassicollis* in rats,[21] and *Taenia saginata* in oxen.[22] Resistance to reinfection with *Hymenolepis fraterna* also has been shown in mice and in rats.[23] Little or no resistance to reinfection is acquired by hosts which are infected only with adult cestodes residing exclusively in the intestinal lumen, such as *Taenia crassicollis* in the cat,[24]

[13] M. F. Boyd and S. F. Kitchen, *Am. J. Trop. Med.,* 16: 447 (1936); M. Ciuca, L. Ballif, M. Vieru, and A. Stirbu, *Compt. rend. Soc. de biol.,* 102: 189 (1929); C. Milani and E. Cuboni, *Soc. internaz. di microbiol., Boll. d. sez. ital.,* 3: 521 (1931); F. Pistoni, *Arch. ital. di sc. med. colon.,* 18: 138 (1937).

[14] D. F. Milam and L. T. Coggeshall, *Am. J. Trop. Med.,* 18: 331 (1938).

[15] H. W. Mulligan and J. A. Sinton, *Records Malaria Survey of India,* 3: 529 (1933).

[16] W. H. Taliaferro and L. G. Taliaferro, *Am. J. Hyg.,* 20: 60 (1934).

[17] F. Wolfson and O. R. Causey, *J. Parasitol.,* 25: 510 (1939); R. D. Manwell, *Proc. Soc. Exper. Biol. & Med.,* 32: 391 (1934); R. D. Manwell, *Am. J. Hyg.,* 27: 196 (1938); R. D. Manwell and F. Goldstein, *Am. J. Hyg.,* 30: 115 (1939, sec. C).

[18] T. L. Jahn and L. R. Kuhn, *Biol. Bull.,* 62: 89 (1932); R. F. Nigrelli and C. M. Breder, Jr., *J. Parasitol.,* 20: 259 (1934).

[19] N. H. Fairley, F. P. Mackie, and F. Jasudasan, *Ind. Med. Res. Mem. Supp. Ser. to Ind. J. Med. Res.,* Part IV (1930).

[20] K. B. Kerr, *Am. J. Hyg.,* 22: 169 (1935); A. B. Leonard and A. E. Smith, *J. Parasitol. (Suppl.),* 25: 30 (1939).

[21] H. M. Miller, Jr., *Proc. Soc. Exper. Biol. & Med.,* 28: 467 (1931).

[22] W. J. Penfold, H. B. Penfold, and M. Phillips, *M. J. Australia,* 1: 417 (1936).

[23] D. A. Shorb, *Am. J. Hyg.,* 18: 74 (1933); A. V. Hunninen, *Am. J. Hyg.,* 22: 414 (1935).

[24] H. M. Miller, Jr., *J. Prevent. Med.,* 6: 17 (1932).

Multiceps glomeratus in the dog,[25] and *Hymenolepis diminuta* in the rat.[26]

Comparatively little resistance to reinfection is acquired by man against *Ascaris lumbricoides*,[27] but mice and guinea pigs resist reinfection with the somatic phase of this worm.[28] Likewise, cats resist reinfection with *Toxocara cati*,[29] rats resist *Heterakis spumosa*,[30] and chicks resist *Ascaridia lineata*.[31] Some measure of resistance to reinfection follows hookworm disease in man,[32] and dogs [33] and mice [34] likewise resist reinfection with the animal hookworms. Immunity is also acquired to forms related to hookworms, such as *Nippostrongylus muris* in rats,[35] the trichostrongylid parasites in sheep [36] and rabbits,[37] *Metastrongylus elongatus* in pigs,[38] and *Dictyocaulus filaria* in lambs.[39] Immunity has also been demonstrated in rats after infection with *Strongyloides ratti* and *Trichinella spiralis*.[40]

PREMUNITION

The term "premunition" was proposed by Sergent [41] in 1924 to describe a form of resistance which depends on the mutual tolerance of the host and parasite. The host is enabled to mollify a superimposed infection if the parasites from an initial infection

[25] P. A. Clapham, *J. Helminthol.*, 18: 45 (1940).

[26] A. C. Chandler, *Am. J. Hyg.*, 29: 105 (1939, sec. D).

[27] G. F. Otto and W. W. Cort, *J. Parasitol.*, 20: 245 (1934); E. Roman, *Compt. rend. Soc. de biol.*, 130: 1168 (1939).

[28] O. Wagner, *Ztschr. f. Immunitätsforsch. u. exper. Therap.*, 78: 372 (1933); K. B. Kerr, *Am. J. Hyg.*, 27: 28 (1938).

[29] M. P. Sarles and N. R. Stoll, *J. Parasitol.*, 21: 277 (1935).

[30] G. F. Winfield, *Am. J. Hyg.*, 17: 168 (1933).

[31] G. L. Graham, J. E. Ackert, and R. W. Jones, *Am. J. Hyg.*, 15: 726 (1932).

[32] W. W. Cort, *J. Parasitol.*, 19: 142 (1932).

[33] O. R. McCoy, *Am. J. Hyg.*, 14: 268 (1931); G. F. Otto and K. B. Kerr, *Am. J. Hyg.*, 29: 25 (1939, sec. D).

[34] K. B. Kerr, *Am. J. Hyg.*, 24: 381 (1936).

[35] C. M. Africa, *J. Parasitol.*, 18: 1 (1931); G. L. Graham, *Am. J. Hyg.*, 20: 352 (1934); A. C. Chandler, *Am. J. Hyg.*, 22: 243 (1935).

[36] E. L. Taylor, *J. Helminthol.*, 12: 143 (1934); J. S. Andrews, *J. Agric. Res.*, 58: 761 (1939).

[37] M. P. Sarles, *J. Parasitol.*, 19: 61 (1932).

[38] B. Schwartz and J. T. Lucker, *J. Parasitol.*, 21: 432 (1935).

[39] G. Kauzal, *Australian Vet. J.*, 10: 100 (1934).

[40] A. J. Sheldon, *Am. J. Hyg.*, 25: 53 (1937); O. R. McCoy, *Am. J. Hyg.*, 14: 484 (1931).

[41] E. Sergent, *Riv. di Malariol.* (*Suppl. to No. 3*), 14: 5 (1935).

have persisted in latent form in its tissues. In premunition the resistant state is contemporaneous with the latent infection and ceases with cure. Premunition differs from true immunity, therefore, in that it represents a co-infected state, whereas true immunity is a post-infection (or post-vaccination) state. In most cases, however, premunition is followed by a true absolute immunity which lasts for at least a brief period.[42]

Protozoan infections.—In many protozoan infections, acquired resistance is always of the nature of premunition, requiring the persistence of the causal agent in latent form. With respect to others, a true immunity is, at least ultimately, developed. In human amoebiasis resistance lasts only so long as the controlled infection continues. When amoebiasis is cured, either spontaneously or by drug treatment, the person is again as susceptible to infection as a normal individual.

Among the trypanosomiases the resistance observed following infection with *Trypanosoma brucei*[43] and *Trypanosoma congolense*[44] in cattle, *Trypanosoma marocanum* in camels,[45] and *Trypanosoma cruzi*[46] in various animals represents premunition. On the other hand an absolute and complete immunity is displayed by recovered rats to *Trypanosoma lewisi* and by recovered mice to *Trypanosoma duttoni*.

Resistance to reinfection with the malarias of monkeys,[47] birds,[48] and dogs[49] have all been shown to depend in part on premunization. In the case of human malaria premunition prob-

[42] E. Sergent and others, *Tr. Roy. Soc. Trop. Med. & Hyg.*, 27: 277 (1933); G. Sicault and A. Messerlin, *Bull. Soc. path. exot.*, 31: 911 (1938).

[43] E. W. Bevan, *Tr. Roy. Soc. Trop. Med. & Hyg.*, 30: 199 (1936); C. Schilling, *Deutsche med. Wchnschr.*, 61: 832 (1935).

[44] R. Van Saceghem, *Bull. Ag. Congo Belge*, 27: 47 (1936); C. Schilling, *Ztschr. f. Immunitätsforsch. u. exper. Therap.*, 89: 306 (1936).

[45] E. Sergent, *Bull. Soc. path. exot.*, 22: 887 (1929).

[46] W. A. Collier, *Ztschr. f. Hyg. u. Infektionskr.*, 112: 88 (1931).

[47] W. H. Taliaferro and L. G. Taliaferro, *Am. J. Hyg.*, 20: 60 (1934); K. V. Krishnan, R. O. A. Smith, and C. Lal, *Indian J. M. Research*, 21: 639 (1934); H. E. Shortt and others, *Indian J. M. Research*, 25: 763 (1938).

[48] W. H. Taliaferro, *South. M. J.*, 24: 405 (1931); W. Gingrich, *J. Prevent. Med.*, 6: 197 (1932); Z. W. Jermoljewa and I. S. Bujanouskaja, *Ztschr. f. Immunitätsforsch. u. exper. Therap.*, 73: 276 (1932); E. Sergent, E. Sergent, and A. Catanei, *Ann. Inst. Past.*, 53: 101 (1934).

[49] H. E. Shortt and others, *Indian J. M. Research*, 25: 763 (1938).

ably is responsible for the earlier resistance to reinfection,[50] but a state of complete immunity finally develops which lasts for an indefinite period.[51] Sergent [52] considers that the resistance to malaria manifested by Negroes as a race in the tropics is accounted for by premunition, the Negroes being first infected at an early age and repeatedly reinfected thereafter.

In coccidiosis premunition has not been experimentally demonstrated.[53] True immunity in coccidiosis is of such extraordinarily brief duration, however, that more or less constant reinfection is required to prolong the immune state.

Helminth infections.—Because of the nature of the helminth infections, the occurrence of premunition in the helminthiases is difficult to determine. In the case of the purely intestinal adult cestodes, acquired immunity has been described by some investigators,[54] although others have demonstrated no such refractoriness to reinfection.[55] Those who believe resistance to reinfection to these intestinal parasites is manifested consider that the animals are premunized and that so long as forms from the initial infection persist new worms cannot be established. Recently, however, experimental studies have indicated that the mere crowding of intestinal parasites, involving competition for both the available space and food in the intestine, plays a larger part in preventing reinfection than does an immune response by the host. For example, if the worms of an initial infection with *Hymenolepis diminuta* are removed by an anthelminthic, reinfection can promptly occur.[56]

[50] E. Sergent, *Bull. Soc. path. exot.*, 22: 887 (1929) ; W. A. P. Schüffner and others, *Zentralbl. f. Bakt.*, 125: 1 (1932) ; M. Ciuca, L. Ballif, and M. C. Vieru, *Bull. Soc. path. exot.*, 26: 300 (1933) ; P. Daleas, *Bull. Soc. med.-chir. de L'Indochine,* 13: 432 (1935).

[51] M. F. Boyd, W. K. Stratman-Thomas, and S. F. Kitchen, *Am. J. Trop. Med.,* 16: 311 (1936) ; M. Ciuca, L. Ballif, and M. Chelarescu-Vieru, *Tr. Roy. Soc. Trop. Med. & Hyg.,* 27: 619 (1934) ; M. Ciuca, L. Ballif, and M. Vieru, *Arch. roumaines de path. expér. et de microbiol.,* 1: 577 (1928).

[52] E. Sergent, *Riv. di Malariol.,* 14 (Suppl. to No. 3): 5–25 (1935).

[53] N. F. Morehouse, *J. Parasitol.,* 24: 311 (1938) ; E. E. Tyzzer, H. Theiler, and E. E. Jones, *Am. J. Hyg.,* 15: 319 (1932).

[54] C. Joyeux and J. G. Baer, *Marseille-méd.,* 68: 493 (1931) ; M. Palais, *Compt. rend. Soc. de biol.,* 117: 1016 (1934).

[55] H. M. Miller, Jr., *J. Prevent. Med.,* 6: 17 (1932) ; G. W. Luttermoser, *J. Parasitol. (Suppl.),* 24: 14 (1938).

[56] A. C. Chandler, *Am. J. Hyg.,* 29: 105 (1939, sec. D).

In the case of larval cestodes, which usually invade somatic tissue, an immune response certainly accounts for the resistance to reinfection.[57] It is especially difficult in these cases, however, to prove whether premunition or a true immunity is responsible for this resistance, since, once present in the somatic tissues, these larvae—particularly those of the cestodes—are never dislodged naturally so long as the host survives. However, rats from which the cysticerci of *Taenia crassicollis* are surgically removed have been shown to remain immune for at least two months.[58] In this case the immunity to the cestode larvae must not have depended on the persistence of the organisms of the initial infection.

In certain nematode infections essentially the same problems exist concerning premunition as with the cestodiases. With many nematodes, however, an added difficulty must be dealt with, since the parasite may characteristically reside successively in the somatic tissue as a larva and in the intestine of the same individual as an adult. A second infection with *Ascaris* or hookworm is seldom superimposed on one already existing. Premunition probably has relatively little to do with this apparent resistance, because of the considerable competition for space and food in the host's intestine. If the adult stage of *Ascaris* or of the hookworms is removed by anthelminthics, reinfection usually promptly recurs unless the initial infection has been extraordinarily severe. In trichiniasis an animal certainly resists reinfection with *Trichinella spiralis*.[59] It is impossible, however, to determine how much of this resistance is due to premunition and how much to true immunity, for the larvae cannot be removed from the body of the living animal or destroyed by any known means.

Some light is thrown on the general problem of premunition in the helminthiases by the fact that immunity against infection can be developed by vaccination with the antigens of killed helminths, a matter which will be discussed in some detail presently. During such vaccination, no infection whatsoever develops, yet the vac-

[57] H. M. Miller, Jr., *Proc. Soc. Exper. Biol. & Med.*, 28: 467 (1931); K. B. Kerr, *Am. J. Hyg.*, 22: 169 (1935); W. J. Penfold, H. B. Penfold, and M. Phillips, *M. J. Australia*, 1: 417 (1936).

[58] H. M. Miller, Jr., and E. Massie, *J. Prevent. Med.*, 6: 31 (1932).

[59] O. R. McCoy, *Am. J. Hyg.*, 14: 484 (1931); *Proc. Soc. Exper. Biol. & Med.*, 30: 85 (1932).

cinated animals become resistant. In these cases a true immunity certainly is developed. Probably to at least an equal extent a true immunity also follows actual infection with the same parasite.

IMMUNITY ACQUIRED BY VACCINATION WITH KILLED OR AVIRULENT ORGANISMS

Animals can be rendered immune to several different parasites by vaccination with killed or avirulent organisms. The best effects are seen with somatic tissue parasites or forms which invade somatic tissues during part of their development. Such parasites are most exposed to the defense mechanisms which are developed by vaccination.

Protozoa.—In the case of the trypanosomiases many examples of protection or partial protection by vaccination are known. The best protection is obtained with trypanosomes of the *lewisi* group. Absolute immunity against *Trypanosoma lewisi* can be conferred upon rats by vaccination with killed cultures or suspensions of this organism.[60] Some resistance likewise follows the inoculation of mice with *Trypanosoma duttoni.*[61] Vaccination against the so-called "pathogenic trypanosomes" is much less successful. When the specific immunological strain of trypanosome is used both for vaccination and later infection, some degree of resistance can be demonstrated. This has been shown in various laboratory animals against *Trypanosoma gambiense, Trypanosoma equiperdum, Trypanosoma evansi,* and other pathogenic species.[62] In the field, however, immunization has not proved practical, probably because these pathogenic trypanosomes are more or less constantly changing immunologically, and vaccination with one strain of a species will not protect against others. Furthermore, many immunological strains of these trypanosomes may exist constantly in nature. Attempts to immunize experimental animals against either *Leishmania tropica* or *Leishmania donovani* by

[60] F. G. Novy, W. A. Perkins, and R. Chambers, *J. Infect. Dis.,* 11: 411 (1912); W. H. Taliaferro, *Am. J. Hyg.,* 16: 32 (1932); J. T. Culbertson and W. R. Kessler, *Am. J. Hyg.,* 29: 33 (1939, sec. C).

[61] W. R. Kessler: unpublished experiment.

[62] L. Reiner and S. S. Chao, *Am. J. Trop. Med.,* 13: 525 (1933); I. J. Kligler and R. Comaroff, *Ann. Trop. Med.,* 29: 145 (1935); I. J. Kligler and M. Berman, *Ann. Trop. Med.,* 29: 457 (1935); A. Castellani and I. Jacono, *Policlinico,* 44: 325 (1937).

injecting killed or avirulent organisms have uniformly failed.[63]

In coccidiosis parenteral vaccination with killed coccidian substance does not protect against subsequent infection,[64] although the feeding of oocysts which have been rendered avirulent by heat confers immunity to chicks for at least brief periods.[65]

The vaccination of man against malaria has not been tested significantly, although autogenous vaccines are said to exert in man a therapeutic effect involving enhanced resistance against *Plasmodium vivax*.[66] Monkeys are not protected against *Plasmodium knowlesi* by killed homologous organisms.[67] Canaries, on the other hand, become comparatively resistant after the injection of bird malaria parasites which have been killed with formaldehyde or rendered avirulent by exposure to low temperature.[68]

Helminth.—Rabbits can be partially immunized to *Fasciola hepatica* by injecting the dried substance of this parasite.[69] Likewise, rats and rabbits resist the onchospheres of *Taenia crassicollis* and *Taenia serrata*, respectively, after vaccination with the dried substance of the homologous parasite.[70] The protein fraction of either the adult or the larval form of *Taenia crassicollis* serves as the antigen for vaccinating the rat, although the protein-free polysaccharide is unsatisfactory for the purpose.[71] Rats can also be protected by introducing pieces of *Taenia serrata* intraperitoneally, but injections of the powdered substance of *Taenia saginata, Diphyllobothrium latum, Hymenolepis* sp. or *Dipylidium* sp. provide no protection.[72] Kittens are reported to acquire partial immunity to adult *Taenia crassicollis* after the subcuta-

[63] L. Parrot, *Compt. rend. Soc. de biol.*, 100: 411 (1929) ; T. J. Kurotchkin, *Nat. M. J. China*, 17: 458 (1931) ; B. Malamos, *Arch. f. Schiffs- u. Tropen-Hyg.*, 41: 416 (1937).

[64] E. E. Tyzzer, *Am. J. Hyg.*, 10: 269 (1929) ; E. R. Becker, *Am. J. Hyg.*, 21: 389 (1935).

[65] H. A. Jankiewicz and R. H. Scofield, *J. Am. Vet. M. A.*, 84: 507 (1934).

[66] S. W. Koustansoff, *Zentralbl. f. Bakt.*, 116: 241 (1930).

[67] M. D. Eaton and L. T. Coggeshall, *J. Exper. Med.*, 70: 141 (1939).

[68] W. D. Gingrich, *J. Infect. Dis.*, 68: 46 (1941) ; W. B. Redmond, *J. Parasitol. (Suppl.)*, 25: 28 (1939).

[69] K. B. Kerr and O. L. Petkovich, *J. Parasitol.*, 21: 319 (1935).

[70] H. M. Miller, Jr., *Proc. Soc. Exper. Biol. & Med.*, 27: 926 (1930) ; D. H. Campbell, *Am. J. Hyg.*, 23: 104 (1936) ; L. C. Feng and R. Hoeppli, *China M. J.*, 55: 45 (1939) ; K. B. Kerr, *J. Parasitol.*, 20: 328 (1934).

[71] D. H. Campbell, *Am. J. Hyg.*, 23: 104 (1936) and *J. Infect. Dis.*, 65: 12 (1939).

[72] H. M. Miller, Jr., *Proc. Soc. Exper. Biol. & Med.*, 29: 1125 (1932).

54   SPECIFICALLY ACQUIRED IMMUNITY

neous injection or the feeding of the substance of the larval parasite.[73] Vaccination with hydatid substance protects sheep from
hydatid disease [74] and even the dog against the adult stage of
Echinococcus granulosus.[75] Mice and rabbits, however, are said
not to become immune to *Echinococcus granulosus* as a result of
repeated injections of hydatid membrane.[76] Rats cannot be protected against *Hymenolepis diminuta* by feeding mashed homologous worms or by injecting their substance parenterally.[77]

A partial immunity is developed by vaccinated guinea pigs to
somatic infection with *Ascaris lumbricoides*.[78] Likewise rats can
be immunized to forms such as *Nippostrongylus muris*,[79] *Trichinella spiralis*,[80] and *Strongyloides ratti* [81] by injecting parenterally
the killed larval forms of the respective species. Little or no immunity is conferred, on the other hand, by vaccinating chicks with
Ascaridia lineata.[82]

IMMUNITY ACQUIRED PASSIVELY BY THE INJECTION OF IMMUNE SYSTEM

Immunity can be conferred upon normal animals by injecting
them with the serum of an immune animal. As in actively immune animals, so in those passively immunized the effect is greatest upon parasites of the somatic tissue.

Protozoa.—Only limited evidence is available for the passive
transfer of immunity in leishmaniasis. A specific immune serum
does not cure hamsters of *Leishmania donovani* infection, for example, although it does prolong the disease. Such a serum also will
retard the growth of this parasite in cultures.[83] One report has appeared of the protection of man against cutaneous leishmaniasis

[73] T. Ohira, *Tr. Far East Assoc. Trop. Med., 9th Congress,* 1: 601 (1935).
[74] E. L. Turner, E. W. Dennis, and D. A. Berberian, *J. Parasitol.,* 23: 43 (1937).
[75] E. L. Turner, D. A. Berberian, and E. W. Dennis, *J. Parasitol.,* 22: 14 (1936).
[76] F. Dévé, *Compt. rend. Soc. de biol.,* 115: 1025 (1934).
[77] A. C. Chandler, *Am. J. Hyg.,* 31: 17 (1940, sec. D).
[78] K. B. Kerr, *Am. J. Hyg.,* 27: 52 (1938).
[79] A. C. Chandler, *Am. J. Hyg.,* 16: 750 (1932); 24: 129 (1936).
[80] O. R. McCoy, *Am. J. Hyg.,* 21: 200 (1935); A. Trawinski, *Zentralbl. f. Bakt.,* 134: 145 (1935).
[81] A. J. Sheldon, *Am. J. Hyg.,* 29: 47 (1939, sec. D).
[82] L. L. Eisenbrandt and J. E. Ackert, *Am. J. Hyg.,* 32: 1 (1940, sec. D).
[83] B. Malamos, *Arch. f. Schiffs- u. Tropen-Hyg.,* 41: 416 (1937).

by grafting upon normal persons small pieces of the skin of an individual immune to oriental sore.[84] The studies upon passive immunity in trypanosomiasis are much more successful. An homologous serum acts either prophylactically or therapeutically upon *Trypanosoma lewisi*,[85] *Trypanosoma duttoni*,[86] or some others of the *lewisi* group,[87] as well as upon *Trypanosoma cruzi*.[88] Serum from animals immune to the pathogenic trypanosomes is likewise effective on passive transfer, providing it is tested with the homologous strain of trypanosome.

Passive transfer of immunity has been seldom tried in human malaria. However, the serum from syphilitics who have been treated with malaria abates the symptoms of acute cases of malaria to which it is injected [89] and sometimes effects complete cure.[90] The serum from rabbits which have been injected repeatedly with blood from a case of malaria is said to reduce the number of circulating parasites in an acute case to which it is injected, although this effect may be of a nonspecific character.[91] Better evidence for the passive transfer of immunity is available in the animal malarias. The serum of a specifically immune *Macacus rhesus*, for example, has a depressing effect on fresh infections with *Plasmodium knowlesi* or *Plasmodium inui*,[92] a direct relationship existing between the dose of parasites and the amount of serum needed to protect against it.[93] Likewise, in the bird malarias passive transfer of immunity has been demonstrated, although protective antibodies often occur in the serum in only very low concentration.[94] Nevertheless sometimes perfect protection against the bird malarias is afforded by a

[84] V. K. Lotti, *Ann. Trop. Med.*, 26: 545 (1932).

[85] W. H. Taliaferro, *J. Infect. Dis.*, 62: 98 (1938).

[86] W. H. Taliaferro, *J. Immunol.*, 35: 303 (1938).

[87] J. T. Culbertson, *J. Parasitol.*, 27: 45 (1941).

[88] J. T. Culbertson and M. H. Kolodny, *J. Parasitol.*, 24: 83 (1938).

[89] N. Lorando and D. Sotiriades, *J. Trop. Med.*, 39: 197 (1936); D. Sotiriades, *J. Trop. Med.*, 39: 257 (1936).

[90] N. Lorando and D. Sotiriades, *Tr. Toy. Soc. Trop. Med. & Hyg.*, 31: 227 (1937).

[91] N. T. Koressios, *Riv. di malariol.*, 12: 353 (1933).

[92] L. T. Coggeshall and H. W. Kumm, *J. Exper. Med.*, 66: 177 (1937); E. Mosna, *Riv. di parassitol.*, 2: 327 (1938).

[93] L. T. Coggeshall and M. D. Eaton, *J. Exper. Med.*, 68: 29 (1938).

[94] R. Hegner and L. Eskridge, *Am. J. Hyg.*, 28: 367 (1938); R. Hegner and M. Dobler, *Am. J. Hyg.*, 30: 81 (1939, sec. C); W. H. Taliaferro and L. G. Taliaferro, *J. Parasitol. (Suppl.)*, 25: 29 (1939), and *J. Infect. Dis.*, 66: 153 (1940).

particularly potent serum.[95] Attempts to transfer immunity passively in coccidiosis [96] and in amoebiasis have thus far been ineffectual.

Helminth.—Passive immunity has not been demonstrated in any trematode infection, but among the cestodiases it has been shown in the cysticercosis of rats [97] and rabbits.[98] The serum from rabbits infected with *Coenurus cerebralis* sensitizes guinea pigs passively, so that they can be shocked thereafter, often fatally, with coenurus fluid.[99]

Immunity has also been passively transferred against some nematodes. Dogs suffer less from the dog hookworm if injected with an immune serum at the time of infection,[100] and mice sometimes resist a fatal somatic infection with this parasite if given an immune serum.[101] Passive transfer of immunity also has been successful in rats and mice against *Nippostrongylus muris,*[102] *trichiniasis,*[103] and *Strongyloides* infection.[104]

FACTORS INFLUENCING ACQUIRED IMMUNITY

The potency of the immunity actively acquired by an individual against reinfection with a parasite depends largely upon two factors. One of these is the intensity of the initial infection. An intense infection is more likely than a mild one to elicit a good immune response (see Chapter V). The other factor is the capacity of the tissues of the infected animal to produce an immune response. The tissues which apparently are most concerned in this response are those of the reticulo-endothelial system. When for any reason this

[95] R. D. Manwell and F. Goldstein, *J. Parasitol. (Suppl.),* 24: 19 (1938) ; R. D. Manwell and F. Goldstein, *J. Exper. Med.,* 71: 409 (1940).

[96] G. W. Bachman, *Am. J. Hyg.,* 12: 641 (1930) ; E. R. Becker, *Am. J. Hyg.,* 21: 389 (1935).

[97] H. M. Miller, Jr., and M. L. Gardiner, *J. Prevent. Med.,* 6: 479 (1932) and *Am. J. Hyg.,* 19: 270 (1934), and 20: 424 (1934) ; D. H. Campbell, *J. Immunol.,* 35: 195 (1938).

[98] K. B. Kerr, *Am. J. Hyg.,* 22: 169 (1935).

[99] P. Bosch, *Marseille-méd.,* 71: 291 (1934).

[100] G. F. Otto, *J. Parasitol. (Suppl.),* 24: 10 (1938).

[101] K. B. Kerr, *Am. J. Hyg.,* 27: 60 (1938).

[102] M. P. Sarles and W. H. Taliaferro, *J. Infect. Dis.,* 59: 207 (1936) and *J. Parasitol. (Suppl.),* 24: 35 (1938).

[103] A. Trawinski, *Zentralbl. f. Bakt.,* 134: 145 (1935) ; J. T. Culbertson and S. S. Kaplan, *Parasitology,* 30: 156 (1938).

[104] H. J. Lawlor, *Am. J. Hyg.,* 31: 28 (1940, sec. D).

system of tissues functions inadequately, the immune response is poor. A poor response is generally obtained in very young animals, presumably because the reticulo-endothelial system is immature. This immaturity of tissues seems in part to account for the age resistance noted in some infections [105] (see Chapter III). A poor diet,[106] however, or an intercurrent infection may also undermine an immunity which has already been acquired, and the immune animal may thus become about as susceptible as a normal animal to a given parasite. The removal of a large part of the reticulo-endothelial system, as in splenectomy, also may depress the acquired resistance.[107]

[105] J. T. Culbertson and W. R. Kessler, *Am. J. Hyg.,* 29: 33 (1939, sec. C) ; J. T. Culbertson, *Arch. Path.,* 27: 212 (1939).

[106] D. A. Porter, *Am. J. Hyg.,* 22: 467 (1935).

[107] E. Benhamou, *Bull. Soc. path. exot.,* 25: 685 (1932) ; K. V. Krishnan, R. O. A. Smith, and C. Lal, *Indian J. M. Research,* 21: 343 (1933) and 21: 639 (1934) ; E. G. Nauck and B. Malamos, *Ztschr. f. Immunitätsforsch. u. exper. Therap.,* 84: 337 (1935).

Chapter V

REQUISITES FOR IMMUNE
RESPONSE

NOT ALL THE SPECIES of parasites which invade an animal call
forth an immune response. Often the parasite is more or less
perfectly adjusted to the host, and the effects of its presence are
so slight that the host makes no effort to eradicate the invader. In
other cases the effects of the parasite are so severe and the host is
so poorly able to cope with the invader that death comes before the
host can manifest an effectual immune response. Between these ex-
tremes lie, perhaps, the majority of parasites. Generally some immune response is made to their presence, and usually this response
suffices not only to prevent the death of the host but also, in many
cases, to eradicate the invader and to prevent reinfection with it.

THE CAUSE OF AN IMMUNE RESPONSE

Before an immune response occurs, a host must be stimulated by
the antigens of the parasite. This stimulation usually follows invasion of the host tissue by the parasite itself. Little or no antigenic
stimulation follows most purely intestinal infections or infections in
other sites where tissue is not damaged. Many parasites, however,
characteristically reside within the tissues of specific organs, or
migrate almost at random through various tissues. Others inhabit
the blood. In all of these last cases host tissue is destroyed by the
parasite, and—what is of importance in causing the immune response—antigenic substances from the parasite pass meanwhile
into the host tissue. These antigenic substances may consist of the
parasite body itself or may be the secretions or the metabolites of
the parasite. In any case, their presence in the host tissue is the
cause of the immune response by the host.

When the antigens from a parasite are introduced into the somatic tissues of the infected animal in comparatively small quantity and are not passed into the blood for distribution over the entire body, their effect is localized to tissues in the site occupied by the parasite. The immunity which develops in such cases is correspondingly local both in its origin and in its effect. But, given a sufficient amount of antigen and its general distribution, the immune response of an infected animal involves the participation of its entire body. Any metabolizing tissue or organ can, so far as is known, play a role in the response, especially by producing specific antagonistic substances called antibodies. Usually, however, the greatest activity falls to the cells which are in the best position physically for stimulation by the parasite antigen. Generally the cells of the reticulo-endothelial system seem to occupy such a position, and it is from these cells, therefore, that we observe the greatest immune response. Infections in which the parasite antigens reach these systems in great quantity are those in which the most powerful immune responses occur.

THE SIGNIFICANCE OF THE SEVERITY OF INFECTION

Within limits the potency of the immune response varies in proportion to the intensity of the antigenic stimulation. Animals which suffer severe infections experience the most intense stimulation and respond best with antibody. Such animals are generally more highly resistant to reinfection than animals which suffer only a mild infection with the same parasite. The fact is illustrated especially by infections with protozoans,[1] cestodes,[2] and nematodes.[3] In infections where the parasite does not propagate itself, as in most helminthiases, an especially intense initial infection is required if a powerful response is to be made.

The significance of the severity of infection for an immune response has been brought out especially well in studies concerned with the treatment of human malaria. The final eradication of the

[1] S. P. James, *Tr. Roy. Soc. Trop. Med. & Hyg.*, 24: 477 (1931); M. D. Young, *Am. J. Trop. Med.*, 18: 85 (1938); E. E. Tyzzer, H. Theiler, and E. E. Jones, *Am. J. Hyg.*, 15: 319 (1932).

[2] H. M. Miller, Jr., and M. L. Gardiner, *Am. J. Hyg.*, 20: 424 (1934); D. H. Campbell, *J. Immunol.*, 35: 195 (1938).

[3] C. M. Africa, *J. Parasitol.*, 18: 1 (1931); G. L. Graham, *Am. J. Hyg.*, 20: 352 (1934).

malaria parasite from an individual is known to depend on his immune response to the organism, not on the drugs generally employed for first bringing the disease under control. If drug treatment is withheld from a fresh case of malaria until the disease has become severe, a greater antigenic stimulation will be experienced and a greater immune response made by the patient than if drug treatment is instituted during the first days of infection.[4] The danger of relapse is much less in patients who have experienced severe malaria prior to treatment with drugs, since these persons are, as a result of their severe infection, more highly immune to the malaria parasite. When an active infection does occur in such persons, generally a few small doses of quinine are sufficient clinically to cure the infection, the drug being given to control the parasite until the specific immune mechanism comes into play.

SOMATIC AND INTESTINAL INFECTIONS

As has been stated previously, the immunity acquired against parasites which dwell strictly in the lumen of the intestine is slight compared with that to forms which invade the somatic tissue. This follows because the parasites of the intestinal lumen do little or no damage to the host tissue and because antigens from such parasites are seldom absorbed by the host in sufficient amount to stimulate a vigorous immune response.[5] The parasites of somatic tissues, in contrast, can hardly fail to engender at least some degree of immune response, for their antigens cannot be expelled except into the host tissue.

Somatic tissue parasites and intestinal parasites also differ in their susceptibility to the forces responsible for acquired immunity. The greater effect of these forces is seen upon the somatic tissue forms, these parasites often being immobilized and killed as they pass through the tissue of an immune animal.[6] Once a parasite has developed to a stage which can survive in the intestinal lumen, however, it is largely beyond the influence of the agencies (antibody, defensive cells) which perform the immune function.[7] Never-

[4] S. P. James, *Tr. Roy. Soc. Trop. Med. & Hyg.*, 24: 477 (1931).
[5] A. C. Chandler, *J. Parasitol.*, 23: 558 (1937).
[6] W. H. Taliaferro and M. P. Sarles, *J. Infect. Dis.*, 64: 157 (1939).
[7] A. C. Chandler, *Am. J. Hyg.*, 31: 17 (1940, sec. D); L. L. Eisenbrandt and J. E. Ackert, *Am. J. Hyg.*, 32: 1 (1940).

theless limited effects resulting in slower rate of growth, smaller ultimate size, diminished egg production, and briefer residence impress themselves also upon the lumen-dwelling parasite.[8]

IMMUNE RESPONSE TO KILLED ANTIGENS

Although artificial immunization with killed vaccine does not generally lead to so powerful an immune response as does actual infection with a parasite, the principles underlying artificial immunization and immunization by prior infection are fundamentally identical. In both, antigens from the parasite must stimulate the host to make the immune response. In the infected animal, however, a greater response is generally manifested, because a greater stimulation occurs. The parasite in infected animals is living, growing, and in some cases reproducing—thus actually increasing the amount of constantly available antigenic substances to which the host must respond. In artificial immunization with a killed vaccine, on the other hand, a comparatively small amount of the dead substances of the parasite is injected perhaps every fourth or fifth day, and the effect of one stimulation may largely spend itself by the time the next is given. When the total amount of antigen introduced is large, the potential immune response is often distinctly greater.[9]

A qualitative difference between infection and artificial immunization with a killed vaccine may also exist. In the preparation of the vaccine, significant antigens may be lost or denaturized by the attending physical and chemical conditions. The immune response to such a vaccine would not be so broad, naturally, as that following infection, and might well be too limited for adequate defense against infection on subsequent exposure.

For an effective immune response to a killed vaccine the antigen evidently must be given parenterally. Essentially negative results have followed all attempts to engender immunity by administering the vaccine by mouth, since the antigen apparently is too little absorbed by this route to produce a significant response by the host.[10]

[8] G. L. Graham, J. E. Ackert, and R. W. Jones, *Am. J. Hyg.*, 15: 726 (1932) ; O. R. McCoy, *Am. J. Hyg.*, 32: 105 (1940, sec. D) ; W. H. Taliaferro and M. P. Sarles, *J. Parasitol.*, 23: 561 (1937).

[9] K. B. Kerr, *Am. J. Hyg.*, 27: 52 (1938).

[10] A. C. Chandler, *Am. J. Hyg.*, 24: 129 (1936) ; G. W. Bachman and J. Oliver Gonzalez, *Proc. Soc. Exper. Biol. & Med.*, 35: 215 (1936).

Chapter VI

PARASITES WHICH ELICIT IMMUNITY

B EFORE AN ANIMAL can develop a powerful immunity to a parasite either after infection or after vaccination, it must be stimulated intensely by comparatively large amounts of the parasite antigen. Accordingly the intensity of the immune response after natural infection with a given species of parasite reflects the intensity of the infection experienced and at the same time the extent to which the parasite has stimulated the host antigenically. External parasites have little or no opportunity to elicit immune responses unless they are adapted especially to inoculate some of their body substance beneath the skin of the host, as are most of the blood-sucking arthropods (see Chapter XVII). Parasites which dwell in the intestinal lumen likewise have little chance to cause an immune response in a host unless either before or after they reach this site they penetrate the host tissue. Their antigens are generally absorbed only poorly while they reside in the intestinal lumen. Infections with parasites which spend all or a considerable part of their life cycle in the blood or fixed tissue of the host produce the best immune responses. The immunity acquired from an initial infection with such forms often completely protects the host from reinfection with the homologous parasite.

RELATIVE IMMUNITY DEVELOPED BY DIFFERENT PARASITES

Parasites may conveniently be divided into three groups with respect to their place of residence in a host: (1) those of the somatic tissues; (2) those of the intestinal lumen; and (3) those dwelling in both the somatic tissue and the intestinal lumen. The magnitude of the immune response to any parasite is influenced largely by its place of residence.

PARASITES OF THE SOMATIC TISSUES

The somatic tissue parasites include those which inhabit the blood as well as the fixed tissues. These include the trypanosomes, leishmanias, and malaria organisms among the protozoans, and among helminths the schistosomes, the larval cestodes (plerocercoids, cysticerci, coenuri, and hydatids), and the filarioid nematodes. None of these forms dwells in the intestinal lumen of the host, although certain stages of some (for example, the onchospheres of the helminths) traverse the intestine. All of them are enabled by reason of their position in the host intensively to stimulate an immune response by the host, and to all a vigorous response is characteristically made. Generally an infected animal absolutely resists reinfection with the homologous parasite, and in some cases serum from an immune animal will protect a normal animal to which it is transferred against the infection. It is in infections with these parasites chiefly that diagnosis is possible by detecting specific antibody in the host's serum or by skin tests.

The several varieties of protozoan mentioned all inhabit both the blood and the fixed tissues of many organs, thus providing adequate stimulation for a good immune response. These forms are more or less constantly proliferating, and the host is required to check this proliferation if it is to survive. Generally, in fact, the first evidence of specific resistance to these infections manifests itself as a diminished rate of reproductivity of the parasite.

The larval stage of the cestode parasites generally resides in the somatic tissue of a host, and it is against the antigens of these forms, therefore, that the host makes its principal immune response. The larval and adult stages of each cestode, however, have for the most part the same antigenic constitution, and an immune response engendered by the antigens of one stage can be directed equally— although sometimes with only limited effect—against other stages of the parasite. Therefore a rat can be protected against somatic infection with the cysticerci of *Taenia crassicollis* by inoculating a vaccine prepared from the adult stage of this parasite.[1] Likewise,

[1] H. M. Miller, Jr., *Proc. Soc. Exper. Biol. and Med.*, 27: 926 (1930).

extracts of adult tapeworms can be used in skin tests to detect somatic infection in man with larval tapeworms.[2]

Both the larval and the adult schistosomes inhabit the blood
stream, and both probably stimulate immunity. The adults of the
filarioid nematodes occupy connective tissue, and these are in some
cases, as with *Dracunculus medinensis,* perhaps exclusively responsible for the immune reaction, since larval forms do not exist free
in the host tissue. However, the immune response in the more frequently encountered filarioid nematode infections, such as that
with *Wuchereria bancrofti* or *Loa loa,* probably derives chiefly
from the microfilariae. These larval worms occur in large numbers
in the blood stream—the number being sustained by a fresh daily
production by the adults—and would appear to supply a greater
amount of the antigenic stimulation than the comparatively few
adult worms, which can be found only with great difficulty in re-
cesses of the connective tissue.

PARASITES OF THE INTESTINAL LUMEN

The protozoan parasites of greatest immunological importance
which occupy the intestinal lumen exclusively are the nonpathogenic amoebae, such as *Endamoeba coli, Iodamoeba williamsi,* and
Endolimax nana, and the intestinal flagellates, such as *Trichomonas hominis* and *Chilomastix mesnili.* The most significant
helminths immunologically which occupy this site are several
trematodes (*Fasciolopsis buski* and *Heterophyes heterophyes* of
man), the adult cestodes (*Diphyllobothrium latum, Taenia solium,*
and *Taenia saginata* of man, *Taenia crassicollis* of the cat, *Hymenolepis diminuta* of the rat, and *Raillietina cesticillus* of the chicken),
and a few nematodes (*Enterobius vermicularis* of man and *Heterakis gallinae* of the chicken). One immunological study upon an
acanthocephalid, *Moniliformis dubius* of the rat intestine, has also
appeared.[3] The immune response to all these forms is exceedingly
poor.[4] No specific resistance to reinfection is manifested, although

[2] J. T. Culbertson and H. M. Rose, *J. Clin. Investigation,* 20: 249 (1941).
[3] P. L. Burlingame and A. C. Chandler, *J. Parasitol. (Suppl.),* 26: 18 (1940), and
Am. J. Hyg., 33: 1 (1941, sec. D).
[4] One exception among cestode parasites appears to be the adult stage of *Echinococcus granulosus* in the dog. Dogs were found by E. L. Turner, D. A. Berberian,
and E. W. Dennis (*J. Parasitol.,* 22: 14 [1936]) to be partially resistant to infection

attempts to superimpose infections upon hosts sometimes fail because of the presence already of large numbers of parasites, with consequently insufficient space (crowding) or inadequate food for additional forms. The serum from an animal previously infected with these species will usually not protect a normal animal from infection. Furthermore, antibody is seldom produced, and skin tests with the specific antigen generally are negative.

PARASITES INHABITING BOTH THE SOMATIC
TISSUE AND THE INTESTINAL LUMEN

Among the protozoan parasites the most important forms which reside both in the somatic tissues and in the intestinal lumen are *Endamoeba histolytica, Balantidium coli,* and the coccidians. *Endamoeba histolytica* invades principally the tissues of the intestinal wall, but it can also establish itself in liver, spleen, lung, brain, and other organs. The immune response to *Endamoeba histolytica* is considerable. Exogenous reinfections are quickly checked so long as the old infection persists, and specific immune substances are detectable in the host's serum. *Balantidium coli* infections are confined to the tissues of the intestinal wall. As yet little is known of the immune response to this parasite.

Some species of the coccidians, such as *Eimeria perforans* and *Eimeria stiedae* of the rabbit, usually invade only epithelial cells of the intestine or bile ducts. Others, such as *Eimeria tenella* of the chick, characteristically infect deeper layers of the intestinal wall. To all these coccidians some immune response is made. The response varies with the intensity of the infection and with the depth to which the parasite penetrates into the somatic tissue. The superimposition of infection generally fails, and a small amount of antibody usually appears in the infected host's serum.

Among representative helminths living both in the intestinal lumen and in somatic tissues are the two liver flukes *Clonorchis sinensis* and *Fasciola hepatica,* the cestode *Hymenolepis fraterna,* and such nematodes as *Trichinella spiralis,* the ascarids, the hookworms, and the several species of *Strongyloides.* Usually the two

---

with *Echinococcus granulosus* even after artificial immunization with a killed antigen prepared from the hydatid cyst. Because of the exceptional character of the result, the question requires further investigation.

species of trematodes just named do not actually invade the somatic tissue, but they do ascend to the rather confining lumena of the smaller bile ducts. A marked immune response occurs to their presence in this site. The walls of the bile ducts are thrown into folds, and a distinct inflammatory reaction occurs in the neighborhood of each parasite. Often the parasite is caught in the folds of the wall and is then ultimately destroyed.

In the case of the cestode *Hymenolepis fraterna,* tissue invasion involves only the intestinal villus, where the larval stage dwells. The immune reaction to *Hymenolepis fraterna* is not particularly intense, but it appears nonetheless definite.[5] It is noteworthy that no immune response whatsoever occurs to a closely related species, *Hymenolepis diminuta,* which does not invade the host tissue at all.[6]

The immune response in trichiniasis results either from the somatic infection with the larval forms or from antigens of the adult entering the blood from the intestine,[7] and it often reaches its peak only after all the adult worms are eliminated from the intestine. The immune response to ascarids and hookworms occurs likewise in species of hosts in which intestinal infections with the adult parasites never develop.[8] In the case of one ascarid, *Ascaridia lineata* of the chick, only a comparatively meager immune response follows infection. However, this parasite is known to experience only a minimum of tissue invasion, burrowing only into the mucosa of the intestinal wall. Antibody is seldom produced in this infection.[9]

[5] D. A. Shorb, *Am. J. Hyg.,* 18: 74 (1933).
[6] A. C. Chandler, *Am. J. Hyg.,* 29: 105 (1939, sec. D).
[7] J. Bozicevich and L. Detre, *Pub. Health Rep.,* 55: 683 (1940).
[8] K. B. Kerr, *Am. J. Hyg.,* 27: 28, 1938, and *Am. J. Hyg.,* 24: 381 (1936).
[9] L. L. Eisenbrandt and J. E. Ackert, *Am. J. Hyg.,* 32: 1 (1940, sec. D).

Chapter VII

MECHANISMS OF SPECIFIC
IMMUNITY

THE MECHANISMS by which immunity is manifested against the animal parasites are fundamentally similar to those which are invoked against other types of disease agents, such as bacteria, spirochetes, and filtrable viruses. An animal is equipped to respond immunologically in only a few manners, and it utilizes this equipment with only slight modification, whatever the character of the invader. The immune responses often differ in amount, however, and these quantitative variations are sometimes mistaken for differences in kind.

THE BASES OF SPECIFIC IMMUNITY

The specific immune response of an animal to a parasite involves primarily (1) antibody production and (2) an enhanced function of phagocytic cells. These effects are the result of stimulation of the host tissues by antigens from the parasite. The host is prompted to greatest response by a widespread antigenic stimulation, and sometimes every tissue seems to participate. The tissues of the reticulo-endothelial system are of greatest concern in immunity, however; and if they are stimulated a considerable immune response can generally be expected, no matter what other tissues also are engaged. These reticulo-endothelial tissues are considered primarily responsible for the antibody production by an immune animal.

HUMORAL AGENCIES

The principal role in specific immunity is performed by the antibody. Antibody is found chiefly in the serum of the blood, but also in other serous fluids and possibly even within the tissue cells. It is a specific substance, produced in response to a given antigen, and has the remarkable capacity for uniting chemically with that antigen whenever the two occur together. It occurs exclusively in the globulin fraction of the serum.[1]

Source of antibody.—Probably any body cell which is metabolizing normally and producing globulin is a potential source of antibody. Cells of the reticulo-endothelial system are generally credited with the largest share of antibody-forming function, because they are in the best physical position for antigenic stimulation. The antigen which reaches the body cells is not converted directly to antibody, but instead it acts as a kind of catalyst within those cells which have absorbed it. As a result of the presence of the antigen these cells are induced to produce the modified form of globulin protein—namely, the antibody.

Kinds of antibody.—Antibody can be demonstrated in many ways; these modes of demonstration differ among themselves so much that a distinctive name is often ascribed to the antibody concerned in each reaction. Thus, antibody which clumps a suspension of parasites is an agglutinin; that which precipitates an antigenic extract of the same parasites is called a precipitin; that which lyses or dissolves this parasite is a lysin; and that which under certain conditions unites with the parasite antigens to fix or to absorb a component of serum called complement is called a complement-fixing antibody. Even other names are given to antibody. For example, when antibody prevents infection in animals to which it is inoculated, it is often called a protective antibody. One antibody which occurs especially in the rodent trypanosomiases and which checks the reproduction of the parasites is called an ablastin, or reproduction-inhibiting, antibody.

These different names for antibody are very confusing and often lead to misconceptions as to the nature of the substance itself. It is well to keep in mind, therefore, the fact that no matter in how many ways it can be demonstrated, the total antibody produced against any single parasite is functionally largely a unit, albeit an extraordinarily complex one with manifold potentialities for action.

---

[1] W. H. Taliaferro, *Am. J. Hyg.*, 16: 32 (1932) ; E. A. Mauss, *J. Parasitol. (Suppl.)*, 26: 43 (1940).

It should, however, be further understood that every parasite is constituted physically or chemically of a multiplicity of antigens and that the total antibody produced against each parasite is comprised of many separate antibodies, each the individual response to one of the constituent antigens of the parasite.

Time relations of antibody production.—At least several days are always required after antigenic stimulation—no matter whether this stimulation occurs through infection or through vaccination with antigens from killed parasites—before antibody appears in the serum. Complement-fixing antibodies can be detected in dogs with experimental amoebiasis within three to fourteen days after the animals are infected.[2] The reproduction-inhibiting antibody which is observed in rats infected with *Trypanosoma lewisi* appears about five days after the animals are infected, and increases in concentration thereafter until the end of the infection.[3] A second antibody, of lytic character, terminates these trypanosome infections in rats; the lytic antibody appears only late in the infection and persists in the serum for but a few days after the infection ends. In *Macacus rhesus, Plasmodium knowlesi* infection leads to specific agglutinins in from fifteen to forty-five days after infection, and fixation antibodies against the same parasite are present in relatively high titer after the twenty-first day.[4] Precipitins are detectable in rabbits five days after the last of a series of injections of coccidian vaccine, and they disappear after about fifty days.[5]

Most helminth infections differ from those with protozoa in that the helminths do not multiply after invasion. Accordingly, in the helminthiases antibody production is generally slower and less intensive than in the protozoan infections, although, once underway, continues for long periods. Antibody usually appears in goats experimentally infected with *Schistosoma spindale,* for example, by the second week. It increases in amount till about the third month of infection, and may remain in high concentration during the ensuing year. Sometimes positive tests for antibody against the

---

[2] C. F. Craig, *Proc. Soc. Exper. Biol. & Med.,* 30: 270 (1932).

[3] F. A. Coventry, *Am. J. Hyg.,* 5: 127 (1925).

[4] M. D. Eaton, *J. Exper. Med.,* 67: 857 (1938) ; L. T. Coggeshall and M. D. Eaton, *J. Exper. Med.,* 67: 871 (1938).

[5] G. W. Bachman, *Am. J. Hyg.,* 12: 624 (1930).

schistosomes continue on into the second year after infection.[6] Protective antibody against the cysticerci of *Taenia crassicollis* appears in the blood of infected rats by the fifteenth day and increases thereafter until at least the end of the fourth week.[7] Precipitins against *Trichinella spiralis* (one of the few helminths which do multiply in the mammalian host) appear in infected rabbits in from five to twenty days. Often they are detected while adults are still in the intestine and before larvae have entered the blood.[8] Fixation antibodies against *Trichinella* have been detected in rabbits even as early as the third day, although their titer is not great enough for practical value in diagnosis till about the twenty-fifth day after infection.[9] In human infections with *Trichinella* precipitin tests are seldom positive before the fifth week, although in a few instances by the third.[10] The serum of rabbits infected with the somatic stages of *Ascaris megalocephala* shows maximum fixation of complement about the fifteenth day after infection.[11]

From these examples it is clear that antibody usually can be expected in from two to three weeks after infection with most parasites, although with some intensive infections an earlier response occurs. The maximum antibody response is attained in from one to three months, and after prolonged infection traces of antibody persist during the ensuing year. Antibody appears between the fifth and the tenth day after the last of a series of injections of killed antigen, reaches its peak in two or three weeks, and then decreases rather quickly, seldom being detectable after three or four months unless more antigen is injected.

Specific function of antibody.—Antibody has the specific and invariable function to unite with antigen, and all its effects stem from this activity. Usually antigen-antibody reactions can be demonstrated in vitro, but sometimes they can be shown in the animal body as well. As a result of union of antibody with the antigens of a parasite the life processes of the parasite are seriously interfered

[6] N. H. Fairley, *Arch. f. Schiffs- u. Tropen-Hyg.*, 30: 372 (1926); N. H. Fairley and F. Jasudasan, *Indian M. Research Mem., Supp. to Indian J. M. Research* (1930).
[7] D. H. Campbell, *J. Immunol.*, 35: 195 (1938).
[8] G. W. Bachman, *J. Prevent. Med.*, 3: 465 (1929).
[9] G. W. Bachman and P. E. Menendez, *J. Prevent. Med.*, 3: 471 (1929).
[10] W. W. Spink, *New England J. Med.*, 216: 5 (1937); W. W. Spink and D. L. Augustine, *J. A. M. A.*, 104: 1801 (1935).
[11] W. K. Blackie, *J. Helminthol.*, 9: 91 (1931).

with and the organism is sometimes immobilized or killed.[12] In the case of infections with the protozoans, such as the trypanosomes, the power of reproduction may first be lost by the parasite, and then, as the complete immune response is attained, the parasites may be destroyed by lysis.[13] Both these effects are directly due to the antibody and to the union of antibody with the parasite antigens.

In the cases of the trematode and cestode parasites the precise role of antibody has not yet been thoroughly studied, although the presence of the antibody—whether as the result of active or of passive immunization—certainly interferes with the normal development of the parasite. In certain nematode infections, however, the role of specific antibody in immunity has been clearly exposed. This function has been shown most strikingly in the case of *Nippostrongylus muris* infection of rats, in the classic studies by Taliaferro and Sarles, who have described first how the worm stimulates the rat to produce the antibody and then how this antibody reacts upon the worm. With regard to the migrating larval forms Taliaferro [14] has stated, "The worm's secretions and excretions . . . appear to be the main effective inflammatory stimuli and the effective antigens involved in immunization. Precipitins are formed by the immune host against the excretions and secretions of the worm and react with them to cause visible precipitation in the gut of the worm and around its extremities." Following the union of the antibody with the worm antigens, the worms appear to have difficulty in feeding and in assimilating food, and as a result they may become immobilized in the host tissues. Subsequently the parasite may suffer death and experience complete disintegration.

Taliaferro and Sarles [15] have found also that the adult *Nippostrongylus* induces immunity and is subject to the immune response in essentially the same way as the larva. This follows because the adult worm pierces the intestinal epithelium repeatedly during residence in the intestine. At such times it not only introduces its secretions and excretions into the host tissue but also feeds on blood and tissue fluid of the host. The antibody which finally develops in the

[12] M. Robertson, *J. Path. & Bact.*, 38: 363 (1934).
[13] W. H. Taliaferro, *Am. J. Hyg.*, 16: 32 (1932).
[14] W. H. Taliaferro, *Am. J. Trop. Med.*, 20: 169 (1940).
[15] W. H. Taliaferro and M. P. Sarles, *J. Infect. Dis.*, 64: 157 (1939).

immune host will therefore be ingested by the adult and will combine with the antigens of the adult worm just as with those of the larva. The final effect upon the adult is its elimination from the intestine. The elimination occurs because the normal function of the adult worm suffers as a result of antibody combining with the worm antigen, and the worm is then more easily dislodged by the peristaltic movements of the intestine.

The affinity of antibody for the antigens of *Nippostrongylus* has also been demonstrated in vitro by immersing the larval forms during several days in the serum from a highly immune rat. A precipitate forms about the mouth of the worms, as well as about their excretory pores. Precipitates are laid down also about the genital pores of adult females similarly immersed in the immune serum. The depression of egg production by female worms in immune hosts may be explained by the occlusion of the genital pore with precipitate. Precipitate also is formed within the oesophagus and the intestine of the worm, thus interfering with the digestion and the assimilation of food.[16] Essentially similar observations to those just described have been made with other nematode parasites, such as hookworms [17] and *Trichinella spiralis*,[18] although these have not yet been investigated in full detail (see Figure 1).

CELLULAR AGENCIES

The body cells, beyond having the very significant function of antibody production, play largely an accessory role in specific immunity. Those cells with phagocytic capacities are of chief impor-

[16] M. P. Sarles, *J. Parasitol.*, 23: 560 (1937).
[17] G. F. Otto, *J. Parasitol. (Suppl.)*, 25: 29 (1939).
[18] E. L. Mauss, *Am. J. Hyg.*, 32: 80 (1940, sec. D); J. Oliver Gonzalez, *J. Infect. Dis.*, 67: 292 (1940).

CAPTION FOR FIGURE ON FACING PAGE

THE ACTION OF IMMUNE SERUM IN VITRO UPON THE
INFECTIVE LARVAE OF *NIPPOSTRONGYLUS MURIS*

Note the antibody precipitated about and within the worms. Abbreviations are: ExP, excretory pore; GA, genital anlage; Int, intestine; M, mouth; NR, nerve ring; PBE, posterior bulb of oesophagus; R, rectum; Cut Ppt, cuticular precipitate; Ex Ppt, excretory precipitate; Int Ppt, intestinal precipitate; Or Ppt, oral precipitate; Misc Ppt, miscellaneous precipitate.

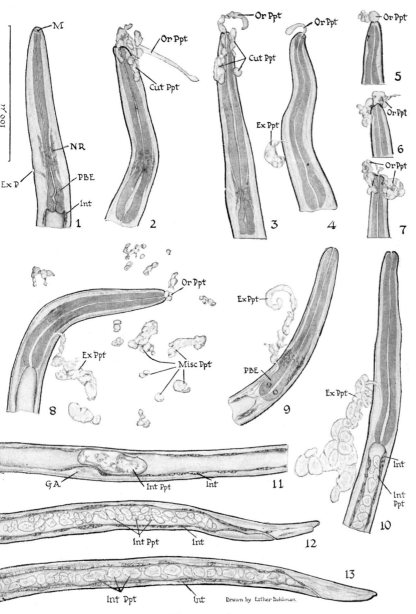

Drawn by Esther Bohlman.

FIGURE 1

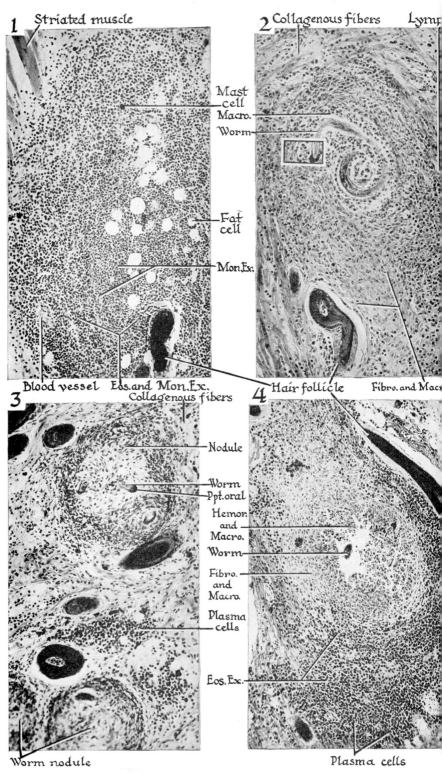

1　Striated muscle

Mast cell
Macro.
Worm

Fat cell

Mon.Ex.

Blood vessel　Eos.and Mon.Ex.
Collagenous fibers

2　Collagenous fibers　　Lymp

Hair follicle　　Fibro. and Mac.

3

Nodule

Worm
Ppt.oral

Hemor.
and
Macro.

Worm

Fibro.
and
Macro.

Plasma
cells

Eos. Ex.

Worm nodule

Plasma cells

FIGURE 2

tance. The phagocytic cells may directly attack parasites, but usually this occurs in an effective degree only after the parasites have been opsonized or sensitized with antibody. For example, the cells of a normal animal generally respond but little to parasites until either an immune serum specific for these parasites also is inoculated or else the animal itself has produced antibody. When antibody is present, however, the cells immediately spring into action and engulf smaller species of parasites or, through the collective action of many cells, immobilize the larger parasite in the tissues.

Cell types of significance in specific immunity.—The same cells of the blood and the connective tissues function in immune animals against parasites as against other types of infectious organisms. Those first mobilized to repel an invading parasite are the polymorphonuclear leucocytes. The macrophages, however, including the mononuclear cells of the blood, the clasmatocytes of the connective tissue, and the Kupffer cells of the liver, which are later called into play, perform much more effectively. All these defensive cells increase sharply in number after parasitic infection, and some of them probably take on the added function of specific antibody production.[19] In certain of the helminth infections a sharp rise in the percentage of eosinophiles in the circulating blood is a usual and conspicuous response.

Time of response.—The time which must elapse before a cellular response is made by a host to a parasite varies with the specific cell type, with the tissue involved, and with the character of the

[19] W. H. Taliaferro, *J. Parasitol.,* 20: 149 (1934).

CAPTION FOR FIGURE ON FACING PAGE

CELLULAR RESPONSE TO *NIPPOSTRONGYLUS MURIS* IN
IMMUNE RATS

The skin and subcutaneous tissue of immune rats after reinfection showing intense inflammation and late stages in the formation of a nodule (x 125).

1: Localized concentration of leucocytes 36 hours after reinfection, from which worm has escaped. 2: Worm with oral cap of precipitate and intestinal precipitate in fully formed compact nodule 7 weeks after a third reinfection. Note precipitate about tip of worm in rectangle. 3: Worms in fully formed compact nodules. Outside the nodules occur islands of plasma cells and a general infiltration of eosinophils (see cells with ring-shaped nuclei). 4: Worm in fully occupied compact nodule. At the periphery of the nodule occur eosinophils and plasma cells. The active worm had caused fresh hemorrhage and is surrounded by macrophages filled with erythrocytes.

invader. A rat infected with *Trypanosoma lewisi,* for example, develops a monocytosis with the peak of cell count on about the fifth day after infection. In *Nippostrongylus* infection of normal rats, on the other hand, connective tissue mast cells, eosinophiles, and macrophages increase in number in the lamina propria of the intestine not until about ten days following infection.[20] In trichiniasis of man a rise in circulating eosinophiles is the most conspicuous cellular response, this being noted during the second week, before antibody tests are generally positive. An eosinophilia is also noted in trichiniasis of pigs; this begins a few days after infection and reaches its peak during the fourth week. In rats with *Trichinella* an eosinopenia is sometimes noted during the first several days after infection, eosinophiles at this time being concentrated in the intestinal mucosa. An eosinophilia usually develops, however, one or two weeks later.[21]

Specific function.—The cells function in specific immunity against protozoans both indirectly through antibody production and directly by attacking the invader. In many cases, especially in leishmaniasis [22] and trypanosomiasis,[23] the response in macrophages so closely parallels the appearance of serum antibody that a relationship between the two phenomena seems likely. In malaria, also, the monocytes may be concerned with specific antibody formation.

With certain protozoa, convincing evidence of the function of the cells through phagocytizing parasites is available. Perhaps the best examples are seen in the malarias. The fixed tissue phagocytes of the spleen and the liver are especially active in these infections, not only of man [24] but also of monkeys [25] and birds.[26] Circulat-

[20] W. H. Taliaferro and M. P. Sarles, *J. Parasitol.,* 23: 561 (1937).

[21] V. D. van Someren, *J. Helminthol.,* 16: 83 (1938); E. H. Beahm and C. M. Downs, *J. Parasitol.,* 25: 405 (1939).

[22] L. E. Napier, K. V. Krishnan, and C. Lal, *Indian M. Gaz.,* 68: 75 (1933).

[23] D. F. Gowe, *Am. J. Trop. Med.,* 17: 401 (1937); C. J. Duca, *Am. J. Hyg.,* 29: 25 (1939, sec. C).

[24] W. H. Taliaferro and H. W. Mulligan, *Indian M. Research Mem., Suppl. Ser. to Indian J. M. Research,* Mem. No. 29 (1937); P. C. C. Garnham, *Tr. Roy. Soc. Trop. Med. & Hyg.,* 32: 13 (1938); L. G. Thomson, *Tr. Roy. Soc. Trop. Med. & Hyg.,* 26: 483 (1933).

[25] W. H. Taliaferro, *Am. J. Hyg.,* 16: 429 (1932); W. H. Taliaferro and P. R. Cannon, *J. Infect. Dis.,* 59: 72 (1936).

[26] W. H. Taliaferro, *Science,* 75: 619 (1932); W. Gingrich, *J. Prevent. Med.,* 6: 197 (1932) and *J. Infect. Dis.,* 68: 37 (1941).

ing phagocytic cells also may perform the same function.[27]

The role of the cells in helminth infections is fundamentally the same as in protozoan diseases, although because of the size of most worm parasites many cells must function collectively before a significant effect is possible. The role of the cells has been studied particularly in the case of the migrating larvae of the nematode *Nippostrongylus muris* in the rat. In immune animals these larvae experience difficulty throughout their somatic migration. As soon as the infective stage has pierced the skin, a vigorous inflammatory response occurs. Defensive cells infiltrate from the blood to the area surrounding the migrating larva and usually delay its passage. Nodules of cells arise about worms which have been immobilized and finally wall them off completely and prevent their escape. Worms soon die under this circumstance, and the macrophage cells then function by clearing away their remains. Essentially similar responses are noted in other sites, such as the lungs and the intestines, upon parasites which may have successfully negotiated the first line of defense (see Figure 2).[28]

What has just been said may imply that the cells themselves act vigorously in defending the body against parasites. One should remember, however, that usually before parasites become vulnerable to the effects of the cells the parasites must first have been in contact with specific antibody. The cells (omitting their antibody-forming function) are primarily scavengers, lacking in the necessary initiative to engage the fully virulent parasite, but able to complete its destruction after it has been rendered vulnerable by specific antibody. In rather similar manner the body cells are considered to play an accessory or adjunctive role with respect to many drugs employed in the therapy of, particularly, the protozoan diseases.[29]

[27] C. D. de Langen, *Geneesk. Tijdschr. v. Nederl.-Indië,* 72: 793 (1932), and *Tr. Roy. Soc. Trop. Med. & Hyg.,* 26: 523 (1933) ; H. See-Lii, *Arch. f. Schiffs- u. Tropen-Hyg.,* 38: 249 (1934) ; H. Stott, *Indian M. Gaz.,* 68: 507 (1933).

[28] W. H. Taliaferro, *Am. J. Trop. Med.,* 20: 169 (1940) ; W. H. Taliaferro and M. P. Sarles, *J. Infect. Dis.,* 64: 157 (1939).

[29] C. W. Jungeblut, *Ergebn. d. Hyg., Bakt., Immunitätsforsch. u. exp. Therap.,* 11: 1 (1930) ; L. Reiner, C. S. Leonard, and S. S. Chao, *Proc. Soc. Exper. Biol. & Med.,* 27: 791 (1930) ; N. v. Jancsó and H. v. Jancsó, *Ann. Trop. Med.,* 28: 419 (1934) ; 29: 95 (1935) ; J. T. Culbertson, *Am. J. Hyg.,* 29: 73 (1939, sec. C) ; F. Hawking, *Ann. Trop. Med.,* 33: 13 (1939).

LOCAL IMMUNITY

Inasmuch as all metabolizing cells are potentially able to manifest an immune response, such a response may be made by one organ or by one tissue alone, to the exclusion of the remainder of the body. Good examples of such strictly local immunity, however, are rare. Usually what begins as a local immune response finally spreads to include the entire body, since as soon as the parasite antigens are developed in sufficient amount to overflow the local tissue they spread to adjacent areas. All tissues which are stimulated by the antigen then take part in the response to it. If the antigen enters the circulation, it is quickly carried to essentially all parts of the body, and a generalized response is assured.

Even though the immune response involves the entire body, the effect upon the parasite is often exerted only in specific local sites. This sometimes occurs because the parasite invades only certain kinds of cells or only some one organ. In coccidiosis of the rabbit, for example, the parasites are confined to the epithelial cells of the intestine or bile ducts, and although the immune response is probably generalized—since specific antibody occurs in the serum of infected animals—this response impresses itself on the parasite only locally—that is, in these epithelial cells.

The immune response to parasites which occur in or migrate through the various somatic tissues is perhaps always of a generalized character. The effect upon the parasites, however, is often confined largely to strategic local points in which the cells are best able to supplement the action of the antibody. In malaria, for example, the phagocytosis of the parasites occurs best in the liver and the spleen.[30] In the case of *Nippostrongylus* infection of the rat the chief sites for the immune effect are skin, lungs, and intestinal mucosa. In experimental trichiniasis the chief effect is upon the adult worms which inhabit the intestine and which bore superficially into the intestinal wall.[31] Although antibody probably plays the predominant role in the immunity to trichiniasis, since the passive transfer of immunity with the serum is possible,[32] eosinophiles

[30] W. H. Taliaferro and H. W. Mulligan, *Indian M. Research Mem., Suppl. Ser. to Indian J. M. Research*, Mem. No. 29 (1937).
[31] O. R. McCoy, *Vol. Jubil. pro Prof. S. Yoshida*, 2: 629 (1939).
[32] J. T. Culbertson and S. S. Kaplan, *Parasitology*, 30: 156 (1938).

nevertheless collect in the mucosa of immune pigs and rats and seem to form a more-or-less effective barrier to infection.[33] The encapsulation of *Trichinella* larvae in the striated muscle may also be evidence of an immune response. In experimental cysticercosis of rabbits immunity appears to depend in part upon the intestinal wall, the local tissue presenting a more or less mechanical barrier to penetration by embryos.[34] In all these cases the immune response results from the stimulation of all or of many tissues. The immunity is directed against the parasite, however, principally in specific local sites which are strategically disposed.

[33] G. W. Bachman, *Rev. de med. trop. y parasitol., bacteriol., clin. y lab.*, 4: 121 (1938) ; V. D. van Someren, *J. Helminthol.*, 16: 83 (1938).

[34] A. B. Leonard and A. E. Smith, *J. Parasitol. (Suppl.)*, 25: 30 (1939).

Chapter VIII

DEMONSTRATION OF IMMUNITY

SEVERAL DIFFERENT METHODS can be followed to determine whether or not a given person or animal has made an immune response to a given parasite. These generally take one of three forms—namely, (1) tests upon the person or animal himself, (2) tests with the serum from the individual, and (3) tests upon the parasite. The advantage of one method over another in any given case depends on the nature of the parasite and the infection which it causes and the attendant danger to the host of applying the method.

DEMONSTRATION OF IMMUNITY BY TESTS UPON THE HOST

Tests to demonstrate an immune response directly in a person or animal usually involve either (1) exposing the individual to reinfection with the homologous parasite or else (2) inoculating the parasite antigens intradermally to the individual in an effort to elicit a local skin response.

EXPOSURE TO REINFECTION

The most convincing evidence of a specific immune response by a person or an animal is his ability to resist reinfection with the homologous parasite. If the host species is one which is normally susceptible to a parasite, and if it was easily infected on initial exposure, the failure to infect on subsequent exposure is almost certainly the result of an immune response which the animal has made to that parasite. Sometimes complete resistance to reinfection is manifested. Among experimental protozoan infections, perhaps the best example of such complete resistance is *Trypanosoma lewisi* infection in rats. Once the rat has recovered from infection with this parasite, it is apparently absolutely resistant thereafter and will quickly overcome even tremendous doses of the homologous organism subsequently introduced. The best experimental helminth infection which can be cited is cysticercosis of rats due to *Taenia crassicollis*.[1] Often, however, the immune response, although definite, is inadequate completely to prevent subsequent reinfection. Mild infections may then follow reinoculation with the parasite. In human malaria,[2] for example, as well as in the malarias of birds and in coccidiosis,[3] second and third infections with the homologous parasite usually occur, although they are of low intensity as to parasite numbers and are often without clinical symptoms. Likewise in hydatid disease of sheep,[4] somatic ascariasis in guinea pigs,[5] *Ascaridia* infection in chickens,[6] hookworm disease in dogs [7] and mice,[8] and in rat infections with *Nippostrongylus muris*,[9] *Trichinella spiralis*,[10] and *Strongyloides ratti*,[11] partial resistance to reinfection is manifested.

SKIN RESPONSE

Another mode of demonstrating an immune response directly in the host himself is by testing the skin of the individual with antigens of the homologous parasite. Man generally manifests both an immediate and a delayed skin reaction. Animals usually show only a delayed type of reaction. A few species, such as the rat, are unsatisfactory subjects for skin tests, since their skins are

---

[1] H. M. Miller, Jr., *Proc. Soc. Exper. Biol. & Med.*, 28: 467 (1931).

[2] M. F. Boyd and L. T. Coggeshall, *Tr. Third Internat. Congr. Trop. Med. and Malaria*, 2: 292 (1938); M. F. Boyd, W. K. Stratman-Thomas, and H. Muench, *Am. J. Hyg.*, 20: 482 (1934); M. F. Boyd, W. H. Kupper, and C. B. Matthews, *Am. J. Trop. Med.*, 18: 521 (1938).

[3] D. P. Henry, *Proc. Soc. Exper. Biol. & Med.*, 28: 831 (1931); E. E. Tyzzer, H. Theiler, and E. E. Jones, *Am. J. Hyg.*, 15: 319 (1932); Wilson, Va. Agric. Exper. Sta., *Tech. Bull.*, No. 42: 1 (1931); H. E. Biester and L. H. Schwarte, *J. Am. Vet. M. A.*, 81: 358 (1932).

[4] E. L. Turner, E. W. Dennis, and D. A. Berberian, *J. Parasitol.*, 23: 43 (1937).

[5] K. B. Kerr, *Am. J. Hyg.*, 27: 28 (1938).

[6] G. L. Graham, J. E. Ackert, and R. W. Jones, *Am. J. Hyg.*, 15: 726 (1932).

[7] O. R. McCoy, *Am. J. Hyg.*, 14: 268 (1931); G. F. Otto and K. B. Kerr, *Am. J. Hyg.*, 29: 25 (1939, sec. D).

[8] K. B. Kerr, *Am. J. Hyg.*, 24: 381 (1936).

[9] C. M. Africa, *J. Parasitol.*, 18: 1 (1931); B. Schwartz, J. E. Alicata, and J. T. Lucker, *J. Washington Acad. Sci.*, 21: 259 (1931).

[10] O. R. McCoy, *Am. J. Hyg.*, 14: 484 (1931).

[11] A. J. Sheldon, *Am. J. Hyg.*, 25: 53 (1937).

TABLE 2

COMPARATIVE IMMUNE RESPONSE AGAINST VARIOUS ANIMAL PARASITES

Quality of Immune Response	Parasite	Host	Resistance to Reinfection	Serum Protects Passively	Skin Reaction	Antibody Demonstrable in Vitro
Good	Trypanosoma lewisi	Rat	+	+		+
	Trypanosoma duttoni	Mouse	+	+		+
	Trypanosoma cruzi	Rat	+	+		+
	Trypanosoma cruzi	Mouse	+	+		+
	Trypanosoma cruzi	Man				+
	Plasmodium vivax	Man	+			+
	Plasmodium ovale	Man	+			+(?)
	Plasmodium malariae	Man	+			+
	Fasciola hepatica	Cattle			+	+
	Fasciola hepatica	Rabbit	+			
	Schistosoma japonicum	Man			+	+
	Schistosoma japonicum	Dog	+			
	Echinococcus granulosus (hydatid)	Man			+	+
	Echinococcus granulosus (hydatid)	Sheep	+			
	Taenia crassicollis (Cyst. faciolaris)	Rat	+	+		
	Taenia serrata (Cyst. pisiformis)	Rabbit	+	+	+	+
	Trichinella spiralis	Man			+	+
	Trichinella spiralis	Rodents	+	+(?)	+	+
	Nippostrongylus muris	Rat	+	+		
	Cordylobia anthropophaga	Guinea pig	+		+	+
	Dermacentor variabilis	Guinea pig	+		+	+
Fair	Leishmania tropica	Man	+			
	Trypanosoma equiperdum	Rodents		+(?)		+
	Endamoeba histolytica	Man			+(?)	+
	Plasmodium falciparum	Man				+
	Plasmodium knowlesi	Monkey		+		+
	Plasmodium cathemerium P. circumflexum, P. rouxi P. relictum	Canary		+		
	Eimeria stiedae	Rabbit	+			+
	Eimeria tenella	Chicken	+			
	Schistosoma hematobium	Man			+	+
	Schistosoma mansoni	Man			+	+
	Taenia saginata (Cyst. bovis)	Cattle	+			

Quality of Immune Response	Parasite	Host	Resistance to Reinfection	Serum Protects Passively	Skin Reaction	Antibody Demonstrable in Vitro
r	Taenia solium (Cyst. cellulosae)	Pig				+
	Taenia solium (Cyst. cellulosae)	Man				+
	Hymenolepis fraterna	Mouse	+			
	Ancylostoma caninum	Dog	+	+		+
	Ancylostoma caninum	Mouse	+			
	Ancylostoma braziliense	Dog	+			
	Ancylostoma braziliense	Cat	+			
	Haemonchus contortus	Sheep	+			
	Ascaridia lineata	Chicken	+			
	Toxocara cati	Cat	+			
	Strongyloides ratti	Rat	+			
	Trichostrongylus calcaratus	Rabbit	+			
	Loa loa	Man			+	+
	Wuchereria bancrofti	Man			+	+
	Onchocerca volvulus	Man			+	+
	Mosquito (bite)	Man			+	
	Bee (sting)	Man			+	
	Psocoptes communis cuniculi	Rabbit				+
or	Trypanosoma gambiense	Man				+
	Trypanosoma rhodesiense	Man				+
	Leishmania donovani	Man				+
	Paragonimus westermanni	Man				+
	Taenia solium (adult)	Man			+(?)	
	Taenia saginata	Man			+(?)	
	Necator americanus	Man			+	
	Ascaris lumbricoides	Man			+	
ne	Endamoeba gingivalis	Man				
	Endamoeba coli	Man				
	Endolimax nana	Man				
	Iodamoeba williamsi	Man				
	Dientamoeba fragilis	Man				
	Trichomonas hominis	Man				
	Giardia intestinalis	Man				
	Chilomastix mesnili	Man				
	Fasciolopsis buski	Man				
	Clonorchis sinensis	Man				
	Heterophyes heterophyes	Man				
	Metagonimus yokogawai	Man				
	Taenia crassicollis	Cat				
	Taenia spp. (adults)	Dog				

of such a texture that despite a potent immunity in the animal no skin reaction can be elicited. Among human infections, particularly, skin tests are of extraordinarily high value in demonstrating an immune response. Such tests are utilized especially in the somatic helminth infections of man, including schistosomiasis,[12] cysticercosis,[13] hydatid disease,[14] filariasis,[15] and trichiniasis.[16]

DEMONSTRATION OF IMMUNE RESPONSE BY TESTS WITH SERUM FROM THE ANIMAL

Serum from the host can be employed in two ways to determine whether the host has made an immune response to a given parasite: (1) by passive transfer of the serum to a susceptible animal in order to test its protective value against the homologous parasite and (2) by testing the serum in vitro for specific antibodies.

PASSIVE TRANSFER

The serum from animals which have suffered from any of several parasitic infections will protect susceptible animals from the homologous parasite. This is seen particularly in trypanosomiasis and malaria, among protozoan infections. In trypanosomiasis the best effects are observed with members of the *lewisi* group of trypanosomes [17] and with *Trypanosoma cruzi,*[18] although when absolutely strain specific serums are used evidence for protection against the pathogenic trypanosomes also is obtained. With the malarias the best success has been obtained in infections of monkeys [19] and of birds.[20] Protection by the transfer of serum also is

[12] N. H. Fairley and F. E. Williams, *M. J. Australia,* 2: 811 (1937); W. H. Taliaferro, W. A. Hoffman, and D. H. Cook, *J. Prevent. Med.,* 2: 395 (1928).

[13] D. R. A. Wharton, *Am. J. Hyg.,* 14: 477 (1931).

[14] K. D. Fairley, *M. J. Australia,* 1: 472 (1929), and 2: 320 (1929).

[15] W. H. Taliaferro and W. A. Hoffman, *J. Prevent. Med.,* 4: 261 (1930); N. H. Fairley, *Tr. Roy. Soc. Trop. Med. & Hyg.,* 25: 220 (1932).

[16] G. W. Bachman, *J. Prevent. Med.,* 2: 513 (1928); D. L. Augustine and H. Theiler, *Parasitology,* 24: 60 (1932).

[17] F. A. Coventry, *Am. J. Hyg.,* 5: 127 (1925); W. H. Taliaferro, *J. Immunol.,* 35: 303 (1938).

[18] J. T. Culbertson and M. H. Kolodny, *J. Parasitol.,* 24: 83 (1938).

[19] L. T. Coggeshall and H. W. Kumm, *J. Exper. Med.,* 66: 177 (1937), and 68: 17 (1938).

[20] R. Hegner and L. Eskridge, *Am. J. Hyg.,* 28: 367 (1938); R. D. Manwell and F. Goldstein, *J. Exper. Med.,* 71: 409 (1940).

seen among such helminth infections as cysticercosis of rats [21] and rabbits,[22] hookworm disease of dogs,[23] *Nippostrongylus* infection of rats,[24] trichiniasis of rodents,[25] and *Strongyloides* infection of rats.[26]

The resistance manifested by a passively immunized animal is usually less than that manifested by one which has been actively immunized. Yet evidence for resistance in animals given serum is undeniable, since subsequent infections are generally comparatively milder and of brief duration. The effectiveness of the serum, however, depends on its antibody content. If the serum used is rich in antibody, passively immunized animals may be completely protected. Serum will not confer resistance to a susceptible animal unless taken from a donor which has been infected intensely enough and for a sufficient time to develop antibodies. In one study upon cysticercosis of rats, for example, serum taken seven days after infection of the donors had little protective value, but that taken fourteen days after infection conferred considerable protection, and that taken twenty-one or twenty-eight days after infection conferred perfect resistance upon the recipient.[27] Rats infected with *Trypanosoma lewisi* usually have but little antibody in their serum before the sixth or seventh day of their infection. Serums must, therefore, be drawn after this time to be effective for the transfer of immunity to *Trypanosoma lewisi* passively to other animals.

IN VITRO TESTS FOR ANTIBODY

The principal in vitro serum antibody tests are those for agglutinins, precipitins, complement-fixing substances, and adhesins. Because of the physical state of the various parasites one type of test is often preferred to others. For example, agglutinin tests are

[21] H. M. Miller, Jr., *Am. J. Hyg.*, 19: 270 (1934) ; D. H. Campbell, *J. Immunol.*, 35: 195 (1938).
[22] K. B. Kerr, *Am. J. Hyg.*, 22: 169 (1935).
[23] G. F. Otto, *J. Parasitol.* (*Suppl.*), 24: 10 (1938).
[24] M. P. Sarles and W. H. Taliaferro, *J. Parasitol.* (*Suppl.*), 24: 35 (1938).
[25] A. Trawinski, *Zentralbl. f. Bakt.*, 134: 145 (1935) ; J. T. Culbertson and S. S. Kaplan, *Parasitology*, 30: 156 (1938).
[26] H. J. Lawlor, *Am. J. Hyg.*, 31: 28 (1940, sec. D).
[27] D. H. Campbell, *J. Immunol.*, 35: 195 (1938).

possible in trypanosomiasis and in malaria, for the parasites involved can somewhat easily be obtained as an agglutinable suspension. With infections by the larger helminths, on the other hand, agglutination tests cannot be performed. With them precipitin tests are somewhat more easily carried out, since the helminth antigens can best be extracted from the parasite. Complement fixation tests can be done in nearly all infections, and adhesin tests in a select few. In each case a positive reaction of the serum shows that the individual has responded by the production of antibody against the parasite antigens.

Agglutination.—The serum of a rat recovered from an infection with *Trypanosoma lewisi* or vaccinated with the antigens of *Trypanosoma lewisi* [28] or *Trypanosoma equiperdum* [29] will agglutinate a suspension of the homologous organism. Likewise the serum of monkeys or birds infected, respectively, with *Plasmodium knowlesi* [30] or *Plasmodium circumflexum,*[31] will clump suspensions of the corresponding parasites. Although the agglutination test is not adaptable to many helminth infections, the filariform larvae of *Strongyloides* are said to be agglutinated by the serum of an animal recovered from strongyloidiasis.[32]

Precipitation.—The presence of precipitins has been reported in the serum of persons or animals with amoebiasis,[33] coccidiosis,[34] and malaria,[35] among protozoan infections. Precipitins have also been demonstrated in such helminth infections as fascioliasis of cattle,[36] in schistosomiasis,[37] cysticercosis of man [38] and pigs,[39]

[28] J. T. Culbertson and W. R. Kessler, *Am. J. Hyg.*, 29: 33 (1939, sec. C).

[29] L. Reiner and S. S. Chao, *Am. J. Trop. Med.*, 13: 525 (1933).

[30] M. D. Eaton, *J. Exper. Med.*, 67: 857 (1938) ; B. Malamos, *Riv. di malariol.*, 16: 91 (1937).

[31] R. D. Manwell and F. Goldstein, *J. Exper. Med.*, 71: 409 (1940).

[32] S. Sato, *Fukuoka-Ikwadaigaku-Zasshi*, 26: 88 (1933).

[33] E. H. Wagener, *Univ. California Publ., Zoology*, 26: 15 (1924).

[34] G. W. Bachman, *Am. J. Hyg.*, 12: 624 (1930).

[35] W. H. Taliaferro and L. G. Taliaferro, *J. Prevent. Med.*, 2: 147 (1928).

[36] W. A. Hoffman and T. Rivero, *Porto Rico Rev. Pub. Health & Trop. Med.*, 4: 589 (1929).

[37] B. Imai, *Japan M. World*, 8: 273 (1928) ; S. Miyaji and B. Imai, *Zentralbl. f. Bakt.*, 106: 237 (1928) ; W. H. Taliaferro, W. A. Hoffman, and D. H. Cook, *J. Prevent. Med.*, 2: 395 (1928).

[38] J. Rothfeld, *Deutsche Ztschr. f. Nervenh.*, 137: 93 (1935) ; A. Trawinski and J. Rothfeld, *Zentralbl. f. Bakt.*, 134: 472 (1935).

[39] A. Trawinski, *Zentralbl. f. Bakt.*, 136: 116 (1936).

echinococcus disease,[40] ascariasis,[41] *Ascaridia* infection of chicks,[42] hookworm disease of dogs,[43] *Nippostrongylus* infection of rats,[44] and trichiniasis.[45]

Complement fixation.—Complement-fixing antibodies have been detected in amoebiasis,[46] leishmaniasis,[47] trypanosomiasis,[48] coccidiosis [49] and malaria,[50] and among helminth infections in fascioliasis,[51] schistosomiasis,[52] *Diphyllobothrium* infection of monkeys,[53] cysticercosis,[54] echinococcus disease,[55] ascariasis,[56] filariasis,[57] and trichiniasis.[58] The complement fixation test is probably the most delicate of all the antibody tests and at once the most delicate test for detecting an immune response by an animal against a parasite. It is, however, an exceedingly difficult test to perform, and unless all the details of its performance are carefully checked incorrect results are often obtained.

Adhesin tests.—The adhesin antibody has been detected only

[40] P. Bonelli, *Gior. di batteriol. e immunol.*, 12: 681 (1934) ; F. Hoder, *Fortschr. d. Med.*, 51: 959 (1933).

[41] F. A. Coventry, *J. Prevent. Med.*, 3: 43 (1929).

[42] L. L. Eisenbrandt and J. E. Ackert, *Am. J. Hyg.*, 32: 1 (1940, sec. D).

[43] G. F. Otto, *Am. J. Hyg.*, 31: 23 (1940, sec. D).

[44] M. P. Sarles, *J. Parasitol.*, 23: 560 (1937).

[45] G. W. Bachman, *J. Prevent. Med.*, 3: 465 (1929) ; D. L. Augustine and H. Theiler, *Parasitology*, 24: 60 (1932) ; W. W. Spink and D. L. Augustine, *J. A. M. A.*, 104: 1801 (1935).

[46] C. F. Craig, *Am. J. Pub. Health*, 27: 689 (1937) ; T. B. Magath and H. E. Meleney, *Am. J. Trop. Med.*, 20: 211 (1940).

[47] S. D. S. Greval, P. C. Sen Gupta, and L. E. Napier, *Indian J. M. Research*, 27: 181 (1939) ; A. M. da Cunha and E. Dias, *Brasil-med.*, 53: 89 (1939) ; P. Zdrodowski and B. Woskressenski, *Bull. Soc. path. exot.*, 23: 1028 (1930).

[48] H. C. Clark and J. Benavides, *Am. J. Trop. Med.*, 15: 285 (1935) ; C. M. Johnson and R. A. Kelser, *Am. J. Trop. Med.*, 17: 385 (1937).

[49] G. W. Bachman, *Am. J. Hyg.*, 12: 624 (1930) ; J. Chapman, *Am. J. Hyg.*, 9: 389 (1929).

[50] M. Massa, *Pathologica*, 21: 8 (1929) ; A. Radosavljević, *Arch. f. Schiffs- u. Tropen-Hyg.*, 34: 629 (1930) ; L. T. Coggeshall and M. D. Eaton, *J. Exper. Med.*, 67: 871 (1938).

[51] O. Wagner, *Ztschr. f. Immunitätsforsch. u. exper. Therap.*, 84: 225 (1935).

[52] B. Imai, *Japan M. World*, 8: 273 (1928) ; N. H. Fairley, *J. Helminthol.*, 11: 181 (1933) ; M. N. Andrews, *J. Helminthol.*, 13: 25 (1935).

[53] J. F. Mueller and O. D. Chapman, *J. Parasitol.*, 23: 561 (1937).

[54] W. P. MacArthur, *Tr. Roy. Soc. Trop. Med. & Hyg.*, 26: 525 (1933).

[55] K. D. Fairley and C. H. Kellaway, *Australian and New Zealand J. Surg.*, 2: 236 (1933) ; J. Outerino, *Ann. de méd.*, 38: 493 (1935).

[56] W. K. Blackie, *J. Helminthol.*, 9: 91 (1931).

[57] N. H. Fairley, *Tr. Roy. Soc. Trop. Med. & Hyg.*, 25: 220 (1932) ; L. van Hoof, *Tr. Roy. Soc. Trop. Med. & Hyg.*, 27: 609 (1934).

[58] G. W. Bachman and P. E. Menendez, *J. Prevent. Med.*, 3: 471 (1929).

in a few parasitic infections. It is present in trypanosomiasis,[59] as well as in leishmaniasis and filariasis.[60]

DEMONSTRATION OF IMMUNITY BY EFFECTS UPON THE PARASITES

An immune response by an animal to a given parasite may be detected by the effect which subsequent residence in that animal has upon the parasite. The actual number of parasites which develop in the immune animal is often less than in the normal animal, the immune animal sometimes manifesting complete resistance to infection. When the parasite does develop in the immune animal, it is often of smaller size than in the normal host and gives evidence either of retarded development or of an inability to reach full maturity. In the case of helminths the egg production by parasites is often significantly reduced in the immune host. These various effects upon the parasites result perhaps chiefly from the action of specific antibody to which the parasites are exposed in the immune host.

Number of parasites.—The number of parasites which develop in immune hosts after reinfection with protozoans is definitely less in the natural trypanosomiases of rodents and in *Trypanosoma cruzi* infection of these animals, as well as in coccidiosis [61] and in the malarias of man,[62] monkey,[63] and bird.[64] An effect upon the number of helminth parasites, likewise, is seen in hosts immune to *Schistosoma japonicum*,[65] the cysticerci of *Taenia serrata* [66] and *Taenia crassicollis*,[67] the hydatid of sheep,[68] the cysticercoids of

---

[59] H. L. Duke and J. M. Wallace, *Parasitology*, 22: 414 (1930); S. Raffel, *Am. J. Hyg.*, 19: 416 (1934); M. Adant, *Ann. Soc. belge de méd. trop.*, 9: 159 (1929); H. C. Brown and J. C. Broom, *Tr. Roy. Soc. Trop. Med. & Hyg.*, 32: 209 (1938).

[60] E. A. Mills and C. Machattie, *Tr. Roy. Soc. Trop. Med. & Hyg.*, 25: 205 (1931); M. T. Balasheva, *Med. Par. and Parasit. Dis.*, 4: 19 (1935); C. G. Pandit, S. R. Pandit, and P. V. S. Iyer, *Indian J. M. Research,* 16: 946 (1929).

[61] H. E. Biester and L. H. Schwarte, *J. Am. Vet. M. A.*, 81: 358 (1932); Wilson, Va. Agric. Exper. Sta., *Tech. Bull.*, No. 42: 1 (1931).

[62] M. F. Boyd and L. T. Coggeshall, *Third Internat. Congr. Trop. Med. and Malaria*, 2: 292 (1938); M. F. Boyd, W. K. Stratman-Thomas, and H. Muench, *Am. J. Hyg.*, 20: 482 (1934).

[63] W. H. Taliaferro and L. G. Taliaferro, *Am. J. Hyg.*, 20: 60 (1934).

[64] R. D. Manwell and F. Goldstein, *Am. J. Hyg.*, 30: 115 (1939, sec. C).

[65] M. Ozawa, *Jap. J. Exper. Med.*, 8: 79 (1930).

[66] K. B. Kerr, *Am. J. Hyg.*, 22: 169 (1935).

[67] H. M. Miller, Jr., *Proc. Soc. Exper. Biol. & Med.*, 28: 467 (1931); D. H. Campbell, *J. Immunol.*, 35: 195 (1938).

[68] E. L. Turner, E. W. Dennis, and D. A. Berberian, *J. Parasitol.*, 23: 43 (1937).

Hymenolepis fraterna,[69] and in trichiniasis,[70] *Ancylostoma caninum* of dogs,[71] *Ascaridia lineata* of chicks,[72] and *Nippostrongylus muris* of rats.[73] In many cases, particularly with the protozoans, infection is sometimes completely prevented.

Size of parasites.—Immune effects upon the size of parasites are observed chiefly with the helminths. Schistosomes which develop in immune dogs are diminutive,[74] and both the larvae [75] and adults [76] of *Taenia crassicollis* in immune rats and kittens, respectively, are smaller than when developed in normal animals. *Nippostrongylus muris* also is stunted in immune rats,[77] and *Ascaridia lineata* is shorter in immune chicks.[78]

Development of parasites.—Helminths often grow more slowly when residing in an immune host, and sometimes they fail to reach maturity. Such retardation has been observed in *Schistosoma japonicum* in immune dogs,[79] in *Taenia crassicollis* in immune cats,[80] and in *Nippostrongylus muris* in immune rats.[81] Furthermore, egg production is less in the case of *Hymenolepis fraterna*,[82] *Ancylostoma caninum*,[83] *Haemonchus contortus*,[84] and *Nippostrongylus muris*,[85] when these are in immune animals. Fewer larvae are produced by each female *Trichinella* in immune rats.[86] When transferred to a normal host from an immune host, the worms often resume development and reach maturity. The production of eggs may then be resumed.[87]

Persistence of parasites.—Parasites persist in immune animals

[69] A. O. Foster, *Am. J. Hyg.*, 22: 65 (1935).
[70] O. R. McCoy, *Am. J. Hyg.*, 14: 484 (1931).
[71] G. F. Otto and K. B. Kerr, *Am. J. Hyg.*, 29: 25 (1939, sec. D).
[72] G. L. Graham, J. E. Ackert, and R. W. Jones, *Am. J. Hyg.*, 15: 726 (1932).
[73] B. Schwartz, J. E. Alicata, and J. T. Lucker, *J. Washington Acad. Sci.*, 21: 259 (1931).
[74] M. Ozawa, *Jap. J. Exper. Med.*, 8: 79 (1930).
[75] H. M. Miller, Jr., *Proc. Soc. Exper. Biol. & Med.*, 27: 926 (1930).
[76] T. Ohira, *Tr. Far East Assoc. Trop. Med., 9th Congr.*, 1: 601 (1935).
[77] A. C. Chandler, *Am. J. Hyg.*, 23: 46 (1936).
[78] G. L. Graham, J. E. Ackert, and R. W. Jones, *Am. J. Hyg.*, 15: 726 (1932).
[79] M. Ozawa, *Jap. J. Exper. Med.*, 8: 79 (1930).
[80] T. Ohira, *Tr. Far East Assoc. Trop. Med., 9th Congr.*, 1: 601 (1935).
[81] A. C. Chandler, *Am. J. Hyg.*, 23: 46 (1936).
[82] A. V. Hunninen, *Am. J. Hyg.*, 22: 414 (1935).
[83] O. R. McCoy, *Am. J. Hyg.*, 14: 268 (1931).
[84] E. L. Taylor, *J. Helminthol.*, 12: 143 (1934).
[85] A. C. Chandler, *Am. J. Hyg.*, 16: 750 (1932).
[86] O. R. McCoy, *Am. J. Hyg.*, 21: 200 (1935).
[87] A. C. Chandler, *Am. J. Hyg.*, 23: 46 (1936).

for shorter periods than in normal animals. *Trypanosoma lewisi,* for example, will usually persist for two or three weeks in the normal rat. Large doses inoculated to the immune rat, however, will be destroyed in a few hours.[88] A second infection with malaria in an immune man, likewise, will survive only a week or less, whereas a primary infection endures for months. Helminths also persist for shorter periods in immune hosts. If *Trichinella* larvae be fed to immune rats, for example, they are passed directly through the intestine in from eight to eighteen hours, mostly with no development.[89] In the normal rat these larvae persist for from three days to several weeks, depending on the number administered.[90]

[88] W. H. Taliaferro, *J. Infect. Dis.,* 62: 98 (1938).
[89] O. R. McCoy, *J. Parasitol. (Suppl.),* 24: 35 (1938) and *Am. J. Hyg.,* 32: 105 (1940, sec. D).
[90] O. R. McCoy, *Science,* 75: 364 (1932).

Part Two

IMMUNITY IN SPECIFIC DISEASES

Chapter IX

THE AMOEBIASES

THE ONLY PARASITIC AMOEBA significant as the cause of disease in either man or animals is *Endamoeba histolytica*. Essentially all to be said on the immunology of amoebiasis will, therefore, refer to this form. *Endamoeba histolytica* is generally regarded as primarily a human parasite, which produces in a small percentage of the general population the very serious diseases, amoebic dysentery and amoebic abscess. Morphologically identical amoebas have been found in several animals.

NATURAL RESISTANCE

HOST RESTRICTION

Although *Endamoeba histolytica* is primarily a human parasite, it will, nevertheless, also infect a number of lower animals. The *Macacus rhesus* is believed to be a natural host of the parasite,[1] and the rat also appears significant as an agency for its transmission. Dogs, cats, monkeys, and rats can all be experimentally infected, and intestinal lesions develop in infections of the first three of these species.[2] Lesions in the cat are not of the undermining character seen in human infections, but are of simpler form and are generally surrounded by areas of inflammation, which suggest the possible intervention of bacterial infection.[3] Cysts are not usually formed in infections of cats or dogs, although they are found in men and monkeys and often in rats. Generally the parasite succeeds in es-

[1] C. Dobell, *Parasitology,* 23: 1 (1931).
[2] F. O. Atchley, *Am. J. Hyg.,* 23: 410 (1936) ; C. F. Craig and J. C. Swartzwelder, *Proc. Soc. Exper. Biol. & Med.,* 37: 671 (1938) ; H. Tsuchiya, *Am. J. Trop. Med.,* 19: 151 (1939) ; R. Hegner, C. M. Johnson, and R. M. Stabler, *Am. J. Hyg.,* 15: 394 (1932) ; H. L. Ratcliffe, *Am. J. Hyg.,* 14: 337 (1931) ; E. C. Faust, *Am. J. Trop. Med.,* 12: 37 (1932).
[3] H. Tsuchiya, *Am. J. Trop. Med.,* 19: 151 (1939).

tablishing itself in only part of a group of animals to which it is administered experimentally, although a strain once passed through a given animal species gradually adapts itself to that host and on subsequent passages will infect a higher percentage of individuals.[4]

Most human beings are naturally resistant to infection with *Endamoeba histolytica*. Evidence for this lies chiefly in the fact that the great majority of persons never contract infection with this parasite, even though almost certainly they are repeatedly exposed to it. Those individuals who do acquire the infection generally keep it comparatively well controlled, and old lesions heal about as rapidly as new ones are formed. Usually in such resistant persons symptoms are never observed, and occasionally spontaneous cures occur.

The basis for the absolute natural resistance of most species of animals to infection with *Endamoeba histolytica* is still obscure, but some experimental evidence has been presented which seems largely to explain why generally only a rather small percentage of individuals within a susceptible species can be infected. The resistance of the individual animal appears to be related to the degree of gastric acidity. If, for example, cysts of *Endamoeba histolytica* are fed to rats with little or no food in their stomachs, the infection rate is higher than in rats with full stomachs, presumably because passage through the full stomach is delayed, with consequently greater, or even complete, destruction of the parasites from prolonged contact with the stomach acid. The infection rate likewise can be increased by neutralizing the stomach acid by the addition of alkali.[5] Unless free hydrochloric acid is present in the gastric juice, even the trophozoites of *Endamoeba histolytica* fed to dogs pass unharmed through the stomach and set up colonic infections.[6]

FACTORS INFLUENCING NATURAL RESISTANCE

Age.—Young dogs and cats are more susceptible to experimental infection with *Endamoeba histolytica* than are older animals, the older ones not infrequently remaining wholly symptomless. The susceptibility of dogs is said to decrease more rapidly than that of

[4] F. O. Atchley, *Am. J. Hyg.*, 23: 410 (1936); H. Tsuchiya, *Am. J. Trop. Med.*, 19: 151 (1939); E. Faust, *Am. J. Trop. Med.*, 12: 37 (1932).
[5] H. Tsuchiya, *Am. J. Trop. Med.*, 19: 151 (1939).
[6] J. C. Swartzwelder, *Pub. Health Rep.*, 52: 1447 (1937).

cats as age and weight advance.[7] In man the greatest incidence of infection, as found in one extensive survey,[8] occurs between the ages of twenty-six and thirty-five years. Children below five years are seldom infected, not because of an inherent resistance, but probably because they are less exposed to infection. Persons above thirty-five years may owe their comparative resistance to a specific immunity acquired from prior infection. In a second survey, covering more than twenty thousand persons in rural Tennessee, the age incidence with *Endamoeba histolytica* was found to rise rapidly in childhood, increase slightly in middle adult life, and decline in those more than sixty years of age.[9] However, the clinician must never lose sight of the fact that persons of any age are potentially susceptible to infection with this parasite.

Sex.—A larger percentage of males than of females contract infection with *Endamoeba histolytica,* and of these a higher percentage of the males suffer symptoms of amoebic dysentery. Likewise, males contract amoebic liver abscess much more frequently than females, this condition seldom being encountered among women.

Race.—While all races are susceptible to infection with *Endamoeba histolytica,* the white race appears to suffer more than others from symptoms of the disease. This is noted particularly among those individuals newly arrived in the tropics, such persons suffering infection and symptoms more frequently than do the natives. However, the possibility of previous exposure or infection with the parasite among natives is generally not given due consideration in these comparisons of racial resistance, and the chance for the building up through prior infection of a specific immunity by the native races is sometimes wholly lost sight of.

Climate.—Climate seems to be a significant factor in natural resistance to amoebic infection. Infection with amoebae has its greatest incidence and symptoms are most frequently encountered among persons in the tropics. Furthermore, individuals who have the infection often improve on removal from the tropics to temperate zones. Climate per se may not deserve, however, quite all the significance usually attached to it as a factor in resistance to

---

[7] O. Wagner, *Arch. f. Schiffs- u. Tropen-Hyg.,* 39: 1 (1935).

[8] E. C. Faust, *J. Pediat.,* 2: 53 (1933).

[9] H. E. Meleney, E. L. Bishop, and W. S. Leathers, *Am. J. Hyg.,* 16: 523 (1932).

amoebiasis. The diet, the use of alcohol, and the general tempo of life are different in the tropics, compared with the temperate zone, and these may largely explain the difference seen in resistance to the infection in the two regions. On the other hand, the climate doubtless has great significance in the natural survival and transmission of the parasite. Conditions of moisture and temperature in the tropics are more or less ideally suited to its survival and facilitate its dissemination. The chance for exposure to the parasite is, then, greater in the tropics, and since this exposure may also involve larger numbers of parasites, the chance for more severe infections would be greater.

Diet.—The character of the diet exerts a profound effect upon the natural resistance to amoebic infection, especially as to the severity of the accompanying symptoms. A study of two rural communities of Tennessee revealed a higher incidence of dysentery in the one with a generally poor diet than in the other with a better diet, even though 40 percent of the population in the latter community harbored the parasite.[10] Dogs that are resistant to experimental amoebic infection so long as they are kept on a balanced diet lose their resistance if placed on a poor diet, such as one of canned salmon exclusively.[11] Liver products, on the other hand, seem to improve the condition of dogs after experimental *Endamoeba histolytica* infections.[12] Raw liver is the most effective substance,[13] although liver extract also is helpful if given by mouth.[14] Following the administration of raw liver, the amoebic lesion is arrested, and often the parasite development is completely prevented. Liver seems to play an amoebostatic rather than an amoebocidal role, and at the same time it lessens the danger of secondary bacterial invasion.[15]

A high carbohydrate diet, that is, one favoring Gram-negative bacteria, creates conditions in the rat caecum which favor *Enda-*

[10] F. D. Alexander and H. E. Meleney, *Am. J. Hyg.*, 22: 704 (1935).

[11] E. C. Faust, L. C. Scott, and J. C. Swartzwelder, *Proc. Soc. Exper. Biol. & Med.*, 32: 540 (1934).

[12] E. C. Faust, *Am. J. Trop. Med.*, 12: 37 (1932); E. C. Faust, L. C. Scott, and J. C. Swartzwelder, *Proc. Soc. Exper. Biol. & Med.*, 32: 540 (1934).

[13] E. C. Faust and E. S. Kagy, *Am. J. Trop. Med.*, 14: 235 (1934).

[14] E. C. Faust and J. C. Swartzwelder, *Proc. Soc. Exper. Biol. & Med.*, 33: 514 (1936).

[15] E. C. Faust and E. S. Kagy, *Am. J. Trop. Med.*, 14: 235 (1934).

moeba muris, a natural protozoan of the rat. These parasites survive hardly at all in rats fed a diet high in protein and low in carbohydrate.[16] The absence of vitamin A from the diet or the condition of vitamin A deficiency does not render the rat caecum unfavorable for *Endamoeba muris*.[17]

ACQUIRED IMMUNITY

RESISTANCE TO REINFECTION

No adequate experimental evidence is available for the acquisition of immunity by man through recovery from infection with *Endamoeba histolytica*, although on epidemiological grounds the reinfection of man seems seldom to result in symptoms. Natives in the tropics, where *Endamoeba histolytica* occurs widely, seldom suffer from amoebic dysentery even though the parasite occurs in their colon, whereas persons recently come from temperate zones must guard constantly against contracting severe dysentery when visiting these same tropical areas. The relative susceptibility of the visitor is generally explained by his not having previously been exposed, or at least his not having suffered a prior infection with *Endamoeba histolytica*. The comparative resistance of the native is believed to result from his recovery from an earlier acute infection, the immunity thus acquired being fortified through the years by repeated exposure.

Some animal experimentation with *Endamoeba histolytica* infection provides data which suggests that recovery from acute infection protects against reinfection,[18] although often two or three infections must be experienced before the immunity rises to a significant level.[19]

Premunition.—Immunity after recovery from amoebic infection appears to last only so long as the causal parasite persists as a latent form of infection in the body of the patient. Persons in whom this latent infection is ended, either by spontaneous recovery or by means of drug treatment, are as susceptible as normal persons to a fresh infection with the organism. In this respect immunity in

[16] R. Hegner and L. Eskridge, *J. Parasitol.*, 23: 105 (1937); H. L. Ratcliffe, *J. Parasitol.*, 16: 75 (1929).
[17] W. W. Frye and H. E. Meleney, *J. Parasitol.*, 23: 228 (1937).
[18] C. F. Craig, *Am. J. Trop. Med.*, 7: 225 (1927).
[19] O. Wagner, *Arch. f. Schiffs- u. Tropen-Hyg.*, 39: 1 (1935).

amoebic infection is largely analogous to that in malaria, which will be discussed in a later chapter.

ANTIBODY PRODUCTION

Antibodies can be demonstrated in the serum of both human beings and animals after infection with amoebae. The antibodies are best detected through the complement fixation test.[20] In experimental infection of dogs the fixation antibody has been demonstrated as early as the third day after infection, and most animals are positive by the fifteenth day. After animals recover, the antibodies gradually disappear. Antibodies also are developed in rabbits injected with cultures of *Endamoeba histolytica*.[21]

PASSIVE IMMUNITY

Immunity to amoebic infection has not been shown to be passively transferable in the serum of recovered persons or animals.

MECHANISM OF IMMUNITY

Although it is thoroughly established that immunity in amoebiasis depends upon the persistence of a latent infection with the homologous parasite, the actual mechanism of the immunity is obscure. Nevertheless, it is clear that the entire body becomes sensitized as the result of an infection with amoebae, since antibody specific for the amoeba substance promptly appears in the serum of an infected person or animal. Eventually some role in resistance to reinfection may be assigned this antibody, although none has yet been proved. Furthermore, no role may yet be assigned the leucocytes or other protective cells of the body, since such cells do not even infiltrate the area surrounding an uncomplicated amoebic lesion. The possibility remains that the immunity in amoebiasis is strictly local in character and is maintained by continuation of the infection in certain strategic organs and tissues. The resistance acquired as a local response to infection may, then, be effective locally and may keep the parasite in check thereafter. Organs other than the colon seem to share in this immunity, however. The infrequency with which liver lesions develop in persons with intestinal amoe-

[20] T. Simić, *Ann. de parasitol.*, 13: 345 (1935).
[21] P. E. Menendez, *Am. J. Hyg.*, 15: 785 (1932).

biasis, for example, suggests that the liver also has some capacity for specific resistance against the parasite.

PROPHYLAXIS

Immune phenomena have not been applied in the prophylaxis of amoebic infections.

DIAGNOSIS

The most notable contribution of immunology thus far in amoebic infection is the development of the complement fixation test for diagnosing the disease. Although other workers had previously demonstrated the complement-fixing antibody in serum from amoebic cases,[22] it remained for Craig to develop the test to a point of utility.[23] An alcoholic extract of cultures of *Endamoeba histolytica* has generally been used as the antigen in the fixation test,[24] although an extract of scrapings from colonic ulcers or of intestinal mucus containing amoebae also has been tried successfully.[25] A positive test is given by active cases of amoebic dysentery and by carriers of *Endamoeba histolytica,* as well as by cases with amoebic liver abscess. Extraordinarily severe infections often give negative tests, whereas the strongest reactions are given by individuals with mild or symptomless cases.[26] Persons cured of their infection by treatment give a negative fixation test within a few days or weeks,[27] although the test again becomes positive in those whose infections relapse.[28] The fixation reaction is specific, no fixation occurring with the serum of normal individuals, persons with non-pathogenic intestinal protozoans or persons with most other diseases. Cases of chronic ulcerative colitis, however, usually give a positive fixation test,[29] a result which leads some authorities to be-

[22] G. Izar, *Arch. f. Schiffs- u. Tropen-Hyg.,* 18: 36 (1914); I. Scalas, *Riforma med.,* 37: 103 (1921).
[23] C. F. Craig, *Am. J. Trop. Med.,* 7: 225 (1927).
[24] C. F. Craig, *Proc. Nat. Acad. Sc.,* 14: 520 (1928).
[25] C. F. Craig, *Amebiasis and Amebic Dysentery,* Springfield, Thomas (1934).
[26] C. F. Craig, *J. Lab. and Clin. Med.,* 18: 873 (1933).
[27] C. F. Craig, *Proc. Nat. Acad. Sc.,* 14: 520 (1928); C. F. Craig, *Am. J. Trop. Med.,* 9: 277 (1929); Y. Yamamoto, *J. Orient. Med.,* 24: 969 (1936).
[28] C. F. Craig, *J. Lab. and Clin. Med.,* 18: 873 (1933).
[29] E. D. Kiefer, *Am. J. M. Sci.,* 183: 624 (1932); N. P. Sherwood and L. Heathman, *Am. J. Hyg.,* 16: 124 (1932); H. Tsuchiya, *J. Lab. and Clin. Med.,* 19: 495 (1934).

lieve that this affliction represents a pyogenic infection superimposed on an original amoebic ulceration.[30]

It is obvious from what has been said that the fixation test is very helpful as an aid in the diagnosis of amoebiasis.[31] Nevertheless, there are some who feel that the technical difficulties entailed in its performance render older and simpler methods of diagnosis, for example, fecal examination and stool cultivation, preferable.[32]

A positive complement fixation test is given also by experimentally infected dogs [33] and monkeys,[34] although not by rats. Presumably, some degree of tissue invasion must occur before a test can be positive, and none occurs in rat infections. Experimentally infected dogs sometimes give a positive test after only three or four days, and most infected dogs will give the test within fifteen days. After recovery or successful treatment, dogs give a negative test.[35]

Only very poor results have yet been obtained with other immunological procedures in the diagnosis of amoebic dysentery. Precipitins have been detected in the blood of infected cats by mixing their serum with antigen derived from colonic lesion scrapings by extraction with Coca's fluid,[36] but the method has not been used in human infections. A similar antigen has also elicited skin tests in patients,[37] but such tests have not had extensive trial.

[30] E. D. Kiefer, *Am. J. M. Sci.*, 183: 624 (1932).

[31] T. B. Magath and H. E. Meleney, *Am. J. Trop. Med.*, 20: 211 (1940).

[32] M. Paulson and J. Andrews, *Arch. Int. Med.*, 61: 562 (1938); B. K. Spector, *J. Prevent. Med.*, 6: 117 (1932).

[33] H. E. Meleney and W. W. Frye, *Am. J. Pub. Health*, 27: 505 (1937); C. F. Craig, *Proc. Soc. Exper. Biol. & Med.*, 30: 270 (1932).

[34] C. F. Craig and J. C. Swartzwelder, *Proc. Soc. Exper. Biol. & Med.*, 37: 671 (1938).

[35] H. E. Meleney and W. W. Frye, *Am. J. Pub. Health*, 27: 505 (1937); C. F. Craig and E. Kagy, *Am. J. Hyg.*, 18: 202 (1933).

[36] E. H. Wagener, Univ. California, *Publ., Zoology*, 26: 15 (1924).

[37] R. Bieling, *Arch. f. Schiffs- u. Tropen-Hyg.*, 39: 49 (1935); I. Scalas, *Riforma med.*, 39: 967 (1923).

Chapter X

THE LEISHMANIASES

O NE OF THE most notable contributions of immunology to the study of the leishmania infections lies in the classification of the organisms causing these diseases.[1] The parasites of the several clinical entities are indistinguishable in morphology and physiology, and they can be differentiated only through immune reactions. At the present time three distinct human species are usually acknowledged: *Leishmania donovani* in kala azar, *Leishmania tropica* in oriental sore, and *Leishmania brasiliensis* in espundia, although the last is often treated as a variety of *Leishmania tropica*.[2] The systematic position of other leishmanias is comparatively uncertain, although forms found in clinically similar diseases of the dog—an animal often incriminated as playing some role in the epidemiology of the human leishmaniases—are believed identical immunologically with the corresponding human pathogens [3] and are sometimes assigned the same specific designations. For a more extended discussion, see Chapter XVIII.

The problem of immunity in infection with the leishmanias is rendered peculiarly difficult from the outset by the fact that the causal organisms naturally reside and multiply almost exclusively within cells of the reticulo-endothelial system where immune responses against most infectious agents are believed to be initiated.[4] One would suspect that such responses as were made to an agent which succeeded in reaching the seat of the immune process, and

[1] H. Noguchi, *Proc. Int. Confer. on Health Probs. in Trop. America,* United Fruit Co., Boston, 455 (1924).

[2] F. Da Fonseca, *Am. J. Trop. Med.,* 13: 113 (1933) ; A. Laurinsich: *Pediatria,* 39: 345 (1931) ; P. E. Mesik, *Gior. di batteriol. e. immunol.,* 3: 225 (1928).

[3] N. I. Chodukin, *Suppl. to Pensée med. d'Usbequistane et de Turqumenistane* (1928–29).

[4] L. Bogliolo, *Pathologica,* 26: 735 (1934).

there persisted and proliferated with no difficulty, would be comparatively poor and ineffectual for overcoming that invader. For the most part, this suspicion is borne out by the observed facts, although much of the available information is inconclusive and contradictory. Opposing this view is the almost legendary knowledge that human recovery from an oriental sore insures freedom from subsequent infection with the same disease. Knowledge of this fact has been applied since early times by mothers in endemic areas, who have guarded the facial beauty of their daughters against disfiguration by deliberately inducing a sore on some hidden part of the girls when young.

NATURAL IMMUNITY

HOST RESTRICTION

Leishmania donovani has been found in natural infections of only dogs and cats, besides man. Infections with it have been experimentally induced, however, in a rather wide range of animals. Most studies have been carried on in *Macacus* monkeys, mice, and hamsters, although guinea pigs, rabbits, rats, jerboas, and gerbilles among rodents, and jackals and flying foxes all have been infected. Experimental infection often fails, however, even in hamsters, which are probably the best experimental animal for this protozoan.[5]

Leishmania tropica also can invade many animals. It has been recovered from natural infections in the skin of dogs, and infections can be induced in monkeys, dogs, cats, rats, mice, and guinea pigs. Not infrequently, especially in mice, generalized visceral infections with *Leishmania tropica* ensue if the parasite be injected deeply into the skin. *Leishmania brasiliensis* resembles *Leishmania tropica* in its infectivity in essentially all respects. It is also found naturally in the dog.

FACTORS INFLUENCING NATURAL RESISTANCE

The circumstances of natural infection with all the leishmaniases is so obscure that as yet factors which influence natural resistance have not been determined. Persons of all age groups are apparently susceptible to infection, and even adults may succumb to the vis-

[5] E. Hindle, *Tr. Roy. Soc. Trop. Med. & Hyg.*, 24: 97 (1930).

ceral disease if untreated. However, in the Mediterranean area and in China children are the chief sufferers, those infected in Mediterranean countries being usually less than four years old. Males are more frequently infected than females, possibly because of greater exposure. Undernourishment is a serious predisposing cause, although no specific element of the diet is known to play a role in resistance. Another predisposing factor may be malarial infection. At least monkeys (*Macacus cynomolgus*) with plasmodial infection are believed more susceptible to *Leishmania donovani* than normal monkeys.[6] During human infection with kala azar positive tuberculin tests become negative temporarily.[7]

The reticulo-endothelial system probably plays a significant part in natural resistance. Splenectomy, treatment with benzol,[8] or X ray irradiation [9]—all of which materially depress the function of the reticulo-endothelial system—have been reported to lower the resistance of hamsters to experimental infection with *Leishmania donovani*. On the other hand, the removal of the spleen is said not to enhance the susceptibility of mice to experimental infections.[10] Splenectomy is often resorted to in man, however, as a therapeutic measure, since early in an infection parasites collect in the spleen and can be removed en masse along with that organ.[11]

ACQUIRED IMMUNITY

RESISTANCE TO REINFECTION

Human beings who have recovered from either kala azar or oriental sore are considered immune to reinfection, since second attacks are seldom encountered. Recent experimental studies upon the cutaneous infection have confirmed this view, and the inoculation of hidden parts of persons in endemic areas is recommended as a precautionary measure against later facial lesions.[12] Among experimental animals, mice appear to acquire little or no immunity by

[6] L. E. Napier, R. O. A. Smith, and K. V. Krishnan, *Indian J. M. Research*, 21: 1553 (1934).

[7] D'Oelsnitz, *Bull. et mém. Soc. méd. hôp. de Paris*, 50th yr., 409 (1934).

[8] C. W. Wang and H.-L. Chung, *Proc. Soc. Exper. Biol. & Med.*, 44: 35 (1940).

[9] H.-L. Chung, C. W. Wang, and C.-L. Hsu, unpublished experiments.

[10] K. V. Krishnan, *Ind. Med. Res. Mem., Supp. Ser. to Indian J. M. Research*, No. 25, 109 (1932).

[11] P. Timpano, *Policlinico*, 37: 1710 (1930).

[12] D. A. Berberian, *Tr. Roy. Soc. Trop. Med. & Hyg.*, 33: 87 (1939).

recovery from an earlier infection with *Leishmania tropica*,[13] although dogs do experience some enhancement of resistance. Monkeys, on the other hand, become rather highly resistant to a second infection, thus resembling man.[14] Some cross immunity seems to occur between kala azar and oriental sore. For example, a dog which is immune to kala azar resists the parasites of oriental sore, and a monkey recovered from oriental sore is partially resistant to those of kala azar.[15] Likewise, Chinese hamsters which have been cured of *Leishmania donovani* infection by neostibosan are immune to the dog form, *Leishmania canis*.[16] Whether a latent infection must persist in order that immunity continue in recovered animals or man has not been determined.

ANTIBODY PRODUCTION

Antibody is produced rather poorly in leishmania infections. The presence of the parasite in the haemopoietic tissues themselves, where antibody is believed formed in large amount, may be chiefly responsible for this, since the parasites may so damage the tissue that antibody production cannot proceed normally. Such a point of view is supported by the observation that persons with kala azar produce antibody poorly to other introduced antigens (for example, triple typhoid vaccine), compared with normal persons, resembling in this respect persons with myelogenous leukaemias.[17] Some investigators, however, are unable to confirm this finding.[18] Antibody is usually formed in patients in an amount sufficient to be detected by the complement fixation test. In addition a leishmanicidal antibody also occurs in the serum of patients, which inhibits the growth of the specific leishmanias in cultures to which the serum is added.

PASSIVE IMMUNITY

Attempts passively to transfer immunity have not been successful in the leishmaniases. Only very few such attempts have yet been made, however, because the comparatively poor antibody produc-

[13] A. Laveran, *Bull. Soc. path. exot.*, 8: 680 (1915).

[14] A. Laveran, *Compt. rend. Acad. de Sc.*, 165: 306, 1918, and *Bull. Soc. path. exot.*, 11: 130 (1918).

[15] C. Nicolle and L. Manceaux, *Ann. Inst. Past.*, 24: 673 (1910).

[16] H.-L. Chung and C. W. Wang, *Chinese M. J.*, 56: 519 (1939).

[17] H.-L. Chung and H. A. Reimann, *Arch. Int. Med.*, 46: 782 (1930).

[18] G. Murano and F. Vecchio, *Pediatria*, 47: 861 (1939).

tion in these diseases coupled with the meager evidence for active immunity after recovery from infection suggests that attempts at passive transmission are almost certainly doomed to fail. Serum prepared in rabbits repeatedly injected with cultures of *Leishmania donovani* has not been successful in treating experimental infections in hamsters, although the disease is somewhat prolonged by such treatment.[19]

MECHANISM OF IMMUNITY

Immunity in the leishmaniases depends on the presence of both phagocytic cells and specific antibody in the blood and tissues. A histiocyte response is one of the most characteristic reactions in kala azar, an increase in histiocytes occurring particularly in the spleen and its sinusoids. The presence of large numbers of monocytes in the peripheral blood is an especially favorable prognostic sign, since an increase in these cells is usually coincidental with the development of specific antibody. It is only when antibody is present in the blood and fixed tissues that the protective cells can adequately perform their phagocytic function.[20] The maximum defensive effort of the patient or animal requires, then, the coöperation of both the humoral and the cellular defense agencies.

PROPHYLAXIS

Efforts to protect animals against *Leishmania donovani* through administering killed cultures, living avirulent organisms, or living virulent organisms [21] have been so regularly unsuccessful that they have not been employed in man. In oriental sore, however, prophylaxis through injecting virulent living organisms has long been practised, although the use of controlled methods of vaccination for this purpose is still in its experimental stages.[22] One authority believes, chiefly from results obtained upon himself, that immunity acquired through prophylactic vaccination endures for about seven years.[23] Experimental studies with *Leishmania tropica* vaccine in

[19] B. Malamos, *Arch. f. Schiffs- u. Tropen-Hyg.*, 41: 416 (1937).

[20] L. E. Napier, K. V. Krishnan, and C. Lal, *Indian M. Gaz.*, 68: 75 (1933).

[21] T. J. Kurotchkin, *Nat. Med. J. China,* 17: 458 (1931); B. Malamos, *Arch. f. Schiffs- u. Tropen-Hyg.*, 41: 416 (1937).

[22] A. P. Lawrow and P. A. Dubowskoj, *Arch. f. Schiffs- u. Tropen-Hyg.*, 41: 374 (1937).

[23] E. I. Marzinowsky, *Bull. Soc. path. exot.*, 21: 638 (1928).

Macacus monkeys, however, do not support very strongly the injection of either killed, avirulent, or fully virulent organisms as a prophylactic measure.[24] Nevertheless, the inoculation of man with living virulent organisms is recommended for prophylaxis in endemic areas.

The successful use of a phenolated *Leishmania tropica* vaccine for the cure of oriental sore has recently been reported. A series of injections of the vaccine was considered by one investigator to have cured 151 cases out of 187 treated, and definite improvement was noted in twenty-four of the remainder.[25] Whether or not this effect was of a specific character was not established.

DIAGNOSIS

The complement fixation test is a fairly accurate means of diagnosing human infection with the leishmaniases and is useful particularly when the parasites themselves cannot be seen by direct procedures.[26] In one study, involving 132 known cases of kala azar, none gave a negative reaction, whereas among seventy-five controls, only six patients—and all of these with pulmonary tuberculosis—were positive.[27] In experimental canine infections, however, results with the test are often irregular.[28] Confusion sometimes occurs in human cases because the patient tested also has a positive Wassermann reaction, although when the leishmania antigen is prepared from cultures [29] rather than from heavily infected organs, this difficulty can largely be avoided.[30] A "reverse" complement fixation test has also been devised, the leishmania antigen being detected in the patient's serum with antibody coming from a rabbit repeatedly injected with cultures of *Leishmania donovani*.[31] The method has not as yet been extensively applied.

Skin tests can be elicited in patients with leishmaniasis, cultures

[24] L. Parrot, *Compt. rend. Soc. de biol.*, 100: 411 (1929).

[25] J. C. Ray, *Indian J. Pediat.*, 2: 149 (1935).

[26] A. M. da Cunha and E. Dias, *Compt. rend. Soc. de biol.*, 129: 991 (1938).

[27] S. D. S. Greval, P. C. Sen Gupta, and L. E. Napier, *Indian J. M. Research*, 27: 181 (1939).

[28] P. Zdrodowski and B. Woskressenski, *Bull. Soc. path. exot.*, 23: 1028 (1930).

[29] A. M. da Cunha and E. Dias, *Brasil-med.*, 53: 89 (1939).

[30] A. Georgiewsky, *Pensée Med. d'Usbekistane*, No. 3: 80 (1927); R. B. Lloyd, L. E. Napier, and G. C. Mitra, *Indian J. M. Research*, 17: 957 (1930).

[31] L. Nattan-Larrier and L. Grimard-Richard, *Compt. rend. Soc. de biol.*, 113: 1489 (1933); and *Bull. Soc. path. exot.*, 28: 658 (1935).

of the causal organisms serving as antigen.[32] Generally, better reactions to *Leishmania donovani* antigen occur in kala azar than in
oriental sore; the reverse is true with *Leishmania tropica* antigen.[33]
Nevertheless, the skin response in leishmaniasis seems always to be
definitely a group reaction, persons with South American leishmaniasis reacting even to *Trypanosoma equiperdum* antigen.[34] Skin
reactions involving leishmania antigens were first elicited in rabbits
which had been injected with cultures of *Leishmania donovani* and
Leishmania tropica.[35]

The Rieckenberg adhesin test has been tried with limited success,
especially for the diagnosis of oriental sore.[36] It seems not to serve,
however, in canine leishmaniasis.[37]

[32] G. Buss, *Arch. f. Schiffs- u. Tropen-Hyg.*, 33: 65 (1929); A. Dostrovsky, *Ann. Trop. Med.*, 29: 123 (1935); L. de S. Gomes: *Brasil-med.*, 53: 1079 (1939).

[33] B. Malamos, *Arch. f. Schiffs- u. Tropen-Hyg.*, 41: 240 (1937).

[34] A. M. da Cunha, *Rev. Med.-Cirurg. do Brasil*, 39: 37 (1930).

[35] E. H. Wagener, Univ. California *Publ., Zoology*, 20: 477 (1923).

[36] E. A. Mills and C. Machattie, *Tr. Roy. Soc. Trop. Med. & Hyg.*, 25: 205 (1931).

[37] M. T. Balasheva, *Med. Par. and Parasit. Dis.*, 4: 19 (1935).

Chapter XI

THE TRYPANOSOMIASES

COMPARATIVELY LITTLE of our knowledge of the immunology of trypanosomiasis has been learned directly from the human infections with trypanosomes. The principles which are established from the extensive studies of the animal trypanosomiases, however, probably often apply as well in the human diseases. Because the trypanosomes of man also infect many animals, some of the experimental studies in animals have employed the human parasites, although many other investigations have been concerned with species of trypanosomes which occur naturally only in animals. Thus far practically all the available information upon immunity in trypanosomiasis has involved representatives of three groups of trypanosomes: (1) the pathogenic trypanosomes, (2) the natural trypanosomes of rodents, and (3) the trypanosome of man in South America.

THE PATHOGENIC TRYPANOSOMES

Four groups of the pathogenic trypanosomes are generally recognized—namely, the *brucei, congolense, vivax,* and *evansi* groups. The type species of these groups are, respectively, *Trypanosoma brucei, Trypanosoma congolense, Trypanosoma vivax,* and *Trypanosoma evansi.* A number of species are found in each group. Thus, *Trypanosoma gambiense* and *Trypanosoma rhodesiense* (the human trypanosomes of Africa) are included in the *brucei* group, *Trypanosoma simiae* is placed in the *congolense* group, *Trypanosoma caprae* and *Trypanosoma uniforme* are found in the *vivax* group, and *Trypanosoma equiperdum, Trypanosoma hippicum,* and *Trypanosoma equinum* in the *evansi* group.

The criteria for the classification of the pathogenic trypanosomes are in part morphologic characters and in part the elements of the life cycle in the invertebrate host.[1] However, the individual species as well as the several groups can also be differentiated through immunologic methods (see Chapter XVIII).

NATURAL RESISTANCE

HOST RESTRICTION

Of all the pathogenic trypanosomes those of the *brucei* group have the broadest potential host range. The type species, *Trypanosoma brucei,* for example, will establish itself in representatives of practically all orders of mammals and survives for a time also in some birds. The host range of the human members of this group (*Trypanosoma gambiense* and *Trypanosoma rhodesiense*) is about as great as that of *Trypanosoma brucei.* The Rhodesian parasite, for example, has been reported also to persist briefly in fowls.[2]

Species of trypanosomes in the other groups have more limited host range than those of the *brucei* group. Members of the *congolense* group, for example, infect only ungulates, carnivores, rodents, and certain monkeys, and those of the *vivax* group are confined almost exclusively to the ungulates and certain carnivores. The *evansi* group enjoys a somewhat wider host choice, although even so its choice is narrower than that of the *brucei* group of trypanosomes. The type species of the *evansi* group, *Trypanosoma evansi,* for example, is known to infect only ungulates, carnivores, rodents, and certain primates, as well as the elephant.

FACTORS INFLUENCING NATURAL RESISTANCE

Various factors influence the natural resistance of hosts to trypanosomes, although the specific roles of the separate factors is as yet poorly understood. With the pathogenic trypanosomes infection leads almost invariably to death unless interrupted by specific treatment. On the other hand, when an animal is naturally completely resistant to a given species, little can be done to render it susceptible.

Age and sex.—Age and sex are not very significant factors in the natural resistance of animals to the pathogenic trypanosomes. Usually, if an animal species is susceptible at all, either sex can be

[1] C. M. Wenyon, *Protozoology,* New York, William Wood (1926).
[2] E. Roubaud and A. Provost, *Bull. Soc. path. exot.,* 32: 807 (1939).

108   THE TRYPANOSOMIASES

infected at any age. However, very young rats often survive infection with these forms for a few days longer than older animals, suggesting a kind of reverse age resistance in these infections.[3]

Diet.—The diet, which plays a prominent role in natural resistance against some other types of parasitic infection, has not yet been shown to have equal importance in the trypanosomiases. The general plane of nutrition does not affect the resistance of cattle to *Trypanosoma congolense*,[4] although pigeons are rendered susceptible to *Trypanosoma brucei* by starvation.[5] Vitamin A does not affect the resistance of rats to *Trypanosoma brucei*,[6] although the administration of vitamin C enhances the resistance of guinea pigs to *Trypanosoma equiperdum*.[7] The carbohydrate level of the blood appears to be of considerable importance, for more intense infections and earlier death from *Trypanosoma equiperdum* occur in guinea pigs given sugar,[8] whereas life is prolonged and the infection sometimes aborted by injections of insulin.[9] Copper added to the diet is said to protect guinea pigs against *Trypanosoma equiperdum*.[10] The administration of alcohol to mice for one or two weeks before infection with *Trypanosoma gambiense* is said to hasten their death.[11]

Intercurrent infection.—In double trypanosome infections one species often interferes with another. *Trypanosoma brucei* suppresses *Trypanosoma congolense* in rats and mice, but in cattle *Trypanosoma congolense* is the dominant form.[12] Double infections of *Trypanosoma brucei* and *Trypanosoma lewisi* in rats cause no change in the course of either parasite,[13] but *Trypanosoma gambiense* and *Trypanosoma duttoni* given simultaneously to mice result in intense and fatal infections with both forms.[14]

[3] H. A. Poindexter, *Am. J. Hyg.*, 29: 111 (1939, sec. C).
[4] M. H. French and H. E. Hornby, Tangany. Terr. *Rep., Dept. Vet. Sci. and Animal Husb.*, Part V (1934).
[5] G. Sollazzo, *Ztschr. f. Immunitätsforsch. u. exper. Therap.*, 60: 239 (1929).
[6] J. Fine, *J. Hyg.*, 34: 154 (1934).
[7] D. Perla, *Am. J. Hyg.*, 26: 374 (1937).
[8] H. A. Poindexter, *Am. J. Trop. Med.*, 13: 555 (1933).
[9] H. A. Poindexter, *J. Parasitol.*, 21: 292 (1935).
[10] D. Perla, *J. Exper. Med.*, 60: 541 (1934).
[11] L. B. Levinson, *Zentralbl. f. Bakt.*, 114: 488 (1929).
[12] C. Schilling, *Ztschr. f. Immunitätsforsch. u. exper. Therap.*, 87: 482 (1936).
[13] J. Grillo and J. Schmitz, *Ztschr. f. Immunitätsforsch. u. exper. Therap.*, 85: 203 (1935).
[14] H. Galliard, *Ann. de parasitol.*, 12: 273 (1934).

An apparent antagonism between malaria and trypanosomiasis is sometimes noted, particularly in young children. Children below three years of age in Africa are rarely infected with trypanosomes, although they suffer intense and frequent malaria infections.[15] Likewise, prior or simultaneous infection of mice with spirochetes often appears to enhance resistance to trypanosomiasis.[16]

Reticulo-endothelial system.—Practically all the studies carried out thus far to determine the importance of the reticulo-endothelial system in natural resistance to the pathogenic trypanosomes have consisted in determining the effect of splenectomy. Sometimes no effect seems to follow splenectomy,[17] but usually resistance is depressed by the operation.[18]

Other factors.—Exposing rats to low environmental temperatures after infection with *Trypanosoma brucei* is said to prolong the infection, the natural resistance to this parasite thus being enhanced.[19]

ACQUIRED IMMUNITY

RESISTANCE TO INFECTION

Most species of animals do not recover from an initial untreated infection with the pathogenic trypanosomes. Sheep and goats, however, are conspicuous exceptions to this rule. After a prolonged infection, lasting about two years, these animals recover from initial infections with *Trypanosoma brucei, Trypanosoma evansi,* or *Trypanosoma congolense,* and for several years thereafter resist reinfection with the homologous parasite. The immunity acquired is absolutely specific. Similarly the acquisition of resistance after recovery from infection has been reported in cattle with *Trypanosoma congolense,*[20] as well as in *Cercopithecus* monkeys with *Tryp-*

[15] R. E. Barrett, *Tr. Roy. Soc. Trop. Med. & Hyg.,* 25: 191 (1931).

[16] J. G. Thomson and P. De Muro, *J. Trop. Med.,* 35: 33 (1932); K-D Gno, *Zentralbl. f. Bakt.,* 139: 113 (1937).

[17] R. S. Tscherikower, *Ztschr. f. Immunitätsforsch. u. exper. Therap.,* 68: 182 (1930); L. J. Davis, *Ann. Trop. Med.,* 25: 79 (1931).

[18] I. J. Kligler, *Ann. Trop. Med.,* 23: 315 (1929); O. Nieschultz and F. K. Wawo-Roentoe, *Ztschr. f. Immunitätsforsch. u. exper. Therap.,* 65: 312 (1930); J. Schwetz, *Bull. Soc. path. exot.,* 27: 253 (1934).

[19] F. Van den Branden, *Ann. Soc. belge de méd. trop.,* 19: 243 (1939).

[20] R. van Saceghem, *Bull. Ag. Congo Belge,* 27: 47 (1936); *Bull. Soc. path. exot.,* 31: 296 (1938).

anosoma gambiense.[21] Immunity to reinfection is manifested also by animals which have been cured of an initial infection by drugs. In infected mice which have been treated with arsacetin, the immunity to reinfection with *Trypanosoma brucei* reaches its peak in about ten days, and sometimes completely protects the animals for several weeks thereafter.[22]

Premunition.—Animals immune to reinfection with the pathogenic trypanosomes sometimes retain the initial infection in latent form. Cattle acquire a tolerance of the parasite if treated early with suitable drugs, and thereafter survive for long periods in endemic areas in spite of reinfection.[23] They are said also to acquire such a tolerance after very small numbers of virulent trypanosomes are inoculated.[24] Usually the organisms are recoverable in small numbers from the blood throughout the resistant period.

ANTIBODY PRODUCTION

Animals vary greatly in their capacity to produce antibody after infection with the pathogenic trypanosomes. The rat and mouse form none at all against any of these parasites and are quickly killed by them, suffering overwhelming blood stream infections. The guinea pig and many other animals, on the other hand, produce a lytic antibody which—although not interfering with the reproduction of the trypanosomes—finally destroys most of the parasites against which it is specifically developed. Generally a few parasites escape the effects of this lysin, however, after undergoing some degree of biologic alteration, and continue to propagate themselves as a new relapse strain of parasite which is resistant to the original lysin. In a few days a second lysin is developed which destroys the majority of the organisms of the relapse strain. A succession of relapses may occur, with a specific and distinct lysin being developed in turn to each of the relapse strains of trypanosomes. No limit is known for the number of crises and relapses which may occur, but, finally, after its forces of resistance are exhausted, the animal succumbs to the infection.[25] Different relapse

[21] P. Le Gac, *Bull. Soc. path. exot.*, 24: 372 (1931).
[22] C. H. Browning and R. Gulbransen, *J. Path. and Bact.*, 43: 479 (1936).
[23] E. W. Bevan, *Tr. Roy. Soc. Trop. Med. & Hyg.*, 30: 199 (1936).
[24] C. Schilling, *Deutsche med. Wchnschr.*, 61: 832 (1935); *Ztschr. f. Immunitätsforsch. u. exper. Therap.*, 89: 112 and 306 (1936).
[25] H. Russell, *Tr. Roy. Soc. Trop. Med. & Hyg.*, 30: 179 (1936).

strains of the same parent strain of trypanosome once more re-
semble each other closely, however, after passage through the fly
vector.[26] The production of relapse strains is said to be suppressed
by the administration of germanin to infected animals.[27]

PASSIVE IMMUNITY

The passive transfer of immunity in the pathogenic trypanosomiases is largely an academic problem, for neither serum prophylaxis nor serum therapy is used in these diseases. The chief use of
studies on passive transfer has consisted in demonstrating the dis-
tinction immunologically between the relapse strains of trypanosomes as seen in guinea pigs, and the specificity of the action of the
lysins developed to each strain. The determinations are made for
the most part in mice, which themselves neither produce antibody
to the trypanosome nor cause any variation in the organism, the
mouse thus serving as a kind of test tube in which the lytic effect
can be studied.

MECHANISM OF IMMUNITY

The acquired immunity against the pathogenic trypanosomes
operates chiefly through the action of the lytic antibody of the
serum, which destroys the circulating trypanosomes after they are
formed. The antibody does not affect the rate of the trypanosome
reproduction. At the time of crisis the complement titer of the
serum of the infected animal is about one-third or one-fourth the
normal value.[28]

The effective antibody probably has its origin largely in the
reticulo-endothelial system, although thus far there is little proof
for this.[29] An increase in the number of monocytic cells occurs soon
after infection and may help to account for the antibody production.[30] Antibody production is less in young animals, this deficiency

[26] J. C. Broom and H. C. Brown, *Tr. Roy. Soc. Trop. Med. & Hyg.*, 34: 53 (1940).
[27] I. L. Kritschewski and S. S. Kaganova, *Ztschr. f. Immunitätsforsch. u. exper. Therap.*, 61: 478 (1929).
[28] I. Horner, *J. Immunol.*, 37: 85 (1939).
[29] I. Kritschewski and L. Schwarzmann, *Ztschr. f. Immunitätsforsch. u. exper. Therap.*, 56: 322 (1928); M. Zolog and O. Comsia, *Compt. rend. Soc. de biol.*, 122: 1135, 1138 (1936).
[30] D. F. Gowe, *Am. J. Trop. Med.*, 17: 401 (1937).

probably explaining the more frequent relapse seen in young animals after chemotherapy.[31]

PROPHYLAXIS

The resistance of experimental animals to the pathogenic trypanosomes can be enhanced by vaccination with dead trypanosomes.[32] Usually complete protection is not afforded by vaccination, although vaccinated animals generally live longer than untreated animals.[33] Such resistance as is developed by vaccination is absolutely specific.[34]

Vaccines have been prepared by various methods. Sometimes the trypanosomes are killed by incubation in the refrigerator in saline,[35] by treatment with parabenzoquinone,[36] or by treatment with bile.[37] Purified lipoid or protein fractions of the pathogenic trypanosomes—for example, *Trypanosoma evansi*—are not effectual as vaccine in prophylaxis.[38]

In endemic areas cattle can be protected by inoculating very small doses of living trypanosomes (*Trypanosoma brucei*), not more than fifty organisms generally being introduced.[39] Animals so treated live longer than untreated animals, but eventually succumb to the infection.[40]

The greatest difficulty with all the biologic methods of prophylaxis follows from the fact that immunization with one strain will not protect against infection with any of the other species or immunologically distinct strains of pathogenic trypanosomes which exist in nature. As yet it appears impracticable to prepare a polyvalent vaccine which would be effective against all such species and strains.

[31] H. Neumann, *Ztschr. f. Immunitätsforsch. u. exper. Therap.*, 74: 177 (1932).

[32] I. J. Kligler, L. Olitzki, and H. Kligler, *J. Immunol.*, 38: 317 (1940).

[33] L. Reiner and S. S. Chao, *Am. J. Trop. Med.*, 13: 525 (1933); E. Biocca, *Soc. internz. di microbiol., Boll. d. sez. ital.*, 11: 136 (1939).

[34] V. Zavagli, *Arch. ital. di sc. med. colon*, 10: 30 (1929); I. J. Kligler and M. Berman, *Ann. Trop. Med.*, 29: 457 (1933).

[35] I. J. Kligler and M. Berman, *Ann. Trop. Med.*, 29: 457 (1933).

[36] L. Reiner and S. S. Chao, *Am. J. Trop. Med.*, 13: 525 (1933).

[37] A. Castellani and I. Jacono, *Policlinico*, 44: 325 (1937).

[38] I. J. Kligler, L. Olitzki, and H. Kligler, *J. Immunol.*, 38: 317 (1940).

[39] C. Schilling, *Deutsche med. Wchnschr.*, 61: 832 (1935).

[40] C. Schilling, *Ztschr. f. Immunitätsforsch. u. exper. Therap.*, 89: 112 (1936); 96: 521 (1939).

DIAGNOSIS

The method of choice for the diagnosis of the pathogenic trypanosomiases is the detection of the causal organism in the blood, lymph gland juice, or spinal fluid. Many attempts have been made, however, to diagnose them by serological reactions.[41] *Trypanosoma equiperdum* infection (dourine) of horses has been most extensively studied, and a fair measure of success has been attained, particularly with the complement fixation test. Comparatively little value is yet attached to these tests in diagnosing human trypanosomiases.

A thermoprecipitation test for antigen has also been described in experimental trypanosomiasis. Extracts of various organs and tissues of rats, guinea pigs, and rabbits infected with *Trypanosoma equiperdum* contain an antigen reactive with the serum of recovered animals. The antigen is of protein character, although it is commingled with a carbohydrate. It occurs in largest amount in tissues active in blood formation and blood destruction.[42]

An in vitro reaction known as the red-cell adhesin test has been developed in recent years for the diagnosis of human trypanosomiasis, and from the application made thus far, appears especially promising. It is a specific serological test in which a suspension of trypanosomes, human red cells, complement, and serum from the patient suspected of trypanosomiasis are incubated together. In positive cases the red cells are caused to adhere firmly to the trypanosomes.[43] The red cells serve merely a passive role, however, since the cells of other primate animals can be substituted for the human erythrocytes.

THE NONPATHOGENIC TRYPANOSOMES OF RODENTS

Many immunological studies have been performed with the natural trypanosomes of rodents, although most of these are concerned with *Trypanosoma lewisi* in rats or *Trypanosoma duttoni* in mice.

[41] C. Richet and G. Antoine, *Bull. Acad. Méd.*, 122: 471 (1939).

[42] H. A. Poindexter, *J. Exper. Med.*, 60: 575 (1934), and *Am. J. Trop. Med.*, 16: 485 (1936).

[43] J. M. Wallace and A. Wormall, *Parasitology*, 23: 346 (1931) ; G. F. T. Saunders, *West African M. J.*, 5: 28 (1931) ; A. F. Brown, *Tr. Roy. Soc. Trop. Med. & Hyg.*, 26: 471 (1933) ; H. C. Brown and J. C. Broom, *Tr. Roy. Soc. Trop. Med. & Hyg.*, 32: 209 (1938).

Recently, a natural trypanosome of the Florida cotton rat, *Trypanosoma sigmodoni,* has also been studied immunologically.

NATURAL RESISTANCE

HOST RESTRICTION

The nonpathogenic trypanosomes of rodents differ sharply from the pathogenic forms in host range, since they are generally restricted to very few closely related hosts. *Trypanosoma lewisi,* the type species of the *lewisi* group, for example, occurs in the rat and can be inoculated to the guinea pig, but will infect no other animal. Other members of the *lewisi* group are also confined strictly to their natural hosts, usually infecting no other animal even within the same order. The natural trypanosomes of chiropterans and edentates also have a narrow host range.

FACTORS INFLUENCING NATURAL RESISTANCE

Age.—If an animal is susceptible at one age to infection with the rodent trypanosomes, it can generally be infected at any age. However, susceptible animals often manifest a relative resistance as they grow older. This "age resistance," which has been discussed at some length in Chapter III, is seen in rodent infections such as that of rats with *Trypanosoma lewisi.*[44] Young rats are usually killed by these parasites, many organisms developing in the blood, whereas older rats usually survive and experience relatively mild infections. Similarly, young mice suffer distinctly heavier infections with *Trypanosoma duttoni* than do older mice.[45] From this it is obvious that age is significant in the natural resistance to these parasites.

Sex.—No difference in natural resistance to the nonpathogenic trypanosomes is known to be related to the sex of the host.

Intercurrent infection.—The effects of an intercurrent infection on the course of the nonpathogenic trypanosomiases is comparatively slight,[46] although some evidence for an effect has been reported. Rats with *Bartonella* infection or with other disabling con-

[44] C. A. Herrick and S. X. Cross, *J. Parasitol.,* 22: 126 (1936) ; C. J. Duca, *Am. J. Hyg.,* 29: 25 (1939, sec. C).

[45] J. T. Culbertson, unpublished experiments.

[46] J. Grillo and J. Schmitz, *Ztschr. f. Immunitätsforsch. u. exper. Therap.,* 85: 203 (1935).

ditions, such as paratyphoid infection, suffer after splenectomy more severe infections with *Trypanosoma lewisi* than do rats without these intercurrent infections.[47] In mice *Trypanosoma duttoni* may cause intense or even fatal infections if the animals suffer also with *Trypanosoma gambiense*.[48]

Reticulo-endothelial system.—Most of the studies designed to show the significance of the reticulo-endothelial system in natural resistance to the nonpathogenic trypanosomes have involved the removal of the spleen. Rats and guinea pigs are not rendered more susceptible to *Trypanosoma lewisi* by splenectomy than normal animals,[49] but splenectomized mice suffer heavier infections with *Trypanosoma duttoni* than normal mice.[50] Harvest mice can even be infected with *Trypanosoma lewisi* if their spleens be extirpated.[51]

ACQUIRED IMMUNITY

RESISTANCE TO REINFECTION

Once animals recover from infection with the nonpathogenic trypanosomes, they are immune to reinfection. The immunity is particularly durable, probably lasting for the life of the animal. The acquisition of immunity through recovery from an initial infection has been demonstrated conclusively in the case of rats infected with *Trypanosoma lewisi* and of mice infected with *Trypanosoma duttoni*. The cotton rat also acquires immunity by recovery from a natural infection with *Trypanosoma sigmodoni*. Albino rats which have recovered from an experimental infection with *Trypanosoma sigmodoni* are thereafter resistant to *Trypanosoma lewisi*.[52]

Premunition.—The immunity acquired by recovery from the trypanosomes of the *lewisi* group is complete and absolute, not re-

[47] W. H. Taliaferro, P. R. Cannon, and S. Goodloe, *Am. J. Hyg.*, 14: 1 (1931).
[48] H. Galliard, *Ann. de parasitol.*, 12: 273 (1934).
[49] O. Nieschultz and F. K. Wawo-Roentoe, *Ztschr. f. Immunitätsforsch. u. exper. Therap.*, 2: 294 (1929) ; W. H. Taliaferro, P. R. Cannon, and S. Goodloe, *Am. J. Hyg.*, 14: 1 (1931) ; J. Schwetz, *Ann. de parasitol.*, 9: 10 (1931) ; *Bull. Soc. path. exot.*, 27: 62 (1934).
[50] H. Galliard, *Bull. Soc. path. exot.*, 26: 609 (1933) ; W. H. Taliaferro and Y. Pavlinova, *J. Parasitol.*, 22: 29 (1936).
[51] R. Bruynoghe and P. Vassiliadis, *Ann. Soc. belge de méd. trop.*, 9: 191 (1929) ; P. Vassiliadis, *Arch. internat. de méd. éxper.*, 6: 89 (1930).
[52] J. T. Culbertson, *J. Parasitol.*, 27: 45 (1941).

quiring the persistence of the infection in latent form. Blood taken from recovered animals does not reveal the parasite by microscopic examination, and culture media or animals inoculated with such blood remain sterile.

ANTIBODY PRODUCTION

Two antibodies are produced by rats after infection with *Trypanosoma lewisi*. One of them is a lytic substance similar in function to the antibody elaborated by guinea pigs after infection with pathogenic trypanosomes. The other, known as an ablastin, has primarily the property of inhibiting the reproduction of the trypanosomes but also probably the capacity to destroy by lysis immature trypanosomes present when it appears. The ablastin appears comparatively early in the course of the infection, usually about the fifth or sixth day, and gradually increases in concentration during the ensuing days. It declines in concentration after all the parasites have finally disappeared, but is believed to persist in small amount for the remaining life of the rat and to account for the resistance of the animal to reinfection. The lytic antibody appears rather explosively only after the infection has gone on for some time and lyses almost at once all the trypanosomes then in the blood. A few days later it disappears from the blood, although it can be recalled by reinfecting the rat or by inoculating a vaccine prepared of the homologous organisms.

Antibodies entirely similar to those in rats against *Trypanosoma lewisi* are produced in mice infected with *Trypanosoma duttoni*.[53] The *duttoni* infection, however, progresses more slowly and usually does not attain the intensity characteristic of *Trypanosoma lewisi* in the rat. The ablastin generally appears between the tenth and the fifteenth day of the *Trypanosoma duttoni* disease, and the lysin often is developed only after six or eight weeks. Probably other species of nonpathogenic trypanosomes also produce similar antibodies, although no information is yet available concerning them.

PASSIVE IMMUNITY

The serum from animals which have recovered from infections with the *lewisi* group of trypanosomes after transfer to normal ani-

[53] W. H. Taliaferro, *J. Immunol.*, 35: 303 (1938).

mals will protect them against infection with the homologous para-site. This is well established in the case of *Trypanosoma lewisi* infection of rats and has recently been shown also for *Trypanosoma duttoni* of mice [54] and for *Trypanosoma sigmodoni* of the cotton rat.[55] A considerable group specificity occurs in the action of the serum, for anti-*lewisi* rat serum will also protect mice against *Trypanosoma duttoni,* and anti-*duttoni* mouse serum will protect rats against *Trypanosoma lewisi.*[56]

MECHANISM OF IMMUNITY

Immunity against trypanosomes of the *lewisi* group depends al-most exclusively on the function of the two serum antibodies (an ablastin and a lysin), although possibly phagocytic cells or other elements of the reticulo-endothelial system play a small role. The ablastin antibody checks the propagation of the parasite and lyses the younger immature forms, thus causing the sharp drop in para-site number usually seen about the seventh day of the infection. The lytic antibody terminates the infection, eliminating all the surviving parasites. Studies on passive immunity have indicated strongly that the serum alone is capable of conferring protection to an animal, for rats which are splenectomized and blockaded with India ink are about as well protected by the serum as are normal rats.[57]

PROPHYLAXIS

Rats can be rendered immune to *Trypanosoma lewisi* [58] and mice can be protected against *Trypanosoma duttoni* [59] by the repeated injection of a killed suspension of the homologous parasites. Ap-parently the reaction is one with group specificity, for mice also can be protected against *Trypanosoma duttoni* by prior injections of the *lewisi* vaccine. The antigen for prophylactic vaccination has been prepared in different ways by various investigators. The

[54] W. H. Taliaferro, *J. Immunol.,* 35: 303 (1938).
[55] J. T. Culbertson, *J. Parasitol.,* 27: 45 (1941).
[56] W. H. Taliaferro, *J. Immunol.,* 35: 303 (1938).   [57] *Ibid.*
[58] F. G. Novy, *Proc. Soc. Exper. Biol. & Med.,* 4: 42 (1907); W. H. Taliaferro, *Am. J. Hyg.,* 16: 32 (1932); C. Schilling and B. Borghi, *Ztschr. f. Hyg. u. Infek-tionskr.,* 113: 586 (1932); J. T. Culbertson and W. R. Kessler, *Am. J. Hyg.,* 29: 33 (1939, sec. C).
[59] W. R. Kessler, unpublished experiments.

formolization of concentrated cultures or of trypanosomes isolated from the blood of heavily infected animals generally provides a good vaccine and is a comparatively simple procedure.[60]

DIAGNOSIS

Immunological procedures are not usually invoked in diagnosing the trypanosomiases caused by members of the *lewisi* group, because the parasites themselves can be observed easily in blood by the microscope. Complement-fixing and agglutinating antibodies are nevertheless produced.[61]

THE TRYPANOSOME OF MAN IN SOUTH AMERICA, TRYPANOSOMA CRUZI

NATURAL RESISTANCE

HOST RESTRICTION

Trypanosoma cruzi, although found in man and in some other primates, is probably a natural parasite of lower orders of mammals. It infects a broad range of host, including rodents, carnivores, chiropterans, marsupials, and edentates, besides the primates.[62] It is not infective for birds or for cold-blooded animals.[63] The parasite will survive in fowl embryos for about one week.[64]

FACTORS INFLUENCING NATURAL RESISTANCE

Age.—Older individuals are more resistant to *Trypanosoma cruzi* than are younger individuals. This is seen both in natural infections of man and in experimental infections of rodents. Young children, for example, suffer intense and frequently fatal infections, whereas older persons experience a chronic form of disease. Young mice and rats quickly succumb to infection, whereas those near mating age suffer but little, if any, and often do not reveal the parasite in their blood stream.[65]

[60] J. T. Culbertson and W. R. Kessler, *Am. J. Hyg.,* 29: 33 (1939, sec. C).
[61] J. Marmorston-Gottesman, D. Perla, and J. Vorzimer, *J. Exper. Med.,* 52: 587 (1930); J. T. Culbertson and W. R. Kessler, *Am. J. Hyg.,* 29: 33 (1939, sec. C).
[62] J. B. Arantes, *Mem. Inst. Oswaldo Cruz,* 6: 233 (1931); H. C. Clark and L. H. Dunn, *Am. J. Trop. Med.,* 12: 49 (1932).
[63] E. Dias, *Compt. rend. Soc. de biol.,* 112: 1474 (1933).
[64] E. Roubaud and J. Romaña, *Bull. Soc. path. exot.,* 32: 874 (1939).
[65] P. Regendanz, *Zentralbl. f. Bakt.,* 116: 256 (1930); J. A. Zuccarini, *Compt. rend. Soc. de biol.,* 105: 113 (1930); S. Niimi, *Jap. J. Exper. Med.,* 13: 543 (1935); M. H. Kolodny, *Am. J. Hyg.,* 29: 13 and 155 (1939, sec. C).

Other factors.—The natural resistance of rats and mice to *Trypanosoma cruzi* is not altered by splenectomy.[66] Resistance is depressed by exposing the animals to a low environmental temperature.[67]

ACQUIRED IMMUNITY

RESISTANCE TO INFECTION

Animals which have recovered from an infection with *Trypanosoma cruzi* are immune to reinfection with the same parasite.[68] Usually the initial infection persists in latent form for at least several months after the animal has recovered from the acute phase of the infection,[69] and the presence of the parasite may be responsible for the resistance which the host manifests, although no proof of this point has yet been offered.

PASSIVE TRANSFER

Serum from rats recovered from *Trypanosoma cruzi* infection will protect normal rats from the homologous parasite.[70] The serum must be injected prophylactically to be effective. When the serum is given therapeutically, little benefit ensues.

MECHANISM OF IMMUNITY

The mechanism of acquired immunity to *Trypanosoma cruzi* is still obscure. Some investigators doubt that the reticulo-endothelial system plays any part in immunity to *Trypanosoma cruzi*,[71] although the spleen characteristically is enlarged and a rise occurs in the number of monocytic cells during *Trypanosoma cruzi* infections.[72]

PROPHYLAXIS

As yet neither persons nor animals have been successfully protected against *Trypanosoma cruzi* by vaccination.

[66] H. Galliard, *Bull. Soc. path. exot.*, 23: 188 (1930) ; F. D. Wood, *Am. J. Trop. Med.*, 14: 497 (1934) ; R. A. Kelser, *Am. J. Trop. Med.*, 16: 405 (1936).
[67] M. H. Kolodny, *Am. J. Hyg.*, 32: 21 (1940, sec. C).
[68] J. T. Culbertson and M. H. Kolodny, *J. Parasitol.*, 24: 83 (1938).
[69] W. A. Collier, *Ztschr. f. Hyg. u. Infektionskr.*, 112: 88 (1931).
[70] J. T. Culbertson and M. H. Kolodny, *J. Parasitol.*, 24: 83 (1938).
[71] I. Kritschewski and L. Schwarzman, *Ztschr. f. Immunitätsforsch. u. exper. Therap.*, 56: 322 (1928).
[72] S. F. Wood, Univ. California *Publ., Zoology*, 41: 389 (1937).

DIAGNOSIS

The complement fixation reaction is useful for the diagnosis of Chagas's disease, it being called in this infection the "Machado reaction." The test has been used in diagnosis with considerable success.[73] The antigen can be prepared from heavily infected hearts of puppies [74] or, more satisfactorily, from pure cultures of the organism.[75] The serum of infected animals will agglutinate formolized cultures of *Trypanosoma cruzi* and will precipitate extracts of such cultures.[76]

ADDITIONAL IMMUNOLOGICAL SUBJECTS

TRYPANOTOXINS

For many years the production of trypanotoxins—toxins peculiar to the pathogenic trypanosome infections—has been postulated. Trypanotoxins were believed to be of the character of endotoxins, originating within the trypanosome body, and being liberated into the plasma where the parasites were lysed or otherwise destroyed. Presumptive evidence for the development of toxins in the trypanosomiases follows from the fact that in most natural infections with the pathogenic trypanosomes—for example, human infection with *Trypanosoma gambiense* and *Trypanosoma equiperdum* infection (dourine) of the horse—comparatively few trypanosomes are demonstrable in the blood at any time, even though the clinical symptoms are those suggesting a generalized toxemia.[77] Furthermore, when the blood of heavily infected rats or mice is transferred to corresponding normal animals, somnolence sometimes occurs, and death follows after two or three days. Comparatively recently the rabbit cornea has been found to be peculiarly susceptible to injections of the substance of *Trypanosoma gambiense* and *Trypanosoma equiperdum,* this presumably containing trypanotoxins. The corneas of previously vaccinated animals or

[73] W. Minning, *Arch. f. Schiffs- u. Tropen-Hyg.,* 39: 315 (1935); R. A. Kelser, *Am. J. Trop. Med.,* 17: 385 (1936); C. M. Johnson and R. A. Kelser, *Am. J. Trop. Med.,* 17: 385 (1937); J. G. Lacorte, *Acta Med. Rio de Janeiro,* 1: 264 (1938).
[74] W. Minning, *Arch. f. Schiffs- u. Tropen-Hyg.,* 39: 315 (1935).
[75] R. A. Kelser, *Am. J. Trop. Med.,* 16: 405 (1936).
[76] A. Packchanian, *J. Immunol.,* 29: 84 (1935); *Pub. Health Rep.,* 55: 2116 (1940).
[77] G. Ledentu, *Bull. Soc. path. exot.,* 21: 544 (1928); P. Regendanz, *Arch. f. Schiffs- u. Tropen-Hyg.,* 37: 196 (1933).

animals injected with an antitrypanosome serum are less susceptible to the action of the toxin, thus suggesting that a true toxin in
the strict immunological sense (that is, in eliciting antitoxin) is
produced by these pathogenic trypanosomes.[78]

The majority of investigators at the present time, however, question that trypanosomes produce a toxin. Those few workers who
have described such substances have found their repeated demonstration exceedingly difficult. It seems possible that the apparent
toxic conditions of infected animals is actually explained on a different basis, for example, by an altered blood chemistry. It has long
been known that in experimental rat infections with the pathogenic
trypanosomes there is terminally a reduced blood sugar, and recently a definitely elevated serum potassium has been described.[79]
Death from these infections in rodents bears such marked resemblance physically to death from hypoglycaemic shock or potassium
poisoning that these conditions rather than trypanotoxins may be
the cause of the fatal end in trypanosomiasis.

TRYPANOCIDAL ACTION OF NORMAL SERUM

The normal serum of several animals has a peculiar antagonistic
action on certain species of trypanosomes. The property is manifested by sheep serum as well as rat serum on *Trypanosoma duttoni*
of the mouse.[80] By far the most completely studied example, however, is the action of the serum of man and of certain other primates
upon the pathogenic trypanosomes. Human serum destroys practically all the pathogenic trypanosomes with the exception of those
found in man, *Trypanosoma gambiense* and *Trypanosoma rhodesiense*. After the latter species has been passed repeatedly through
laboratory rodents it, too, becomes susceptible to human serum,
but *Trypanosoma gambiense* retains its natural resistance for years
after residence in animals. Neither the trypanosomes of the *lewisi*
group nor *Trypanosoma cruzi* are susceptible to the effects of the
primate serums.[81]

The action of the trypanocidal serums is direct and occurs both

[78] N. Tokura, *Igaku Keukyn*, 9: 14 (1935).
[79] R. L. Zwemer and J. T. Culbertson, *Am. J. Hyg.*, 29: 7 (1939, sec. C).
[80] A. Thiroux, *Compt. rend. Acad. de sc.*, 149: 534 (1909); W. H. Taliaferro,
J. Immunol., 35: 303 (1938).
[81] J. T. Culbertson, *Arch. Pathol.*, 20: 767 (1935).

in the animal body and in vitro. The substance in the serum responsible for the action is highly labile, being inactivated by prolonged storage, by heat, or by other agencies which inactivate complement.[82] The trypanocidal substance is found in the globulin fraction of the serum and is antigenic.[83] Susceptible strains of trypanosomes can be rendered resistant to the action of the serum in about the same manner in which they can be made fast to specific drugs.

The trypanocidal substance is absent, or present in reduced amount, in the blood of persons with various liver disorders (amoebic abscess; icterus), in certain dietary deficiency diseases of children, and in hemophilia. It usually occurs in decreased concentration in the blood of young children and is absent from the child at birth.

Since human serum acts only on the pathogenic trypanosomes of animals, not on those infective for man, the trypanocidal action of human serum appears to account for the natural resistance of man to the animal forms. The point is debatable, however, for man remains resistant to the animal trypanosomes even after these are made fast to human serum. Furthermore, man is not infected with the trypanosomes of the *lewisi* group which naturally resist his serum.[84]

NATURAL TRANSFER OF RESISTANCE FROM MOTHERS
TO YOUNG

Immune mother animals transmit to their young specific resistance against homologous trypanosomes. Some evidence for this was presented several years ago by Schilling and his co-workers, who pointed out that very young game animals in Africa are somewhat resistant to the pathogenic trypanosomes. They believed the young acquired their resistance after birth, parasiticidal antibodies reaching the young in the mother's milk.[85]

The question has since been carefully studied in detail with the non-pathogenic group of trypanosomes. Specific protective sub-

[82] J. T. Culbertson and P. S. Strong, *Am. J. Hyg.*, 21: 1 (1935).
[83] B. Handler, *Am. J. Hyg.*, 21: 18 (1935).
[84] J. T. Culbertson, *Ann. Trop. Med.*, 28: 93 (1934).
[85] C. Schilling, *Ztschr. f. Immunitätsforsch. u. exper. Therap.*, 87: 47 (1936), and 96: 521 (1939).

stances pass in the milk to the young of mother rats immune to *Trypanosoma lewisi* [86] and *Trypanosoma cruzi* [87] and of mother mice immune to *Trypanosoma duttoni*.[88] Very little, if any, immunity is acquired by the young through the placenta prior to birth. Mother rats immunized by the inoculation of a formolized *Trypanosoma lewisi* vaccine also transmit resistance to their young in similar manner.[89] The immunity acquired from the mother is in all cases temporary, and several weeks after being weaned the young are as susceptible to infection as the young of a normal mother.

Immunity is developed by the mother and transmitted to the young very rapidly. For example, if a normal mother rat is infected with a trypanosome within a day or so after her litter is delivered, the young which nurse her will acquire complete resistance by the end of the second week of the nursing period. The mother meanwhile has elaborated the protective substance and passed it to the young through her milk. A mother powerfully immune at the time her litter is delivered, however, is often able to transmit enough protective substance to the young during their first twenty-four hours completely to prevent the development of an infection in them subsequently.

[86] J. T. Culbertson, *J. Parasitol.*, 24: 65 (1938), and 25: 182 (1939).
[87] M. H. Kolodny, *Am. J. Hyg.*, 30: 19 (1939, sec. C).
[88] J. T. Culbertson, *J. Immunol.*, 38: 51 (1940).
[89] J. T. Culbertson, *J. Parasitol.*, 27: 75 (1941).

Chapter XII

THE MALARIAS

MALARIA is the most important parasitic disease of man; more people suffer from it than from any other infection. In the tropics, and in many parts of the temperate zones as well, it is so widely prevalent that no resident can expect to escape contracting the disease. The comparative infrequency of death from malaria is explained by the fact that an infected individual usually acquires a specific immunity against the malaria parasite with which he is infected and generally, even if untreated, brings the infection under control. In addition, efficacious drugs are available to treat the disease. The ultimate eradication of the parasite from the body is due mostly to the immune response, however, for the treatment with drugs merely keeps the parasite in check until the patient's own defensive forces have been raised to an effective level. Immune responses essentially similar to those in human malaria are also seen in the malarias of monkeys and of birds.

HUMAN MALARIA

NATURAL RESISTANCE

HOST RESTRICTION

The four species of parasites which cause human malaria produce natural infections only in man. The few experimental infections with the human parasites which have been established in animals have been of only evanescent character. The inoculation of primates has been most successful.[1] *Plasmodium vivax* persists in a chimpanzee for six weeks or so,[2] and *Plasmodium falciparum* about eight days in the howler monkey.[3] Malarial pigment has been

---

[1] J. Schwetz, *Zentralbl. f. Bakt.*, 130: 105 (1933).
[2] J. Rodhain, *Compt. rend. Soc. de biol.*, 132: 69 (1939); J. Rodhain and G. Muylle, *Compt. rend. Soc. de biol.*, 131: 114 (1939).
[3] W. H. Taliaferro and P. R. Cannon, *Am. J. Hyg.*, 19: 335 (1934).

seen in a Java monkey at autopsy twelve days after *Plasmodium malariae* was inoculated. Infections in the lower animals have almost always failed, although ring stages of *Plasmodium vivax* have been reported in very young rodents and puppies for a few days after the injection of infected human blood.[4] Blood withdrawn from these animals during the first hours after inoculation usually is still infective for man,[5] although that taken after several days is not.[6]

In no animal, therefore, does infection with human malarial organisms approximate that usually seen in man. For this reason these parasites are very markedly restricted in the choice of host. Actually their host range is less than that of most other kinds of parasite.

FACTORS INFLUENCING NATURAL RESISTANCE

Infections with human malaria organisms vary markedly because of variations in the resistance of different persons. Many factors influence this resistance; some of these will be briefly described.

Race.—A marked difference in susceptibility to malaria is manifested by different races. Negroes are almost wholly insusceptible to *Plasmodium vivax*[7] and *Plasmodium ovale*. They suffer comparatively mild infections with the malignant parasite *Plasmodium falciparum* and practically never develop the serious complication of *Plasmodium falciparum* infection, blackwater fever.[8] White persons, in contrast, are almost invariably susceptible to all the malarial parasites, and they generally suffer severe symptoms of disease and even death.[9] Negroes often fail to develop the enlarged spleen so characteristic of infection in white persons and those with some white blood.[10] Members of the two races are about equally susceptible to *Plasmodium malariae*.

Some authorities believe that the resistance to *Plasmodium vivax*

[4] M. Yoshino, *Arch. f. Schiffs- u. Tropen-Hyg.*, 30: 624 (1926).
[5] G. Bodechtel, *Klin. Wchnschr.*, 9: 2020 (1930).
[6] J. Ségal, *Ann. de Parasitol.*, 8: 590 (1930).
[7] M. F. Boyd, *South. M. J.*, 27: 155 (1934); M. F. Boyd and W. K. Stratman-Thomas, *Am. J. Hyg.*, 18: 485 (1933).
[8] M. F. Boyd, *South. M. J.*, 27: 155 (1934); G. Giglioli, *Riv. di malariol.*, 11: 27 (1932).
[9] M. F. Boyd, *South. M. J.*, 27: 155 (1934); M. F. Boyd and W. K. Stratman-Thomas, *Am. J. Hyg.*, 19: 541 (1934).
[10] P. S. Carley, *Am. J. Trop. Med.*, 12: 467 (1932).

of Negroes and of other native peoples in the tropics is not congenital or genetic, but occurs only in those individuals who have recovered from a prior infection, perhaps at an early age.[11] Since even very young Negro children resist infection, however, and since Negroes born and reared entirely outside areas in which malaria is endemic are also resistant, a natural resistance dependent upon race must be recognized. The genetic constitution of the host is considered, therefore, to play a very significant role in natural resistance to malaria.[12]

Age.—Persons of the white race who have never previously suffered from the disease can be infected with malaria parasites at any age. However, young persons suffer the most intense infections, are most likely to succumb,[13] and after apparent cure are most prone to relapse. Adults, in contrast, often terminate their infections in a few days without specific treatment.[14] Surveys of the general population in endemic areas reveal a much higher percentage infection of children than of adults, especially with *Plasmodium vivax*.[15] Often as many as 40 percent of children under fifteen years of age are infected with malaria in contrast with from 5 to 15 percent of persons over fifteen years.[16] The greater infection rate among children depends largely on the fact that the young child has not acquired a specific immunity by recovery from a previous infection. It is said, however, that mosquitoes prefer to bite children.[17]

Sex.—Males and females are equally susceptible to malaria, any difference in incidence of infection between the sexes being related to exposure. Infection with malaria is, however, especially serious in the pregnant woman, latent infections flaring up frequently in

[11] E. Sergent, *Riv. di malariol.*, 14 (Suppl. to No. 3): 5 (1935); W. A. P. Schüffner and others, *Zentralbl. f. Bakt.*, 125: 1 (1932).

[12] M. F. Boyd and W. K. Stratman-Thomas, *Am. J. Hyg.*, 18: 485 (1933).

[13] M. Ciuca, L. Ballif, and M. Vieru, *Arch. roumaines de path. expér. et de microbiol.*, 3: 209 (1930).

[14] I. Balteanu, I. Alexa, and E. Alexa, *Arch. roumaines de path. expér. et de microbiol.*, 8: 491 (1935).

[15] M. Rankov, *Arch. f. Schiffs- u. Tropen-Hyg.*, 40: 277 (1936); F. Pistoni, *Arch. ital. di sc. med. colon.*, 18: 138 (1937); L. Piccaluga, *Riv. di malariol.*, 18: 166 (1939); W. C. Earle, *Porto Rico J. Pub. Health and Trop. Med.*, 15: 3 (1939).

[16] I. Balteanu, I. Alexa, and E. Alexa, *Arch. roumaines de path. expér. et de microbiol.*, 8: 491 (1935).

[17] M. F. Boyd, *Introduction to Malariology*, Cambridge, Harvard University Press (1930).

pregnancy as well as during labor or after parturition.[18] Infection with *Plasmodium falciparum* is particularly dangerous during pregnancy and often causes abortion.[19]

Intercurrent infection.—The effect of an intercurrent infection upon the course of malaria is an old problem, but one of which even yet relatively little is well established. Malaria and tuberculosis are sometimes said to be mutually antagonistic,[20] but the better evidence indicates that the infections are independent of each other or else that the contraction of one lowers the natural resistance of the host to the other. For example, cases of tuberculosis are prone to relapse if malaria is superimposed,[21] the tuberculous process meanwhile lighting up and extending.[22] At the same time, the tuberculin test in such persons becomes negative.[23] Conversely, latent malaria can be induced to relapse by injecting tuberculin, one-half milligram usually being sufficient for the purpose.[24] Malaria and typhoid fever have little or no mutual influence,[25] although symptoms in typhoid are sometimes more severe in patients with malaria.[26]

Experimental studies indicate that a simultaneous infection with two species of malaria influences the development of each parasite. When *Plasmodium vivax* and *Plasmodium malariae* are inoculated simultaneously, for example, *Plasmodium vivax* is the dominant species, *Plasmodium malariae* sometimes failing to develop at all.[27] When *Plasmodium vivax* and *Plasmodium falciparum* are inoculated together, *Plasmodium vivax* is eventually the dominant species, although *Plasmodium falciparum* is the more prominent initially.[28]

[18] P. Daleas, *Bull. Soc. med.-chir. de l'Indochine*, 13: 432 (1935); D. S. Karve, *Kenya and East African M. J.*, 6: 43 (1929); G. A. W. Wickramasuriya, *Malaria and Ancylostomiasis in the Pregnant Woman*, London, Oxford University Press (1937).

[19] D. S. Karve, *Kenya and East African M. J.*, 6: 43 (1929).

[20] S. Collari, *Riv. di malariol.*, 11: 308 (1932).

[21] A. Manai, *Riv. di malariol.*, 13: 443 (1934).

[22] B. Boggian, *Riv. di patol. e clin. d. tuberc.*, 8: 513 (1934).

[23] H. Ishioka, *J. M. A., Formosa*, 36: 1502 (1937); B. Boggian, *Riv. di patol. e clin. d. tuberc.*, 8: 513 (1934).

[24] C. A. Mallardo and P. Cotrufo, *Riforma med.*, 52: 1651 (1936).

[25] G. Giglioli, *Riv. di malariol.*, 12: 708 (1933).

[26] R. C. R. Nazario, *Porto Rico Rev. Pub. Health & Trop. Med.*, 4: 365 (1929).

[27] B. Mayne and M. D. Young, *Pub. Health Rep.*, 53: 1289 (1938).

[28] M. F. Boyd and S. F. Kitchen, *Am. J. Trop. Med.*, 17: 855 (1937).

Diet.—The role the diet plays in resistance to malaria is not well established, although often the occurrence of relapse is related to the ingestion of large amounts of sugar.[29]

Reticulo-endothelial system.—Natural resistance against malaria is intimately related to the function of the cells of the reticulo-endothelial system. Parasites are phagocytized especially by the fixed-tissue macrophages, and such organs as the spleen become charged both with malarial parasites and with malarial pigment. A monocytosis occurs during infection, indicating a broad stimulation of the reticulo-endothelial system. Splenectomy, resorted to for one or another reason in man, is said to lead to recrudescence of latent malaria, presumably because of the consequent depression of reticulo-endothelial function.[30] When the spleen has been severely damaged by malaria, however, its removal is often advised, providing the infection has gone on for sufficient time to give other tissues an opportunity to assume the splenic function.

ACQUIRED IMMUNITY

RESISTANCE TO REINFECTION

Persons who have suffered an initial infection with malarial parasites resist reinfection with the same organism. This is observed among individuals newly arrived in endemic areas, in children born in such areas, and in persons specifically inoculated with malaria parasites as a therapeutic measure in neurosyphilis. Generally, the immunity to reinfection is relative rather than absolute. During the initial infection a severe parasitaemia with accompanying symptoms may be experienced. During subsequent infections the symptoms are often entirely omitted and the number of parasites markedly reduced. Finally, after many reinfections no parasites whatsoever may occur in the blood.[31]

[29] W. Bird, *Indian J. M. Research,* 16: 109 (1928).

[30] E. Benhamou, *Bull. Soc. path. exot.,* 25: 685 (1932).

[31] M. Ciuca, L. Ballif, and M. Vieru, *Arch. roumaines de path. expér. et de microbiol.,* 3: 209 (1930) ; M. F. Boyd and L. T. Coggeshall, *Third Int. Congr. Trop. Med. & Malaria,* 2: 292 (1938) ; M. F. Boyd and S. F. Kitchen, *Am. J. Trop. Med.,* 16: 447 (1936) ; M. F. Boyd, *Am. J. Trop. Med.,* 20: 749 (1940) ; C. Milani and E. Cuboni, Soc. internz. di microbiol., *Boll. d. sez. ital.,* 3: 521 (1931) ; M. Ciuca, L. Ballif, and M. Chelarescu-Vieru, *Tr. Roy. Soc. Trop. Med. & Hyg.,* 27: 619 (1934) ; M. Ciuca, L. Ballif, and M. Vieru, *Arch. roumaines de path. expér et de microbiol.,* 1: 577 (1928).

Usually immunity is built up rapidly against *Plasmodium vivax* or *Plasmodium ovale*, less readily against *Plasmodium malariae*, and only very slowly, if at all, against *Plasmodium falciparum*.[32] Children, however, acquire immunity slowly against all species, manifesting little resistance before the sixth year of life and suffering repeated severe infections until that time.[33] Immunity once established is effective either against trophozoites of infective blood introduced by syringe or against sporozoites inoculated by mosquito,[34] although the sporozoites, at least of *Plasmodium ovale*, seem to have greater power to develop in an immune person than do the trophozoites.[35] Immunity lasts longest against *Plasmodium vivax* and *Plasmodium ovale*, and for the briefest period against *Plasmodium falciparum*.[36] Immunity against *Plasmodium vivax* probably endures for at least three years,[37] possibly for as long as seven years.[38]

Species and strain specificity of acquired immunity.—Persons who have recovered from infection with one species of malaria parasite are not immune to others.[39] Indeed, the immunity in malaria is usually effective only against that single homologous strain within a given species which produced the initial infection in that person.[40] For this reason, a malaria epidemic may occur in a com-

[32] F. Pistoni, *Arch. ital. di sc. med. colon.*, 18: 138 (1937); M. Ciuca, L. Ballif, and M. Chelarescu-Vieru, *Tr. Roy. Soc. Trop. Med. & Hyg.*, 27: 619 (1934); P. Dschaparidse, *Nachr. d. trop. Med.*, 2: 260 (1929); J. A. Sinton, E. L. Hutton, and P. G. Shute, *Tr. Roy. Soc. Trop. Med. & Hyg.*, 33: 47 (1939).
[33] I. J. Kligler, *Tr. Roy. Soc. Trop. Med. & Hyg.*, 27: 269 (1933).
[34] M. Ciuca, L. Ballif, and M. Chelarescu-Vieru, *Bull. Soc. path. exot.*, 27: 330 (1934); M. F. Boyd and S. F. Kitchen, *Am. J. Trop. Med.*, 16: 317 (1936).
[35] J. A. Sinton, *Tr. Roy. Soc. Trop. Med. & Hyg.*, 33: 305, 439 (1939–40).
[36] W. C. Earle, *Porto Rico J. Pub. Health and Trop. Med.*, 15: 3 (1939); J. A. Sinton, *Proc. Roy. Soc. Med.*, 31: 1298 (1938).
[37] M. F. Boyd, W. K. Stratman-Thomas, and S. F. Kitchen, *Am. J. Trop. Med.*, 16: 311 (1936).
[38] M. F. Boyd and C. B. Matthews, *Am. J. Trop. Med.*, 19: 63 (1939).
[39] M. Ciuca, L. Ballif, and M. Vieru, *Arch. roumaines de path. et de microbiol.*, 1: 577 (1928); M. F. Boyd, S. F. Kitchen, and C. B. Matthews, *Am. J. Trop. Med.*, 19: 141 (1939); S. P. James, *Tr. Roy. Soc. Trop. Med. & Hyg.*, 24: 477 (1931); S. P. James, W. D. Nicol, and P. G. Shute, *Am. J. Trop. Med.*, 15: 187 (1935).
[40] M. F. Boyd, *Am. J. Trop. Med.*, 20: 69 (1940); M. F. Boyd and W. K. Stratman-Thomas, *Am. J. Hyg.*, 17: 55 (1933), and 18: 482 (1933); M. F. Boyd, W. K. Stratman-Thomas, and S. F. Kitchen, *Am. J. Hyg.*, 21: 364 (1935), and *Am. J. Trop. Med.*, 16: 139 (1936); P. C. Korteweg, *Nederl-Tijdschr. v. Geneesk.*, 77: 4547 (1933); S. P. James, W. D. Nicol, and P. G. Shute, *Proc. Roy. Soc. Med.*, 25: 1153 (1932).

munity which has long been comparatively immune to the disease, providing a new strain of the parasite is introduced either through infected persons or mosquitoes. Sometimes, however, reinfections with heterologous strains within the species result in clinically milder attacks than if there had been no prior experience whatsoever with malaria.[41] When two strains within a given species infect an individual simultaneously, immunity against either is built up only slowly and poorly.[42] Immunologically distinct strains of the *ovale* parasite evidently do not occur, since persons recovered from infection with one strain of *Plasmodium ovale* are protected against the other known strains of the same species of parasite.[43]

Relapse.—Relapse in malaria may be defined as the recurrence of clinical malaria, after the apparent cure of a first infection, in the absence of exogenous reinfection. It is one of the most conspicuous characteristics of malaria. Its causes are many, and what explains the relapse in one case may not apply in another. Relapses are divided into two groups: short-term relapses, which occur within six weeks after apparent recovery, and long-term relapses, which occur after longer periods. Those following an infection with *Plasmodium falciparum* are almost always of the short-term variety. Those following *Plasmodium vivax* and, especially, *Plasmodium malariae* are of the long-term variety, occurring sometimes after two or three years. Reports of relapse with *Plasmodium vivax* after intervals greater than three years, however, should be viewed with caution before every possibility of exogenous reinfection is excluded. Relapse with *Plasmodium malariae,* on the other hand, has been observed even after twenty years or more.[44] Relapses in *Plasmodium ovale* infections are rare.[45]

The many possible causes of relapse in malaria are divisible rather inaccurately into internal and external factors. Among in-

[41] M. F. Boyd, W. K. Stratman-Thomas, and H. Muench, *Am. J. Hyg.*, 20: 482 (1934).

[42] M. F. Boyd, W. H. Kupper, and C. B. Matthews, *Am. J. Trop. Med.*, 18: 521 (1938).

[43] J. A. Sinton, E. L. Hutton, and P. G. Shute, *Tr. Roy. Soc. Trop. Med. & Hyg.*, 33: 47 (1939).

[44] E. McCulloch, *Canad. M. A. J.*, 37: 26 (1937); W. A. Gardner and L. Dexter, *J. A. M. A.*, 111: 2473 (1938).

[45] J. A. Sinton, E. L. Hutton, and P. G. Shute, *Tr. Roy. Soc. Trop. Med. & Hyg.*, 32: 751 (1939).

ternal, or constitutional, factors pregnancy and parturition are probably most important.[46] Relapse also is observed in those who have undergone splenectomy [47] or other operative procedure or who have experienced extraordinary fatigue. The age of the patient also is important, since relapse occurs most frequently in children less than fifteen years old.[48] Among external factors, the character, intensity, and duration of treatment is the most significant. Relapse may occur in any poorly treated case, but is noted especially in those in which treatment was instituted very early, then discontinued after a brief time. If the initial infection is let run on prior to treatment for a period sufficient to permit the patient to respond immunologically, the danger of relapse is greatly reduced. The diet, change of climate, extreme heat or cold, and traumatic shock are also causes contributing to relapse.

Premunition.—The best evidence of immunity in malaria can be elicited in persons still harboring their original infection in latent form.[49] The failure to infect Caucasians on first experimental inoculation is usually explained on the basis of their being premunized.[50] The almost complete resistance of Negroes,[51] Malayans,[52] and other natives of the tropics is also sometimes accounted for on this basis. Premunition is absolutely strain-specific, and if a heterologous strain of the same species of parasite is inoculated an infection will promptly ensue.[53] Absolute immunity, however, probably remains for some time after a latent infection has been wholly eradicated.[54] At least, massive doses of blood from some recovered

[46] D. S. Karve, *Kenya & East African M. J.,* 6: 43 (1929) ; P. C. C. Garnham, *Tr. Roy. Soc. Trop. Med. & Hyg.,* 32: 13 (1938).

[47] E. Benhamou, *Bull. Soc. path. exot.,* 25: 685 (1932).

[48] I. Balteanu, I. Alexa, and E. Alexa, *Arch. roumaines de path. expér. et de microbiol.,* 8: 491 (1935) ; I. J. Kligler, *Tr. Roy. Soc. Trop. Med. & Hyg.,* 27: 269 (1933), and 24: 331 (1930).

[49] E. Sergent, *Riv. di malariol.,* 14 (Suppl. to No. 3): 5 (1935) ; E. Sergent, *Bull. Soc. path. exot.,* 22: 887 (1929) ; E. Sergent, E. Sergent, L. Parrot, and A. Donatien, *Tr. Roy. Soc. Trop. Med. & Hyg.,* 27: 277 (1933).

[50] M. F. Boyd and W. K. Stratman-Thomas, *Am. J. Hyg.,* 19: 541 (1934); M. Ciuca, L. Ballif, and M. Chelarescu-Vieru, *Bull. Soc. path. exot.,* 26: 300 (1933).

[51] E. Sergent, *Riv. di malariol.,* 14 (Suppl. to No. 3): 5 (1935).

[52] W. A. P. Schuffner and others, *Zentralbl. f. Bakt.,* 125: 1 (1932).

[53] M. F. Boyd and W. K. Stratman-Thomas, *Am. J. Hyg.,* 18: 482 (1933).

[54] M. Ciuca, L. Ballif, and M. Vieru, *Arch. roumaines de path. expér. et de microbiol.,* 1: 577 (1928) ; G. Sicault and A. Messerlin, *Bull. Soc. path. exot.,* 31: 911 (1938).

persons often fail to infect normal individuals to which they are injected.[55]

ANTIBODY PRODUCTION

Although antibody is known to be formed by man after infection with malaria, comparatively little has been established about the nature of the antibody formation. The complement fixation test becomes positive after the fifth paroxysm in *Plasmodium vivax* infection in neurosyphilitics and remains so for from ten to thirty days. Thereafter it is negative.[56] Tests for complement fixation and for the precipitin antibody have been developed for use in diagnosis. These will be referred to in the section on diagnosis (see also Chapter XX).

PASSIVE IMMUNITY

The possibility of the passive transfer of immunity against human malaria has not been carefully investigated. A few successful attempts to treat malaria with serum from recovered patients [57] and from rabbits injected with malarial parasites [58] have been reported, but the results in these are not very convincing.

MECHANISM OF IMMUNITY

Immunity in malaria is intimately related to the function of the reticulo-endothelial system. It depends in part upon the defensive cells of this system and in part upon humoral antibodies which probably arise chiefly from these cells. The phagocytic cells of the reticulo-endothelial system in the normal person are able to perform their function of phagocytosis to some extent even when the malarial parasites first enter the blood.[59] But as a result of an infection, these cells as well as all components of the reticulo-endothelial system are stimulated markedly and their function

[55] M. F. Boyd, W. K. Stratman-Thomas, and S. F. Kitchen, *Am. J. Trop. Med.*, 16: 311 (1936).

[56] A. Radosavljević, *Arch. f. Schiffs- u. Tropen-Hyg.*, 34: 629 (1930).

[57] N. Lorando and D. Sotiriades, *J. Trop. Med.*, 39: 197 (1936), and *Tr. Roy. Soc. Trop. Med. & Hyg.*, 31: 227 (1937); D. Sotiriades, *J. Trop. Med.*, 39: 257 (1936).

[58] N. T. Koressios, *Riv. di malariol.*, 12: 353 (1933).

[59] W. H. Taliaferro and H. W. Mulligan, *Indian M. Research Mem.*, *Suppl. Ser. to Indian J. M. Research*, Mem. No. 29 (1937); P. Decourt, *Bull. Soc. path. exot.*, 32: 7 (1939).

thereafter is of a much higher order. The spleen becomes enlarged, the number of monocytic cells of the peripheral blood rises,[60] and specific antibody is developed. The precise function of the antibody is still somewhat obscure, although most probably it behaves as an opsonin, sensitizing the parasites so that they are more readily engulfed by the phagocytic cells.[61] Usually this phagocytosis is largely restricted to the phagocytes of the reticulo-endothelium,[62] although occasionally, especially in heavy infections, phagocytosis by cells in the peripheral blood likewise is observed.[63] The possibility remains that the antibody is also antitoxic in function [64] or directly parasiticidal.[65] One study upon *Plasmodium ovale* infection has suggested that immunity to this parasite is both antitoxic and antiparasitic in its nature. The antitoxic immunity is considered to reach a high level more rapidly than the antiparasitic immunity after repeated reinfection, although the antiparasitic immunity persists longer, once it is established.[66]

The more intense malarial infections seen in children probably occur because the function of the reticulo-endothelial system is deficient in young individuals. During the first several years of life children in endemic areas may suffer repeated infections with malaria, a new infection being contracted as soon as the previous one is ended, with no evidence that an immunity has been developed.[67] Gradually, however, as the child reaches four years or more of age and its reticulo-endothelial system attains a more nearly complete function, the clinical symptoms become progressively less, and eventually a firm resistance is acquired both to the clinical effects and, finally, to the presence of the parasite.

[60] G. A. Winfield, *J. Lab. & Clin. Med.*, 17: 985 (1932).

[61] J. G. Thomson, *Tr. Roy. Soc. Trop. Med. & Hyg.*, 26: 483 (1933).

[62] H. Stott, *Indian M. Gaz.*, 68: 507 (1933).

[63] C. D. DeLangen, *Tr. Roy. Soc. Trop. Med. & Hyg.*, 26: 523 (1933), and *Geneesk. Tijdschr. v. Nederl-Indië*, 72: 793 (1932); H. See-Lii, *Arch. f. Schiffs- u. Tropen-Hyg.*, 38: 249 (1934).

[64] A. Radosavljević, *Arch. f. Schiffs- u. Tropen-Hyg.*, 34: 629 (1930); M. Ashford, *Am. J. Trop. Med.*, 16: 665 (1936).

[65] A. Radosavljević, *Arch. f. Schiffs- u. Tropen-Hyg.*, 34: 629 (1930); H. Neumann, *Riv. di malariol.*, 12: 319 (1933); G. J. Perekropow, *Ztschr. f. Immunitätsforsch. u. exper. Therap.*, 57: 219 (1928).

[66] J. A. Sinton, *Tr. Roy. Soc. Trop. Med. & Hyg.*, 33: 585 (1940).

[67] S. R. Christophers, *Indian J. M. Research*, 12: 273 (1924); G. MacDonald, *Indian J. M. Research*, 18: 1347 (1931); W. C. Earle and others, *Porto Rico J. Pub. Health & Trop. Med.*, 15: 391 (1939).

Relationship to chemotherapy.—Before an individual can develop a vigorous immune response to the malarial parasite, that individual must be injured by his infection. When damage is slight, the immune response is correspondingly slight; but when the injury is great, the immunity developed is of a higher order. When a malarial patient is treated with specific antimalarial drugs, his immediate need for specific immune response becomes less and his effort thus to cure himself is retarded. But it is in just such cases that relapses occur, since the complete eradication of the malarial parasite from the body is seldom accomplished save through the intervention of the host's own specific defense mechanism. The present tendency in endemic areas is, therefore, to withhold treatment after the initial infection until the patient has suffered a number of paroxysms (twenty or so) and thus has had an opportunity to raise his natural defense facilities to an effective level. This schedule is adhered to not only for adults but for children as well, giving only enough drug at any time to prevent the patient's being carried off by the infection.[68] Persons who live outside endemic areas, however, or who are for any other reason unlikely to experience further attacks of malaria are usually given radical drug treatment at the earliest opportunity.[69]

PROPHYLAXIS

Prophylaxis by vaccination has not been tried significantly in malaria. The great difficulty entailed in preparing a suitable antigen has precluded the use of sterile vaccines. As yet the inoculation of attenuated organisms has not been attempted as a prophylactic measure in human malaria, since strains of such parasites are not available. Schilling has reported immunizing persons by repeated injections of very small numbers of living virulent organisms, beginning with one hundred parasites and gradually increasing the number given.[70] One report of the successful use of autovaccines therapeutically has appeared, but as yet it has had no further trial.[71]

[68] S. P. James, *Tr. Roy. Soc. Trop. Med. & Hyg.*, 24: 477 (1931) ; J. A. Sinton, *J. Malaria Institute of India*, 2: 191 (1939); D. B. Wilson, *Tr. Roy. Soc. Trop. Med. & Hyg.*, 32: 435 (1939).
[69] J. A. Sinton, *J. Malaria Institute of India*, 2: 191 (1939).
[70] C. Schilling, *Deutsche med. Wchnschr.*, 65: 1264 (1939).
[71] S. W. Koustansoff, *Zentralbl. f. Bakt.*, 116: 241 (1930).

DIAGNOSIS

The best and simplest method for diagnosing malarial infection is by finding the malarial parasite in blood films from the patient. Immunological tests have in general been extremely troublesome to perform because of the difficulty in procuring a suitable antigen, and at best they have generally given rather poor results. Antigens derived by extraction of infected blood,[72] especially from the placenta,[73] have, however, been used with meager success in the fixation test. Recently decidedly more favorable results have been obtained in the fixation test with an antigen prepared from the monkey malaria parasite, *Plasmodium knowlesi*.[74] Often confusion results in the fixation test from the fact that malaria patients give positive Wassermann tests as well as Kahn tests in the absence of syphilis.[75]

A precipitin test also has been devised for diagnosing malaria, the antigen coming from infected placental blood. Of thirty-two serums from infected persons in one study, thirty-one were positive by this test, whereas only one of thirty-two control serums was positive.[76] Cultures of malaria parasites also have been used as a source of antigen in the precipitin test.[77] Skin tests likewise have been tried in the diagnosis of malaria, but with little success except in the hands of those who devised them.[78]

Henry test.—The Henry test has been quite widely tried for diagnosing malaria and seems to give rather favorable results, although those who have employed it are still in conflict as to its nature, its specificity, and its general practicability. Apparently it is not dependent upon an antigen-antibody union,[79] since distilled

[72] A. Radosavljević, *Arch. f. Schiffs- u. Tropen-Hyg.*, 34: 629 (1930).
[73] M. Massa, *Pathologica*, 21: 18 (1929).
[74] M. D. Eaton and L. T. Coggeshall, *J. Exper. Med.*, 69: 379 (1939).
[75] O. Cherefeddin, *Arch. f. Schiffs- u. Tropen-Hyg.*, 34: 282 (1930); A. Panagia, *Riv. di malariol.*, 12: 873 (1933); G. M. Saunders and T. B. Turner, *South. M. J.*, 28: 542 (1935); A. S. Azzi and A. Del Frade, *Arch. de med. inf.*, 7: 388 (1938); S. F. Kitchen, E. L. Webb, and W. H. Kupper, *J. A. M. A.*, 12: 1443 (1939); A. E. Taussig and M. M. Orgel, *J. Lab. & Clin. Med.*, 22: 614 (1937).
[76] W. H. Taliaferro and L. G. Taliaferro, *J. Prevent. Med.*, 2: 147 (1928).
[77] R. Row, *Tr. Roy. Soc. Trop. Med. & Hyg.*, 24: 623 (1931).
[78] O. Herrmann and M. Lifschitz, *Ztschr. f. Immunitätsforsch. u. exper. Therap.*, 65: 240 (1930); M. M. Tschechnowitzer and W. D. Moldawskaya-Kritschewskaya, *Trop. Med. & Parasitol.*, 9: 261 (1931); F. Rocchi, *Riv. di malariol.*, 10: 161 (1931); F. Trensz, *Compt. rend. Soc. de biol.*, 116: 1082 (1934).
[79] V. Chorine, *Riv. di malariol.*, 13: 807 (1934).

water can be substituted for the melanine pigment or other substance which generally serves as "antigen." [80] The reaction seems to depend upon the relative instability of malarial serums, in which an excess of globulin always occurs.[81] Many investigators consider the test useful as a diagnostic aid,[82] even though it is often positive in such other diseases as leishmaniasis, trypanosomiasis, and typhus fever.[83] After drug treatment of the malarial patient the serum gives a negative Henry test.[84]

MONKEY MALARIA

NATURAL RESISTANCE

HOST RESTRICTION

Many distinct species of malaria occur in monkeys. Comparatively few of these have been studied immunologically, however. The majority of the reported studies have been concerned with *Plasmodium knowlesi*, *Plasmodium cynomolgi*, *Plasmodium inui*, and *Plasmodium brasilianum*. These parasites are restricted almost entirely to monkeys, although *Plasmodium knowlesi* and *Plasmodium inui* also can infect man.[85] One other species, *Plasmodium rodhaini* from the chimpanzee, which resembles *Plasmodium malariae* of man, is also said to infect human beings.[86] Among different species of monkeys, however, these various parasites produce very

[80] R. H. Wiseman, *Lancet*, 2: 543 (1934); V. Chorine and D. Koechlin, *Bull. Soc. path. exot.*, 28: 375 (1935); V. Chorine, R. Prudhomme, and D. Koechlin, *Compt. rend. Soc. de biol.*, 116: 1255 (1934).

[81] E. Benhamou and R. Gille, *Compt. rend. Soc. de biol.*, 118: 1573 (1935); A. F. X. Henry, *Compt. rend. Soc. de biol.*, 107: 1520 (1931).

[82] M. de Alda Calleja, *Med. Paises Calidos*, 9: 203 (1936); A. Badensky and E. Bivol, *Compt. rend. Soc. de biol.*, 114: 224 (1933); M. Biasiotti, *Policlinico*, 40: 557 (1933); R. Brandt and L. Horn, *Klin. Wchnschr.*, 14: 1538 (1935); V. Chorine, *Riv. di malariol.*, 11: 273 (1932); V. Chorine and M. Rodieux, *Bull. Soc. path. exot.*, 26: 1249 (1933); I. Gnochvili, I. Kigueloukhes, and M. Mougiri, *Med. Par. and Parasit. Dis.*, 4: 461 (1935); A. Kappus, *Arch. f. Schiffs- u. Tropen-Hyg.*, 36: 576 (1932); P. R. Lacour, *Henry's Malaria Flocculation*, Paris, Doin et Cie. (1934).

[83] P. Gerbinis, *Bull. Soc. path. exot.*, 27: 19 (1934); A. F. X. Henry, *Compt. rend. Soc. de biol.*, 116: 1237 (1934).

[84] A. Badensky and E. Bivol, *Compt. rend. Soc. de biol.*, 114: 224 (1933); A. Corradetti, *Riv. di malariol.*, 11: 282 (1932); V. Chorine, *Bull. Soc. path. exot.*, 26: 269 (1933).

[85] M. Ciuca and others, *Compt. rend. Soc. de biol.*, 129: 1234 (1938); C. Inoesco-Miahaiesti and others, *Compt. rend. Soc. de biol.*, 115: 1311 (1934); M. D. Eaton and L. T. Coggeshall, *J. Exper. Med.*, 69: 379 (1939); D. F. Milam and L. T. Coggeshall, *Am. J. Trop. Med.*, 18: 331 (1938).

[86] J. Rodhain, *Compt. rend. Soc. de biol.*, 133: 276 (1940).

different types of infection. For example, *Plasmodium knowlesi* causes in *Macacus rhesus* an infection of the greatest severity which always ends fatally. In *Macacus cynomolgus,* on the other hand, the same parasite causes a chronic type of infection requiring no treatment.[87]

FACTORS INFLUENCING NATURAL RESISTANCE

Little is known of the significance of the age or sex of monkeys in their natural resistance to malaria. The significance of race also is uncertain so far as the monkey host is concerned. Among human beings, Negroes are much more resistant than white persons to *Plasmodium knowlesi.*[88] The factor of greatest importance in natural resistance seems to be the reticulo-endothelium, for limiting its function by the blockage of this system or by the extirpation of the spleen promptly lowers the resistance of monkeys to these parasites.[89]

ACQUIRED IMMUNITY

RESISTANCE TO REINFECTION

Monkeys which have suffered an initial infection with *Plasmodium brasilianum, Plasmodium inui,* or *Plasmodium knowlesi* resist reinfection with the same species of parasite.[90] Human beings also acquire resistance to reinfection with *Plasmodium knowlesi* through recovery from an initial infection.[91] However, individuals who have previously suffered infection with human malaria—for example, *Plasmodium vivax*—are as susceptible to *Plasmodium knowlesi* as a normal person.[92]

[87] J. A. Sinton, *Records Malaria Survey of India,* 7: 85 (1937); B. Malamos, *Arch. f. Schiffs- u. Tropen-Hyg.,* 38: 326 (1934).

[88] D. F. Milam and L. T. Coggeshall, *Am. J. Trop. Med.,* 18: 331 (1938).

[89] B. Malamos, *Arch. f. Schiffs- u. Tropen-Hyg.,* 38: 326 (1934); N. Cassuto, *Riv. di malariol.,* 15: 240 (1936); R. Knowles and B. M. das Gupta, *Indian M. Gaz.,* 69: 541 (1934); K. V. Krishnan, R. O. A. Smith, and C. Lal, *Indian J. M. Research,* 21: 343, 639 (1933–34); E. G. Nauck and B. Malamos, *Ztschr. f. Immunitätsforsch. u. exper. Therap.,* 84: 337 (1935); J. A. Sinton, *Records Malaria Survey of India,* 5: 501 (1935).

[90] J. A. Sinton, *Records Malaria Survey of India,* 7: 85 (1937); W. H. Taliaferro and L. G. Taliaferro, *Am. J. Hyg.,* 20: 60 (1934); H. W. Mulligan and J. A. Sinton, *Records Malaria Survey of India,* 3: 529, 809 (1933); B. Malamos, *Arch. f. Schiffs- u. Tropen-Hyg.,* 41: 162 (1937); J. A. Sinton and H. W. Mulligan, *Records Malaria Survey of India,* 5: 307 (1935).

[91] D. F. Milam and L. T. Coggeshall, *Am. J. Trop. Med.,* 18: 331 (1938).

[92] E. D. W. Greig, *J. Trop. Med.,* 42: 378 (1939).

138 THE MALARIAS

Premunition.—The immunity of monkeys to reinfection with *Plasmodium knowlesi* certainly lasts as long as the parasites persist in a latent form of infection [93] and may be manifested even after the infection is completely eliminated,[94] providing the infection had persisted for a sufficient time and with sufficient severity to cause a vigorous immune response. When long persisting *Plasmodium knowlesi* infections in *Macacus rhesus* are cleared completely with sulfanilamide, for example, the animals are still resistant, even though their blood is not infective for other normal monkeys.[95] If an infection is cured in its incipient stages, however, before an immune response has been made by the host, the animal can then be reinfected almost at once. Humans who have acquired immunity to *Plasmodium knowlesi* also retain their resistance, even after their blood is clear of the parasite. In some cases, however, the parasite has been shown to persist in man for several months in the absence of symptoms.[96]

ANTIBODY PRODUCTION

Antibody production in monkey malaria has been studied chiefly in *Macacus rhesus* infections with *Plasmodium knowlesi*. Specific agglutinins, complement-fixing antibodies, and protective antibodies have been described in this host. Agglutinins appear within fifteen to forty-five days after infection. Their titer rises gradually as the infection subsides, and in animals repeatedly reinfected it may reach 1:1000.[97] The complement-fixing antibody appears during the third week and persists for months thereafter, falling in titer after the administration of the controlling drug, but rising again after each relapse.[98] The protective antibody is usually considered distinct from the other antibodies, although its precise characters have not as yet been accurately determined. The complement fixation antibody and the protective antibody have also been demon-

[93] J. A. Sinton, *Records Malaria Survey of India,* 7: 85 (1937); B. M. das Gupta, *Indian M. Gaz.,* 72: 726 (1937).

[94] K. V. Krishnan, R. O. A. Smith, and C. Lal, *Indian J. M. Research,* 21: 639 (1934); E. G. Nauck and B. Malamos, *Ztschr. f. Immunitätsforsch. u. exper. Therap.,* 84: 337 (1935).

[95] L. T. Coggeshall, *Am. J. Trop. Med.,* 18: 715 (1938).

[96] D. F. Milam and L. T. Coggeshall, *Am. J. Trop. Med.,* 18: 331 (1938).

[97] M. D. Eaton, *J. Exper. Med.,* 67: 857 (1938).

[98] L. T. Coggeshall and M. D. Eaton, *J. Exper. Med.,* 67: 871 (1938).

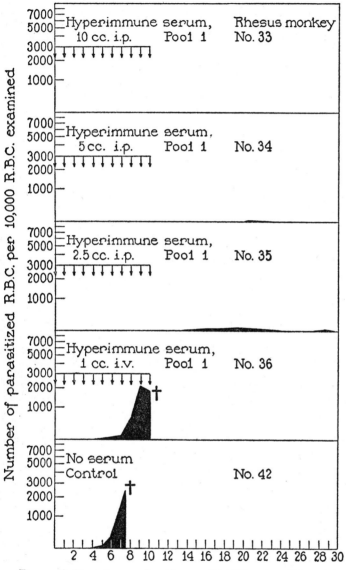

Number of parasitized R.B.C. per 10,000 R.B.C. examined

Hyperimmune serum,   Rhesus monkey
10 cc. i.p.   Pool 1   No. 33

Hyperimmune serum,
5 cc. i.p.   Pool 1   No. 34

Hyperimmune serum,
2.5 cc. i.p.   Pool 1   No. 35

Hyperimmune serum,
1 cc. i.v.   Pool 1   No. 36

No serum
Control   No. 42

Days following infection with *Plasmodium knowlesi*

CHART II

PROTECTIVE ACTION OF IMMUNE SERUM IN
MONKEY MALARIA

strated in the serum of human beings who have been experimentally infected with this parasite.[99]

PASSIVE IMMUNITY

Macacus rhesus is protected against *Plasmodium knowlesi* by the repeated injection of serum from a monkey harboring a chronic infection with this parasite.[100] A direct relationship has been shown to exist between the amount of antiserum required to confer protection and the infective dose of organisms administered.[101] To be useful for the passive transfer of immunity serums evidently must come from infected animals, for those from monkeys artificially immunized with killed antigens are ineffectual (see Chart II).

MECHANISM OF IMMUNITY

The mechanism of the acquired immunity of monkeys against the monkey malarias is fundamentally the same as that of man to human malaria. The elements of the reticulo-endothelial system play the greatest role, either in directly phagocytosing the parasites or in elaborating antibodies which opsonize them preparatory to their engulfment by cells. Soon after infection a distinct stimulation of the reticulo-endothelial system is evident. The spleen enlarges to several times normal size, phagocytic activity becomes enhanced, and eventually antibody appears.[102] In its final analysis, then, resistance against these parasites seems to depend on phagocytosis. However, phagocytosis normally will go on at a rate sufficient to keep the parasites in check and finally to eliminate them only when antibody is present to render simpler the task of the phagocytic cells.

PROPHYLAXIS

As yet monkeys have not been protected against *Plasmodium knowlesi* as a result of vaccination with killed organisms.[103]

[99] L. T. Coggeshall, *J. Exper. Med.*, 72: 21 (1940).

[100] L. T. Coggeshall and H. W. Kumm, *J. Exper. Med.*, 66: 177 (1937) ; E. Mosna, *Riv. di parassitol.*, 2: 327 (1938).

[101] L. T. Coggeshall and M. D. Eaton, *J. Exper. Med.*, 68: 29 (1938).

[102] W. H. Taliaferro, *Am. J. Hyg.*, 16: 429 (1932) ; K. V. Krishnan, C. Lal, and L. E. Napier, *Indian M. Gaz.*, 68: 66 (1933) ; L. T. Coggeshall, *Am. J. Trop. Med.*, 17: 605 (1937) ; T. B. Manon, *Tr. Roy. Soc. Trop. Med. & Hyg.*, 32: 481 (1939).

[103] M. D. Eaton and L. T. Coggeshall, *J. Exper. Med.*, 70: 141 (1939).

The diagnosis of infections with the monkey malarias are routinely performed by the microscopic observation of stained films; yet these infections can be diagnosed by the fixation test and the agglutination test,[104] as well as by an intradermal reaction.[105] The infected red blood cells of *Macacus rhesus* is the source of antigen for all these tests. In the case of the skin test, the antigen is obtained by digesting the infected blood cells with papain. The skin reaction commences in three or four hours after the antigen is injected and reaches its peak in twenty-four hours, with local swelling and central necrosis of the injected site. Antigens prepared from *Plasmodium knowlesi* also are useful in diagnosing by the fixation test human infections with any of the usual human malarias.[106]

A reversed complement fixation test also is possible in acute *Plasmodium knowlesi* monkey infection. In this, circulating malarial antigen is detected by means of a hyperimmune monkey serum.[107]

BIRD MALARIA

NATURAL RESISTANCE

HOST RESTRICTION

Although extensive investigations on the parasites of bird malaria have been carried out, the full limits of the possible host range for each species is still largely undetermined. Usually a variety of birds can be infected with each species, although neither mammals nor cold-blooded hosts are susceptible to any of the bird malarias. One species of parasite, *Plasmodium cathemerium,* has proved infective for, among others, sparrows, wood thrushes,[108] canaries, pigeons, great-horned owls, ducks,[109] and chicks,[110] although infections in the chick are often demonstrable only by the subinoc-

[104] M. D. Eaton, *J. Exper. Med.,* 67: 857 (1938) ; B. Malamos, *Riv. di malariol.,* 16: 91 (1937) ; J. C. Somogyi, *Riv. di parassitol.,* 3: 157 (1939).

[105] J. A. Sinton and H. W. Mulligan, *Indian J. M. Research,* 20: 581 (1932), and *Records Malaria Survey of India,* 3: 323 (1932).

[106] M. D. Eaton, *J. Exper. Med.,* 69: 517 (1939).

[107] M. D. Eaton, *J. Exper. Med.,* 69: 517 (1939).

[108] R. Hegner, *J. Parasitol. (Suppl.),* 26: 28 (1940).

[109] F. Wolfson, *Am. J. Hyg.,* 28: 317 (1938) and 26: 53 (1937).

[110] R. D. Manwell, *Am. J. Trop. Med.,* 13: 97 (1933).

ulation of canaries. At least eight different species of birds are susceptible to *Plasmodium praecox* (*relictum*).[111] Recently the tendency has been to reduce the number of recognized species of malarial parasites in birds. Many of those which were previously reported as distinct species because of their occurrence in new hosts are now considered identical with others.[112] It is, nevertheless, evident that the host range of these parasites is distinctly greater than that of other types of malaria organisms.

These parasites sometimes experience profound modifications on transfer from one host to another. For example, *Plasmodium cathemerium* has a twenty-four hour asexual cycle in the canary and the duck, but a forty-eight hour cycle in the chick. Furthermore, the mean number of merozoites in the segmenters differs in the various hosts, there being 11.2 merozoites in the canary, 7.9 in the duck, and 5.0 in the fowl.[113]

FACTORS INFLUENCING NATURAL RESISTANCE

The factors governing natural resistance in bird malaria have not been much investigated. Age is certainly a factor in the resistance of chickens to *Plasmodium lophurae,* younger birds being definitely more susceptible.[114] The diet also may have some importance in bird malaria,[115] although its precise relationship is yet obscure. Splenectomy affects the natural resistance of birds to these forms very slightly.[116] However, chicks which have received several large doses of carbon ink into the posterior peritoneal cavity are adversely affected. Such birds do not check the reproduction of *Plasmodium lophurae* so quickly as normal birds and hence experience more severe infections.[117] Intercurrent infections are not known to affect the natural resistance. An infection with *Spirocheta*

---

[111] P. A. Démina, *Med. Par. and Parasit. Dis.,* 7: 578 (1938).

[112] R. D. Manwell, *Am. J. Trop. Med.,* 15: 265 (1935); A. Giovannola, *Riv. di parassitol.,* 3: 1 (1939).

[113] R. Hegner, *J. Parasitol.* (*Suppl.*), 26: 28 (1940).

[114] L. T. Coggeshall, *Am. J. Hyg.,* 27: 615 (1938); W. H. Taliaferro and L. G. Taliaferro, *J. Infect. Dis.,* 66: 153 (1940).

[115] G. H. Boyd, *Am. J. Hyg.,* 18: 295 (1933).

[116] O. R. Causey, *Am. J. Hyg.,* 30: 93 (1939, sec. C); C. M. Herman and A. I. Goldfarb, *Am. J. Trop. Med.,* 19: 595 (1939).

[117] W. Trager, *J. Parasitol.* (*Suppl.*), 26: 28 (1940).

gallinarum, for example, does not influence the resistance of fowls to *Plasmodium gallinaceum.*[118]

ACQUIRED IMMUNITY

RESISTANCE TO REINFECTION

The immunity against reinfection of birds which have recovered from an initial attack of malaria has been repeatedly demonstrated. The most satisfactory studies have been carried on in canaries after infection with *Plasmodium cathemerium,*[119] *Plasmodium circumflexum,*[120] *Plasmodium elongatum,*[121] *Plasmodium praecox* (*relictum*),[122] *Plasmodium rouxi,*[123] and *Plasmodium vaughani.*[124] Chickens also develop resistance to reinfection with the pheasant parasite *Plasmodium lophurae.*[125] Very few consistent immunological differences have been seen between different strains of bird malarial parasites belonging to the same species.[126] and a very considerable amount of cross-immunity has been observed among many of the recognized species.[127] As illustrative of this cross-immunity the following examples may be cited: birds with a latent infection of *Plasmodium praecox* or of *Plasmodium cathemerium* are protected against reinfection with respect to both the homologous and the heterologous species of parasite.[128] Recovery from *Plasmodium praecox* infection likewise protects birds against both *Plasmodium praecox* and *Plasmodium vaughani,*[129] and recovery from *Plas-*

[118] M. Lion, *Bull. Soc. path. exot.,* 32: 713 (1939).

[119] W. H. Taliaferro and L. G. Taliaferro, *J. Prevent. Med.,* 3: 197, 209 (1929).

[120] R. D. Manwell and F. Goldstein, *Proc. Soc. Exper. Biol. & Med.,* 39: 426 (1938), and *J. Parasitol. (Suppl.),* 24: 19 (1938).

[121] R. D. Manwell, *Am. J. Hyg.,* 27: 196 (1938).

[122] F. Wolfson, *J. Parasitol. (Suppl.),* 24: 18 (1938).

[123] R. D. Manwell and F. Goldstein, *J. Parasitol. (Suppl.),* 24: 19 (1938).

[124] R. D. Manwell, *Proc. Soc. Exper. Biol. & Med.,* 32: 391 (1934).

[125] L. T. Coggeshall, *Am. J. Hyg.,* 27: 615 (1938); W. H. Taliaferro and L. G. Taliaferro, *J. Infect. Dis.,* 66: 153 (1940).

[126] R. D. Manwell and F. Goldstein, *Proc. Soc. Exper. Biol. & Med.,* 39: 426 (1938), and *J. Parasitol. (Suppl.),* 24: 19 (1938); F. Wolfson and O. R. Causey, *J. Parasitol.,* 25: 510 (1939).

[127] F. Wolfson, *J. Parasitol. (Suppl.),* 24: 18 (1938); R. D. Manwell and F. Goldstein, *J. Parasitol. (Suppl.),* 24: 19 (1938).

[128] E. Sergent, E. Sergent, and A. Catanei, *Bull. Soc. path. exot.,* 24: 327 (1931); W. Gingrich, *J. Prevent. Med.,* 6: 197 (1932).

[129] R. D. Manwell, *Proc. Soc. Exper. Biol. & Med.,* 32: 391 (1934).

modium rouxi protects against both *Plasmodium rouxi* and *Plasmodium circumflexum*.[130] Cross-immunity is observed chiefly between strains of similar virulence or when the original infecting strain has greater virulence than the subsequently superimposed strain. A weakly virulent strain will confer little or no resistance against a powerfully virulent parasite unless the immunity engendered by the poorly virulent organism can be significantly enhanced by multiple superimposed infections with this organism.[131]

Some species of bird malaria appear absolutely distinct immunologically from those generally used in laboratory studies. For example, *Plasmodium elongatum* does not engender resistance to such species as *Plasmodium praecox* (*relictum*), *Plasmodium cathemerium*, or *Plasmodium circumflexum*, and it readily infects birds which have recovered from infections with such forms.[132] The acquisition of immunity following infection is not prevented by the early administration of large doses of the specific drugs.[133]

Premunition.—Immunity to reinfection with bird malaria apparently requires the persistence in latent form of the original infection.[134] This latent infection sometimes lasts many years.[135] Immunity in the absence of a demonstrable latent infection has only rarely been reported.[136] The persistence of immunity, even to a heterologous superimposed strain, however, depends on the establishment of a latent infection with the superimposed form. Such superimposed strains have been shown to remain latent in an immune bird for at least eight months.[137]

Relapse.—Complete recovery seldom occurs in bird malaria, and relapse is not unusual. Both short- and long-term relapses occur, as in human malaria, short-term relapses being much more frequent. The relapse seems to have a seasonal occurrence, being greatest in the fall and winter. Neither the severity of the initial

[130] R. D. Manwell and F. Goldstein, *J. Parasitol.* (*Suppl.*), 24: 19 (1938).

[131] W. B. Redmond, *J. Infect. Dis.*, 64: 273 (1939).

[132] W. Kikuth, *Zentralbl. f. Bakt.*, 121: 401 (1931); W. Gingrich, *J. Prevent. Med.*, 6: 197 (1932); R. D. Manwell, *Am. J. Hyg.*, 27: 196 (1938).

[133] E. M. Lourie, *Ann. Trop. Med.*, 28: 151 (1934); R. D. Manwell, *Am. J. Hyg.*, 9: 308 (1929).

[134] W. Gingrich, *J. Prevent. Med.*, 6: 197 (1932); E. Sergent, E. Sergent, and A. Catanei, *Ann. Inst. Pasteur*, 53: 101 (1934).

[135] W. H. Taliaferro, *South. M. J.*, 24: 407 (1931).

[136] R. D. Manwell, *Proc. Soc. Exper. Biol. & Med.*, 32: 391 (1934).

[137] C. G. Huff and E. Gambrell, *Am. J. Hyg.*, 19: 404 (1934).

infection nor drug treatment is believed to influence the tendency
to relapse.[138]

ANTIBODY PRODUCTION

Until recently, antibodies had not been demonstrated in the bird
malarias by any of the usual in vitro methods. Agglutinins, however, have now been shown in the serum of canaries infected with
Plasmodium circumflexum.[139] Presumably, then, they occur characteristically in these infections.

PASSIVE IMMUNITY

The earlier attempts to transfer immunity passively in the bird
malarias were for the most part unsuccessful,[140] but recent efforts
have resulted more favorably.[141] In some cases merely the clinical
symptoms are allayed by the administration of serum,[142] but in
others the actual number of parasites is reduced. When an especially powerful serum is used, infection cannot infrequently be
completely inhibited.[143] The most satisfactory results thus far
have been obtained with *Plasmodium circumflexum* in canaries [144]
and *Plasmodium lophurae* in chicks.[145]

MECHANISM OF IMMUNITY

The older point of view on the mechanism of acquired immunity
to malaria in birds involved chiefly an increase in the number of
the phagocytic cells—especially in the liver and the spleen—and

[138] R. D. Manwell, *Am. J. Hyg.*, 9: 308 (1929).
[139] R. D. Manwell and F. Goldstein, *J. Exper. Med.*, 71: 409 (1940).
[140] W. H. Taliaferro and L. G. Taliaferro, *J. Prevent. Med.*, 3: 197, 209 (1929);
W. Gingrich, *J. Prevent. Med.*, 6: 197 (1932); E. Sergent, E. Sergent, and A. Catanei,
Ann. Inst. Pasteur, 53: 101 (1934).
[141] R. D. Manwell and F. Goldstein, *Proc. Soc. Exper. Biol. & Med.*, 39: 426
(1938); R. Hegner and L. Eskridge, *Am. J. Hyg.*, 28: 367 (1938); R. Hegner and
M. Dobler, *Am. J. Hyg.*, 30: 81 (1939, sec. C); R. D. Manwell and F. Goldstein,
J. Exper. Med., 71: 409 (1940); W. H. Taliaferro and L. G. Taliaferro, *J. Parasitol.*
(*Suppl.*), 25: 29 (1939).
[142] R. Hegner and L. Eskridge, *Am. J. Hyg.*, 28: 367 (1938).
[143] R. D. Manwell and F. Goldstein, *J. Exper. Med.*, 71: 409 (1940).
[144] R. D. Manwell and F. Goldstein, *Proc. Soc. Exper. Biol. & Med.*, 39: 426
(1938), and *J. Exper. Med.*, 71: 409 (1940).
[145] W. H. Taliaferro and L. G. Taliaferro, *J. Parasitol.* (*Suppl.*), 25: 29 (1939),
and *J. Infect. Dis.*, 66: 153 (1940).

CHART III

THE DISAPPEARANCE OF WASHED MALARIA-PARASITIZED CELLS FROM THE BLOOD OF A BIRD IN THE LATENT INFECTION AND THE SURVIVAL OF THE SAME TYPE OF CELL IN A CONTROL UNINFECTED BIRD

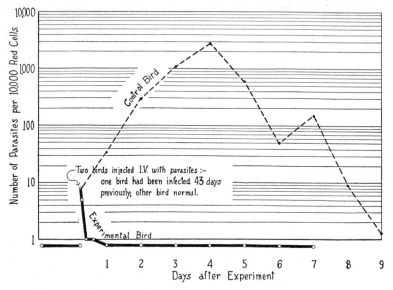

Both birds were injected intravenously with enough washed infected cells so that a few minutes later both showed an infection of about eight parasites per 10,000 red cells. In the bird with the latent infection they were removed from the circulation within twelve hours, but in the uninfected bird they survived and progressively increased in numbers, initiating a typical response.

the enhancement of their capacity to function.[146] Humoral antibody, which had not been demonstrated in these infections at that time, was believed to play only a minor role, if any, in protection. The present viewpoint still assigns the cells the principal defensive function, but this function to be effective is now considered to require the presence in the blood of an opsonizing antibody. A normal bird can check an incipient malarial infection at once if specific antibody is supplied passively to that bird in the form of serum from an immune bird. The mechanism of immunity in these infec-

[146] W. H. Taliaferro, *South. M. J.*, 24: 407 (1931); W. Gingrich, *J. Prevent. Med.*, 6: 197 (1932); E. Sergent, E. Sergent, and A. Catanei, *Ann. Inst. Pasteur*, 53: 101 (1934).

tions is, thus, of a dual character: antibody first combines with the parasite to render it vulnerable to the action of the phagocytic cells,[147] and these cells then actually remove the parasite from the blood stream and destroy it by digestion. It seems possible that the antibody is not present throughout the body in equal concentration, however, but is most available in those strategically placed organs, such as the spleen and the liver, which are best adapted for phagocytosing the malaria parasites and removing them from the circulating blood.[148] Usually, in fact, the peripheral blood serum is distinctly low in content of antibody.

The acquisition of immunity in bird malaria is a progressive phenomenon, not one which develops explosively. Some of the parasites, for example, are destroyed even by the normal bird. The percentage of organisms that are destroyed rises gradually, however, as the immunity begins to develop. Finally, the defensive agencies are able not only to check further increase in the total number of the parasites but even to reduce the number present. Usually, however, a few organisms survive and multiply even in the highly immune bird, although the infection always remains at a low level. Almost certainly a similar progressive development of immunity occurs also in the malarias of man and of monkey.[149]

PROPHYLAXIS

Until recently, attempts to protect birds against malaria with killed organisms have not succeeded.[150] Intense vaccination with formalin-killed parasites has now been shown to confer to canaries a significant degree of resistance against *Phasmodium cathemerium*.[151] When living parasites of attenuated virulence are employed, somewhat better results are obtained,[152] especially when the attenuation is accomplished by exposing the parasites to very low temperature.[153] No success follows the use of small doses of fully

[147] G. M. Findlay and H. C. Brown, *Brit. J. Exper. Path.*, 15: 148 (1934).
[148] W. H. Taliaferro and W. Bloom, *J. Parasitol. (Suppl.)*, 24: 19 (1938).
[149] R. Hegner, *Am. J. Hyg.*, 32: 24 (1940, sec. C).
[150] Z. W. Jermoljewa and I. S. Boujanouskaja, *Ztschr. f. Immunitätsforsch. u. exper. Therap.*, 73: 276 (1932).
[151] W. D. Gingrich, *J. Infect. Dis.*, 68: 46 (1941).
[152] E. Sergent, E. Sergent, and A. Catanei, *Arch. Inst. Pasteur d'algerie*, 12: 10 (1934).
[153] W. B. Redmond, *J. Parasitol. (Suppl.)*, 25: 28 (1939).

virulent organisms, however, since a single parasite is sufficient to establish a heavy infection.

DIAGNOSIS

Immunological procedures have not been used in the diagnosis of bird malaria. The Henry test is said to be positive in some of these infections.[154]

OTHER HAEMOSPORIDIAL INFECTIONS

BABESIA INFECTIONS

The most important *Babesia* infections are those of cattle, sheep and goats, horses, and dogs. The causal organisms of all these infections have only the most limited host range and generally are confined to their natural hosts. Three species are found in cattle, the commonest being *Babesia bigemina,* which causes Texas cattle fever. This infection is of especial interest historically, since it was the first parasitic disease in which the acquisition of immunity to reinfection was demonstrated. It was also the first parasitic disease in which the persistence of the acquired immunity was shown to depend on the continued presence of the parasite in latent form in the blood and fixed tissues of the host (premunition).[155]

Older animals are, peculiarly, more susceptible to Texas cattle fever than young animals (reversed age resistance). If these young animals are inoculated with the parasite, they suffer only mild infection and thereafter successfully resist reinfection with the parasite. This fact has made possible the development of an effective method for vaccinating cattle against Texas fever. It has been widely used and has resulted in extensive saving of life, especially among cattle moved from northern to southern regions in the United States.

Resistance is also developed by dogs through recovery from an initial infection with *Babesia canis.* In this case, too, the persist-

[154] E. Brumpt and V. Chorine, *Ann. de parasitol.,* 15: 372 (1937); I. L. Kritschewsky and L. W. Demidowa, *Ztschr. f. Immunitätsforsch. u. exper. Therap.,* 80: 135 (1933).

[155] T. Smith and F. L. Kilbourne, Bur. Animal Industry (U.S. Dept. Agric.), *Bull.* No. 1, 1–301 (1893).

ence of the immunity depends on the continuance of the original infection in latent form.[156]

THEILERIA INFECTIONS

The *Theileria* are found in cattle, sheep, and some other animals. They are highly specific forms, residing exclusively in their natural host. Several species have been described in cattle, the best known being *Theileria parva*. Cattle which recover from a first infection are thereafter completely resistant to reinfection. The parasite is apparently wholly eradicated from the recovered animal, for ticks fed on such cattle do not become infected. No effective method of vaccination against *Theileria* has yet been devised.

HAEMOPROTEUS INFECTIONS

One of the species of the genus *Haemoproteus* is *Haemoproteus columbae*. This parasite is found in the pigeon, although probably it occurs also in many other birds. No immunity is acquired by the pigeon through recovery from an initial infection, although no reinfection will occur so long as an earlier infection persists.[157] The parasites typically persist for several years in the blood of pigeons.

TOXOPLASMA INFECTIONS

Organisms of uncertain nature and classification, known by the generic name *Toxoplasma*, have been described from various vertebrates, including birds and mammals. They have been recorded several times in man, in whom they are believed to cause an encephalitis. The organisms appear to have a rather broad host range. Human toxoplasma, for example, can infect the mouse and the rabbit as well as the chick, although not the *Macacus* monkey or the rat.[158] Young individuals are more susceptible than older ones. Human infections, for example, are generally confined to young children, although infection of adults also has been reported.[159]

Apparently a considerable immunity is developed by recovery

[156] H. E. Shortt and others, *Indian J. M. Research,* 25: 763 (1938).

[157] G. R. Coatney, *Am. J. Hyg.,* 18: 133 (1933).

[158] A. Wolf and D. Cowen, *Bull. Neur. Inst. New York,* 7: 266 (1938) ; A. Wolf, D. Cowen, and B. Paige, *Science,* 89: 226 (1939).

[159] H. Pinkerton and D. Weinman, *Arch. Path.,* 30: 374 (1940).

from toxoplasma infection. The immunity has a fairly broad specificity, evidently, for animals which have survived an infection with the human toxoplasma thereafter resist reinfection not only with the human form but also with a toxoplasma found naturally in the guinea pig.[160] A humoral antibody is developed in infected animals which protects against percutaneous infection if mixed with the organisms prior to their inoculation. No in vitro effect upon the organisms has been observed.[161]

[160] A. Wolf, D. Cowen, and B. Paige, *J. Exper. Med.*, 71: 187 (1940); A. B. Sabin, *Proc. Soc. Exper. Biol. & Med.*, 41: 75 (1939).

[161] A. B. Sabin and P. K. Olitsky, *Science*, 85: 336 (1937).

Chapter XIII

THE COCCIDIOSES

Coccidiosis is insignificant as a human disease, since only a few hundred human cases altogether have been recorded. Among animals, however, the disease is extraordinarily important, being responsible for great economic loss, especially to raisers of chickens and rabbits. Since the complete life cycle of the human parasite has never been studied, our knowledge of the coccidia and the coccidioses is based chiefly upon observations in animal infections. This is true particularly of the immunology of coccidiosis, since essentially nothing in this field is yet determined with respect to the human infection.

NATURAL RESISTANCE

HOST RESTRICTION

The coccidia are found practically universally in animals of the higher phyla, having been described from nearly all species in which a thoroughgoing search has been made. Individually, however, each species of coccidian has typically a very narrow host range, for generally only two or three species of animal at most, and many times only a single species, are susceptible to infection. When more than one host is susceptible, the hosts are usually very closely related.

The most limited range of host is seen with respect to coccidia of the genus *Eimeria*. For example, the rabbit parasites (*Eimeria perforans* and *Eimeria stiedae*) develop only in the rabbit among all the species of vertebrates. Likewise, the *Eimerias* of the chicken will infect only the chicken, not the pheasant, the turkey, or other birds. However, some members of this genus do infect more than one host, at least when the hosts are near relatives. For example, *Eimeria magna* will infect both the cotton-tail rabbit and the Belgian hare, and *Eimeria miyairii* will infect both the brown and the black rat. Coccidia of the genus *Isospora* appear to have a somewhat broader host choice. For example, *Isospora felis* and *Isospora rivolta* infect both dogs and cats, and similar forms have been recovered from many other carnivores. The possibility remains, however, that many of those morphologically similar parasites found in the other carnivores are distinct species.[1] A recent study upon *Isospora belli* of man has shown that this form will not infect monkeys, puppies, or kittens.[2]

The host restriction among the coccidia appears sometimes to depend on components of the digestive juice of the host. The digestive process of the natural host seems to facilitate the excystation of the parasite. The sporozites thus freed may then infect this host's tissue. In contrast, coccidial cysts pass through the intestine of unreceptive hosts without change.[3]

FACTORS INFLUENCING NATURAL RESISTANCE

Age.—Much of the evidence for age resistance among the coccidioses is inconclusive, because only a few experiments have been carried out in which the possibility of prior infection of the older animals used has been excluded. In *Eimeria tenella* infection of chicks, however, birds of all ages up to fifteen months have been shown to be susceptible to infection, although those over three months old are more resistant to the effects of the disease than those less than this age. In *Eimeria necatrix* infection of chicks, however, very young birds suffer less intense infection than older ones, perhaps because of the disproportionately rapid rate of growth of the intestinal epithelium in the young birds.[4]

Diet.—The diet is of significance in natural resistance against coccidia, although the precise factors which have greatest influence are still somewhat obscure. The most extensive investigations have been concerned with the coccidioses of the chick and of the rat, and these all show that the disease can actually be controlled by means of the diet.[5] Earlier workers recommended adding milk powder to

---

[1] E. R. Becker, *Coccidia and Coccidioses,* Ames, Collegiate Press (1934).
[2] A. Foner, *Tr. Roy. Soc. Trop. Med. & Hyg.,* 33: 357 (1939).
[3] J. M. Andrews, *J. Parasitol.,* 13: 183 (1927).
[4] E. E. Tyzzer, H. Theiler, and E. E. Jones, *Am. J. Hyg.,* 15: 319 (1932).
[5] E. R. Becker, *Science,* 86: 403 (1937).

the diet in order to combat chick coccidiosis,[6] but recent studies show that dried skim milk or dried buttermilk plus wheat middlings in an ordinary chick ration are the components chiefly responsible for a higher death rate in chicks experimentally infected with caecal coccidiosis and it is now recommended, therefore, that these constituents be limited in the diet.[7] Other components of the ration may also play a role. The addition of sulfur to the diet leads to a striking reduction in the mortality in chicks from *Eimeria tenella* infection, although birds fed much sulfur are retarded in growth [8] and often develop rickets.[9] A diet rich in protein as well as in vitamins A and B likewise appears to aid resistance to this parasite.[10] The addition of calcium carbonate to the ration, on the other hand, increases the mortality from *Eimeria tenella*.[11]

The rat coccidian, *Eimeria miyairii*, is hindered in development if the diet is deprived of vitamin G, but stimulated if the diet is rich in this vitamin, particularly when it comes from yeast.[12] Vitamin B_1 (thiamin chloride), on the contrary, exerts a restraining influence on oocyst production by *Eimeria nieschulzi* in the rat.[13] Essentially no restraining role on the development of these coccidians is played by vitamins A or D,[14] however, or by such varied substances as skim milk, lactose, vinegar, iodine, nicotine worm powder, derris, pyrethrum, calomel, sodium bicarbonate, calcium carbonate, calcium chloride, disodium phosphate, or creolin.[15] Careful biological assays carried out upon all the basic diet components indicate that wheat middlings and alfalfa meal are richest in coccidian growth-promoting substance, to which Becker has

---

[6] J. R. Beach and J. C. Corl, *Poult. Sci.*, 4: 83 (1925).

[7] E. R. Becker and P. C. Waters, *Iowa State Coll. J. Sci.*, 12: 405 (1938) ; E. R. Becker and H. L. Wilcke, *Poult. Sci.*, 17: 405 (1938).

[8] C. A. Herrick and C. E. Holmes, *Vet. Med.*, 31: 390 (1936).

[9] C. A. Herrick and C. E. Holmes, Wiscon. Agr. Exp. Sta., *Bull.*, No. 438, 36 (1937) ; C. E. Holmes, H. J. Deobald, and C. A. Herrick, *Poult. Sci.*, 17: 136 (1938).

[10] E. A. Allen, *Am. J. Hyg.*, 15: 163 (1932).

[11] C. E. Holmes, C. A. Herrick, and G. L. Ott, *Poult. Sci.*, 16: 335 (1937).

[12] E. R. Becker and N. F. Morehouse, *Proc. Soc. Exper. Biol. & Med.*, 34: 437 (1936), *J. Parasitol.*, 23: 153 (1937), and *Proc. Soc. Exper. Biol. & Med.*, 33: 487 (1936).

[13] E. R. Becker, *Proc. Soc. Exper. Biol. & Med.*, 42: 597 (1939), and *J. Parasitol.* (*Suppl.*), 26: 26 (1940).

[14] E. R. Becker and N. F. Morehouse, *J. Parasitol.*, 22: 60 (1936).

[15] E. R. Becker and N. F. Morehouse, *Proc. Soc. Exper. Biol. & Med.*, 32: 1039 (1935) ; E. R. Becker and P. S. Spencer, *J. Parasitol.*, 21: 455 (1935).

given the name coccidibios.[16] Coccidibios is probably a complex of factors, but one of the most important seems to be vitamin B_6.[17] Certainly the complex as a whole is water soluble and heat stable.[18] The absence of the coccidibios from the diet is correlated with a decrease in the severity of coccidiosis in the rat.

ACQUIRED IMMUNITY

RESISTANCE TO REINFECTION

If animals once are able to bring under control an initial infection with coccidia, they will resist reinfection for at least short periods thereafter.[19] In one of the earliest experiments thirty-three chickens which had recovered from severe coccidial infection resisted wholly without symptoms a test dose of coccidia which was fatal to sixteen (34 percent) of a control group and produced severe symptoms in all the remainder.[20] Subsequent studies have confirmed this finding. Very light infections, however, often fail to confer any demonstrable resistance to reinfection.[21] The acquired resistance is always rigidly specific.[22] For example, rabbits which have become immune to *Eimeria perforans* remain entirely susceptible to *Eimeria stiedae*.[23]

Immunity to reinfection develops more rapidly against those coccidians which penetrate deeply and are most damaging to the host's tissue.[24] Thus, recovery from a single infection with *Eimeria necatrix* or *Eimeria tenella*, which penetrate deeply into the tissues,

[16] E. R. Becker and R. C. Derbyshire, *Iowa State Coll. J. Sci.*, 12: 211 (1937), and 11: 311 (1937); E. R. Becker and N. F. Morehouse, *J. Parasitol.*, 23: 153 (1937); E. R. Becker and P. C. Waters, *Iowa State Coll. J. Sci.*, 13: 243 (1939).

[17] E. R. Becker, *J. Parasitol. (Suppl.)*, 26: 26 (1940).

[18] E. R. Becker, *Iowa State Coll. J. Sci.*, 14: 317 (1940).

[19] J. R. Beach and J. C. Corl, *Poult. Sci.*, 4: 92 (1925); E. E. Tyzzer, *Am. J. Hyg.*, 10: 269 (1929); E. E. Tyzzer, H. Theiler, and E. E. Jones, *Am. J. Hyg.*, 15: 319 (1932), D. P. Henry, *Univ. Calif. Pub. in Zool.*, 37: 211 (1932), and *Proc. Soc. Exper. Biol. & Med.*, 28: 831 (1931); Wilson, Va. Ag. Exper. St., *Techn. Bull.*, No. 42, 1–42 (1931); C. D. Lee, Iowa State Coll., Ames, Iowa, unpublished thesis (1932); H. E. Biester and L. H. Schwarte, *J. Am. Vet. M. A.*, 81: 358 (1932).

[20] J. R. Beach and J. C. Corl, *Poult. Sci.*, 4: 92 (1925).

[21] E. E. Tyzzer, H. Theiler, and E. E. Jones, *Am. J. Hyg.*, 15: 319 (1932).

[22] E. E. Tyzzer, *Am. J. Hyg.*, 10: 269 (1929); E. E. Tyzzer, H. Theiler, and E. E. Jones, *Am. J. Hyg.*, 15: 319 (1932); E. R. Becker and P. R. Hall, *Am. J. Hyg.*, 18: 220 (1933).

[23] G. W. Bachman, *Am. J. Hyg.*, 12: 641 (1930).

[24] E. E. Tyzzer, *Am. J. Hyg.*, 10: 269 (1929).

suffices to protect chickens from reinfection, whereas repeated infections with *Eimeria mitis* or *Eimeria acervulina* may be required to engender any measure of resistance whatsoever, since these last species induce infection of a more superficial character.

Premunition.—Such studies as have been reported indicate that immunity to reinfection with coccidia is absolute and does not require the persistence in latent form of an earlier infection with the parasite.[25] Yet immunity is maintained only by periodic reinfection, since that which is acquired by recovery from any one infection is comparatively short-lived.[26]

ANTIBODY PRODUCTION

Antibody is produced by animals infected with coccidia, although its formation has not yet been studied very satisfactorily. In artificially immunized animals, complement-fixing antibody can be detected in about five days after the last immunizing injection. This antibody persists for about fifty days.[27]

PASSIVE IMMUNITY

Although antibodies have been demonstrated in animals which are immune to coccidia, the serum of such animals has not been shown to confer resistance to other animals to which it is inoculated.[28]

MECHANISM OF IMMUNITY

Most authorities agree that the serum antibody plays only a minor role, if any, in the immunity of recovered animals to reinfection with coccidia.[29] The widespread reticulo-endothelial system likewise seems of little significance in regard to this immunity, since splenectomy and reticulo-endothelial blockade do not lower resistance. On the contrary, immunity in coccidiosis appears to be of distinctly local nature, having to do only with the epithelial cells

---

[25] N. F. Morehouse, *J. Parasitol.,* 24: 311 (1938) ; E. E. Tyzzer, H. Theiler, and E. E. Jones, *Am. J. Hyg.,* 15: 319 (1932).

[26] C. D. Lee, Iowa State Coll., Ames, Iowa, unpublished thesis (1932).

[27] G. W. Bachman, *Am. J. Hyg.,* 12: 624 (1930).

[28] G. W. Bachman, *Am. J. Hyg.,* 12: 641 (1930) ; E. R. Becker, *Am. J. Hyg.,* 21: 389 (1935) ; E. E. Tyzzer, H. Theiler, and E. E. Jones, *Am. J. Hyg.,* 15: 319 (1932).

[29] J. Chapman, *Am. J. Hyg.,* 9: 389 (1929) ; E. R. Becker, *Am. J. Hyg.,* 21: 389 (1935) ; E. E. Tyzzer, H. Theiler, and E. E. Jones, *Am. J. Hyg.,* 15: 319 (1932).

of the intestine or bile ducts. These cells in the immune animal appear either to protect themselves by preventing sporozoites from entering their cytoplasm or else by providing an unfavorable environment for these sporozoites after they have gained entrance.[30] Probably the two conditions not infrequently supplement each other. Morehouse [31] believes that in rats immune to *Eimeria nieschulzi* the sporozoites are prevented from entering the epithelial cells. However, the sporozoites of *Eimeria tenella* have been found by Tyzzer and his co-workers [32] in the gland cells of immune chicks, where they remain for about twenty-four hours. After entering the cells, however, these parasites experience no further development, but soon die and disintegrate along with the cell which contains them.

PROPHYLAXIS

The vaccination of animals against coccidiosis by the inoculation of specific coccidial substance by various parenteral routes (for example, *Eimeria tenella* in the wing vein of chicks; [33] *Eimeria miyairii* intraperitoneally in rats; [34] *Eimeria perforans* intraperitoneally in rabbits [35]) does not protect the injected animal from subsequent coccidial infection, even though antibodies can be detected in the serum of such vaccinated animals.[36] However, animals can be protected by previous infection through feeding small doses of living coccidia.[37] When small numbers of oocysts are fed daily for about fifteen days, fowls become resistant. This resistance is rigidly specific.[38] Somewhat improved results are obtained if the oocysts are heated prior to administration, since larger doses can then be given and a higher grade immune response elicited.[39] Often

[30] E. R. Becker, *Am. J. Hyg.,* 21: 389 (1935).
[31] N. F. Morehouse, *J. Parasitol.,* 24: 311 (1938).
[32] E. E. Tyzzer, H. Theiler, and E. E. Jones, *Am. J. Hyg.,* 15: 319 (1932).
[33] E. E. Tyzzer, *Am. J. Hyg.,* 10: 269 (1929).
[34] E. R. Becker, *Am. J. Hyg.,* 21: 389 (1935).
[35] G. W. Bachman, *Am. J. Hyg.,* 12: 641 (1930).
[36] *Ibid.*
[37] E. E. Tyzzer, H. Theiler, and E. E. Jones, *Am. J. Hyg.,* 15: 319 (1932) ; H. E. Biester and L. H. Schwarte, *J. Am. Vet. M. A.,* 81: 358 (1932) ; W. T. Johnson, Oregon Agric. Exper. Sta., *Director's Report* (1930).
[38] W. T. Johnson, *J. Parasitol.,* 19: 160 (1932), and Oregon Agric. Exper. Sta., *Director's Report* (1930).
[39] H. A. Jankiewicz and R. H. Scofield, *J. Am. Vet. M. A.,* 84: 507 (1934).

fowls thus immunized are completely resistant to usually fatal doses of the specific parasite subsequently administered.

DIAGNOSIS

Immunological reactions have little promise in the diagnosis of coccidial infections. Antibody cannot be detected in the serum of infected animals by the precipitin test,[40] although its presence is often, though not regularly, revealed by the fixation test.[41] Skin tests also have as yet proved unsatisfactory for practical use,[42] although guinea pigs are said to give a positive skin reaction for some weeks after recovery.[43] However, since oocysts can with comparative ease and regularity be found microscopically in the feces of infected animals, it is seldom or never necessary to resort to biological procedures for aid in the diagnosis of these infections.

[40] G. W. Bachman, *Am. J. Hyg.*, 12: 624 (1930) ; E. E. Tyzzer, H. Theiler, and E. E. Jones, *Am. J. Hyg.*, 15: 319 (1932).

[41] J. Chapman, *Am. J. Hyg.*, 9: 389 (1929), G. W. Bachman, *Am. J. Hyg.*, 12: 624 (1930).

[42] J. Chapman, *Am. J. Hyg.*, 9: 389 (1929).

[43] D. P. Henry, Univ. California *Publ., Zoology*, 37: 211 (1932), and *Proc. Soc. Exper. Biol. & Med.*, 28: 831 (1931).

Chapter XIV

THE TREMATODIASES

THE LIFE CYCLES of most human trematode parasites have been determined only in recent years, and that of several species is still obscure. Experimental infections with these forms have been possible, therefore, only lately and information upon the relevant immunology of the entire group of organisms is even now not abundant. Most of what is known is concerned with human schistosomiasis or with fascioliasis of sheep and cattle. Probably, however, much of the immunological knowledge of these two infections will be shown eventually likewise to apply to the other trematodiases. Two facts stand forth prominently from the studies performed thus far: (1) trematodes in general have somewhat broader vertebrate host range than most other kinds of parasites; and (2) the immunity acquired against those forms (especially blood stream invaders) that produce definite damage to the host tissue is of a more effective level than that against essentially harmless species (those residing in the intestinal lumen).

SCHISTOSOMIASIS

NATURAL RESISTANCE

HOST RESTRICTION

The three species of human schistosomes differ among themselves considerably in their infectivity. *Schistosoma mansoni* has the most restricted range, being found naturally in man exclusively, although it will readily infect a number of other primates experimentally, as well as all of the usual laboratory rodents. *Schistosoma hematobium* is found naturally in monkeys, as well as man, and will also infect many laboratory rodents. In contrast with these forms, *Schistosoma japonicum* is found naturally in human beings, cats, dogs, goats, cattle, and pigs, and will infect experimentally many monkeys, the horse, and the laboratory rodents. All of the human schistosomes have very narrow choice of molluscan host. Usually each species infects only snails of a single genus.

The schistosomes of animals likewise have a comparatively broad host range. *Schistosoma spindale,* for example, is found naturally in cattle, sheep, goats, horses, and antelopes, and has been suspected occasionally of infecting man as well. The species will also infect guinea pigs and perhaps other laboratory animals experimentally.

FACTORS INFLUENCING NATURAL RESISTANCE

Very few factors are yet known to have significance in natural resistance against schistosomiasis. The age of the vertebrate host probably is significant. At least human infections with schistosomiasis are most severe in children between five and eleven years of age and new infections are rarely contracted by persons over forty years old.[1] The absence of the infection from native children below five years of age does not result from an immunity of the young child, but is explained by the fact that their mothers wash the babies only in warmed water. Generally the water is heated sufficiently to destroy the infective stage of the parasite.[2] The significance of the sex of the host, the diet, intercurrent infection, and many other factors on natural resistance of man to schistosomes has not yet been determined. Rats on a vitamin-A-free diet, however, are known to have less resistance to experimental infection with *Schistosoma mansoni* than have normal animals.[3]

ACQUIRED IMMUNITY

RESISTANCE TO REINFECTION

Man has not yet been shown to resist reinfection after experiencing an initial infection with schistosomes. Dogs and monkeys, however, do acquire some measure of resistance following a first ex-

[1] P. K. Dixon, *Tr. Roy. Soc. Trop. Med. & Hyg.,* 27: 505 (1934); A. C. Fisher, *Tr. Roy. Soc. Trop. Med. & Hyg.,* 28: 277 (1934); G. W. St. C. Ramsay, *West African M. J.,* 8: 2 (1934).

[2] P. K. Dixon, *Tr. Roy. Soc. Trop. Med. & Hyg.,* 27: 505 (1934).

[3] C. Krakower, W. A. Hoffman, and J. H. Axtmayer, *Porto Rico J. Pub. Health & Trop. Med.,* 16: 269 (1940).

posure. If dogs are cured of a first infection by means of an injection of stibnal, they will resist fairly well a subsequent infective dose of schistosome cercariae.[4] Monkeys, which are naturally comparatively resistant to initial infection with *Schistosoma spindale*, permitting only partial development of the parasite, acquire an almost complete immunity to subsequent attacks. Practically no development whatsoever of the parasite takes place in the veins of immune monkeys.[5]

ANTIBODY PRODUCTION

Since the schistosomes develop within the blood stream of the host, antibody should always be expected in schistosomiasis. For the most part this expectation is realized. The production of complement-fixing antibody has been studied with especial care in goat infections with *Schistosoma spindale,* the serum having been tested with an antigen derived by alcoholic extraction of the livers of snails heavily infected with the homologous schistosome. Practically all goats develop antibody by the seventh week if they have experienced a significantly intense infection, and they are usually positive within two weeks.[6] The antibody level is generally sustained for at least twelve months thereafter and often well into the second year.

Rabbits and dogs also develop antibody after infection with schistosomes. Dogs may not manifest it before the eighth or the tenth week, but rabbits are usually positive by the third week after infection. Vaccinated rabbits have antibody in their blood within five days or so after the last of a series of immunizing injections.[7] Humans also develop antibodies in schistosomiasis. The test for this antibody is a useful aid in the diagnosis of the disease.

PASSIVE TRANSFER

Immunity to schistosomiasis has not been conferred passively by the inoculation of serum containing antibody.

[4] M. Ozawa, *Jap. J. Exper. Med.*, 8: 79 (1930).
[5] N. H. Fairley, F. P. Mackie, and F. Jasudasan, *Ind. Med. Res. Mem., Suppl. Ser. to Indian J. M. Research*, Mem. No. 17 (1930), Part IV.
[6] N. H. Fairley, *Arch. f. Schiffs-u. Tropen-Hyg.*, 30: 372 (1926).
[7] S. Miyaji and B. Imai, *Zentralbl. f. Bakt.*, 106: 237 (1928).

MECHANISM OF IMMUNITY

The basis of the immunity in schistosomiasis is obscure, since it has not as yet been adequately studied. The immunity would appear to depend largely upon the action of the serum antibody, and this antibody to interfere markedly with the development of the parasites, for parasites which succeed in entering a host whose blood contains antibody usually develop imperfectly and generally fail to reach maturity.[8] What role the body defensive cells play in this immunity is as yet unknown, although they certainly could be expected to act in an auxiliary capacity to the antibody. The formation of pseudotubercles about schistosome eggs which lodge in the liver and elsewhere provides evidence that the cells respond to the presence of the invader.

PROPHYLAXIS

No immunological procedures have been invoked in the prophylaxis of human schistosomiasis. Dogs, however, can be partially immunized against the infection by the injection of a suspension of adult schistosomes.[9]

DIAGNOSIS

Undoubtedly the most valuable contribution of immunology thus far in the study of schistosomiasis is the development of tests which identify the disease. The complement fixation test, the precipitin test, and the skin test all serve well for this purpose. Following the development of an acceptable technic by Fairley,[10] many others have used the fixation test successfully,[11] and this reaction is the one most highly regarded for diagnosis at the present time. Apparently any mammalian schistosome will serve as a source of

[8] M. Ozawa, *Jap. J. Exper. Med.*, 8: 79 (1930); N. H. Fairley, F. P. Mackie, and F. Jasudasan, *Ind. Med. Res. Mem., Suppl. Ser. to Indian J. M. Research,* Mem. No. 17 (1930), Part IV.

[9] M. Ozawa, *Jap. J. Exper. Med.*, 8: 79 (1930).

[10] N. H. Fairley, *Arch. f. Schiffs-u. Tropen-Hyg.,* 30: 372 (1928).

[11] B. Imai, *Japan M. World,* 8: 273 (1928); K. D. Fairley and N. H. Fairley, *M. J. Australia,* 2: 597 (1929); N. H. Fairley, *J. Helminthol.,* 11: 181 (1933); N. H. Fairley and F. Jasudasan, *Ind. Med. Res. Mem., Suppl. Ser. to Indian J. M. Research,* Mem. No. 17 (1930), Parts I and II; M. N. Andrews, *J. Helminthol.,* 13: 25 (1935); A. A. Salam, *J. Egyptian M. A.,* 18: 353 (1935).

antigen for diagnosing any schistosome infection.[12] Generally the antigen is obtained by extracting in alcohol snail livers which are heavily infected with some mammalian schistosome. Positive fixation tests have also been reported in schistosomiasis when extracts of *Fasciola hepatica* have been employed as the antigen.

The precipitin test has had comparatively limited use for diagnosing schistosomiasis,[13] perhaps because it is considered less sensitive than the fixation test. In one series of known cases only 50 percent gave a positive precipitin reaction.[14] Usually saline or Coca's solution extracts of the adult schistosomes or of schistosome-infected snail livers are employed as antigen in precipitin tests.[15]

The skin test is the most promising diagnostic aid in schistosomiasis, because it combines accuracy of result with simplicity of performance. Saline extracts of triturated adult worms or of heavily infected snail livers serve as antigen, and positive reactions provide strong evidence for infection with schistosomes.[16] The test is exclusively of diagnostic value, however, and gives no index of the result of treatment, for positive skin reactions persist for years after the need of treatment is ended.[17] Experimentally infected rabbits also give a positive skin reaction.[18] Prausnitz-Küstner reactions can be performed in the skin of normal persons after local sensitization with serum from an infected individual.[19] Probably any mammalian schistosome will serve as the source of the skin-testing antigen in schistosomiasis.[20] The rather remotely related

[12] N. H. Fairley, *J. Helminthol.*, 11: 181 (1933) ; N. H. Fairley and F. Jasudasan, *Ind. Med. Res. Mem., Suppl. Ser. to Indian J. M. Research*, Mem. No. 17 (1930), Parts I and II; A. A. Salam, *J. Egyptian M. A.*, 18: 353 (1935).

[13] B. Imai, *Japan M. World*, 8: 273 (1928) ; R. Kawamura, *Japan M. World*, 9: 165 (1929) ; W. H. Taliaferro, W. A. Hoffman, and D. H. Cook, *J. Prevent. Med.*, 2: 395 (1928).

[14] B. Imai, *Japan M. World*, 8: 273 (1928).

[15] W. H. Taliaferro, W. A. Hoffman, and D. H. Cook, *J. Prevent. Med.*, 2: 395 (1928).

[16] G. W. St. C. Ramsay, *West African M. J.*, 8: 2 (1934) ; N. H. Fairley and F. E. Williams, *M. J. Australia*, 2: 811 (1927) ; P. Manson-Bahr: *J. Helminthol.*, 7: 99 (1929) ; H. C. Kan, *Chinese M. J.*, Suppl. No. 1: 387 (1936).

[17] N. H. Fairley and F. E. Williams, *M. J. Australia*, 2: 811 (1927).

[18] W. H. Taliaferro, W. A. Hoffman, and D. H. Cook, *J. Prevent. Med.*, 2: 395 (1928).

[19] W. H. Taliaferro and L. G. Taliaferro, *Porto Rico J. Pub. Health & Trop. Med.*, 7: 23 (1931).

[20] M. Khalil and A. Hassan, *J. Egyptian M. A.*, 15: 129 (1932).

cattle liver fluke *Fasciola gigantica* also supplies suitable antigens for the test.[21]

SCHISTOSOME DERMATITIS

Many persons suffer a characteristic dermatitis after cercariae of the schistosomes of animals penetrate their skin.[22] Although only a slight pricking sensation is noticed at the time of penetration, by the next day a distinct papule develops which attains greater size and severity in the ensuing three or four days. The reaction subsides thereafter, although traces of the small lesions are often visible even three or four weeks later. The reaction is not given by all persons. Very severe reactions are seen in those who have been repeatedly exposed to schistosomes.[23] One investigator of the problem, who has been exposed both naturally and experimentally many times since 1934, has reported that his reactions have increased in severity every year.[24]

The cercariae of the animal schistosomes are actually destroyed after penetrating the epithelial layer of the skin of man. Neutrophils and lymphocytes first invade the edematous area about the parasite, and these are followed in a few hours by many eosinophils. These responses are probably markedly accelerated as a result of repeated exposure to cercariae, and in persons who are highly reactive a good cellular response can be expected in about forty-eight hours.[25] It seems possible that the reaction is aided significantly by the natural cercaricidal action which normal human serum has been shown to have for many of the animal schistosomes.[26]

Most investigations upon schistosome dermatitis have been carried on with any of six species of animal schistosomes, and these are all known to elicit the reaction in man. Opinion is divided, however, as to whether the cercariae of the human schistosomes also cause dermatitis when penetrating the skin of man. Most authorities incline to the view that the human schistosome cercariae cannot elicit the reaction in man,[27] and certainly the reaction to the human

[21] A. Hassan and M. Betashe, *J. Egyptian M. A.*, 17: 991 (1934).
[22] W. W. Cort, *J. A. M. A.*, 90: 1027 (1928).
[23] W. W. Cort, *Am. J. Hyg.*, 23: 349 (1936).
[24] S. Brackett, *Arch. Dermat. & Syph.*, 42: 410 (1940).
[25] *Ibid.*   [26] J. T. Culbertson, *J. Parasitol.*, 22: 111 (1936).
[27] J. Watarai, *Jap. J. Exper. Med.*, 14: 1 (1936); H. Vogel, *Arch. f. Schiffs-u. Tropen-Hyg.*, 36: 384 (1932).

schistosomes is comparatively less, if it occurs at all. On the other hand, the human schistosomes, as well as some of the animal forms, do elicit the reaction in animals.[28] In general the reaction can be expected most regularly in strange hosts in which the schistosome cannot continue its development.

FASCIOLIASIS

NATURAL RESISTANCE

Fasciola hepatica has one of the broadest host ranges of all the trematodes. It has been found naturally in sheep, cow, antelope, horse, beaver, squirrel, camel, kangaroo, and still other mammals including man, and can be established experimentally in the rabbit and the guinea pig. Its potential snail host is likewise broad, snails of no less than eight different genera being susceptible to infection. Because this parasite has comparatively little difficulty in finding either vertebrate or invertebrate hosts, it enjoys cosmopolitan distribution. Little is known, however, of the factors which govern the natural resistance of hosts which are insusceptible to infection with it.

ACQUIRED IMMUNITY

Once infected with *Fasciola hepatica,* animals retain the parasites for such protracted periods that studies on the resistance of recovered animals are not feasible. Furthermore, it is not known whether animals while infected will resist a superimposed infection. A partial resistance can be induced artificially, however, in rabbits by vaccinating them with an emulsion of the parasite over a period of three weeks.[29] Flukes which later establish themselves in such immunized rabbits soon become calcified, and they fail to reach maturity. Eggs never appear in the feces of infected immune hosts.

Infections with *Fasciola hepatica* can be identified by the fixation [30] and precipitin reactions,[31] as well as by the skin test.[32] There

[28] H. Vogel, *Arch. f. Schiffs-u. Tropen-Hyg.,* 36: 384 (1932) ; E. C. Herber, *J. Parasitol.,* 24: 474 (1938).

[29] K. B. Kerr and O. L. Petkovich, *J. Parasitol.,* 21: 319 (1935).

[30] O. Wagner, *Ztschr. f. Immunitätsforsch. u. exper. Therap.,* 84: 225 (1935).

[31] W. A. Hoffman and T. Rivers, *Porto Rico Rev. Pub. Health & Trop. Med.,* 4: 589 (1929).

[32] H. K. Sievers and R. Oyarzun, *Compt. rend. Soc. de biol.,* 110: 630 (1932) ; G. Curasson, *Bull. de l'Acad. Vet. de France,* 8: 77 (1935).

is a comparatively broad specificity in the reactions, however, for *Fasciola* antigens will also serve for diagnosing schistosomiasis [33] as well as infection with *Dicrocoelium dendriticum*.[34] Some authorities feel that immunological tests have little place in diagnosing *Fasciola* infections, since eggs of the parasite can be found in the feces of infected animals without difficulty.[35]

OTHER TREMATODIASES

The immunology of only a few other trematode infections has been studied at all, and these involve strictly animal parasites of no great economic importance. Fish acquire a partial immunity to the monogenetic trematode *Epibdella melleni* on being placed in aquarium tanks with the parasite. Initially the fish become intensely infected, but gradually they lose their parasites, and they are not reinfected despite continued exposure.[36] Intestinal infections of fish with various species of *Hamacreadium* do not confer an appreciable resistance to reinfection with the homologous form.[37] Similarly, cloacal infection of herring gulls with *Parorchis acanthus* does not protect these birds against a second infection with the same parasite.[38] The failure of these last infections to elicit a significant immune response in the infected animals is not especially surprising, because when compared with the schistosomes the parasites cause only insignificant damage to their hosts. However, ducks and rats have been shown to acquire resistance to the caecal trematode *Zygocotyle lunata* as a result of a prior infection.[39]

ADDITIONAL IMMUNOLOGICAL SUBJECTS

CERCARICIDAL ACTION OF NORMAL SERUMS

Although the normal blood serums of many animals have long been known to possess bactericidal power and that of certain primates to neutralize filterable viruses or to lyse trypanosomes, no

[33] A. Hassan and M. Betashe, *J. Egyptian M. A.*, 17: 991 (1934).
[34] O. Wagner, *Ztschr. f. Immunitätsforsch. u. exper. Therap.*, 84: 225 (1935).
[35] G. Curasson, *Bull. de l'Acad. Vet. de France*, 8: 77 (1935).
[36] T. L. Jahn and L. R. Kuhn, *Biol. Bull.*, 62: 89 (1932) ; R. F. Nigrelli and C. M. Breder, Jr., *J. Parasitol.*, 20: 259 (1934).
[37] O. R. McCoy, *J. Parasitol.*, 17: 1 (1930).
[38] R. M. Cable, *J. Parasitol.*, 23: 559 (1937).
[39] C. H. Willey, *Zoologica*, June, 1941.

similar action of normal serum upon helminths was known until recently. It has now been established that the fresh serum of many animals, representing all classes of vertebrates, has such an action upon the trematode cercariae, quickly killing these forms and often lysing them. The serums of some animals, however, including the cat and the rabbit, lack the property. The substance responsible for this antagonistic action is highly labile, since it is lost quickly by heating or desiccation and by storage. Agencies which destroy complement also inactivate the cercaricidal power, although the cercaricidal effect is believed to be distinct from complement. The cercaricidal action of the serum may be in part responsible for natural resistance. Infection often fails in animals whose serums possess the cercaricidal property, although in other cases no such correlation is observed.[40] The cercaricidal action of human serum may account in part for the severe local dermatitis in man after exposure to certain animal schistosomes.[41]

The mucus of certain fish manifests an action on monogenetic trematodes essentially similar to that described for the normal serum. Usually the mucus of highly resistant fish exerts the most powerful action, whereas that of very susceptible species affects the parasites only slightly.[42] The mucus is therefore believed to have some significance in the natural resistance of fish to their trematode parasites.

IMMUNITY IN THE MOLLUSCAN HOST

Brief consideration must be given the development of immunity against trematodes by the molluscan host. The problem has been carefully investigated in snails. It is known that cercariae which have been freed from a snail never reinfect the same individual to pass their metacercarial stage, nor do they infect other snails already infected with the same parasite.[43] Furthermore, double infections involving certain species of cercariae seldom or never occur,

[40] J. T. Culbertson and S. B. Talbot, *Science,* 82: 525 (1935); J. T. Culbertson, *J. Parasitol.,* 22: 111 (1936); M. A. Tubangui and V. A. Masilungan, *Philipp. J. Sci.,* 60: 393 (1936).
[41] S. Brackett, *Arch. Dermat. & Syph.,* 42: 410 (1940).
[42] R. F. Nigrelli, *J. Parasitol.,* 21: 438 (1935).
[43] G. F. Winfield, *J. Parasitol.,* 19: 130 (1932); L. O. Nolf and W. W. Cort: *J. Parasitol.,* 19: 38 (1933).

evidently because the immune response made by the snail to one trematode is exerted also against some other species.[44] From these observations it is clear that snails acquire an immunity after infection by trematodes. To this can be added the well-established fact that any species of snail is naturally resistant to many trematodes. In fact, most trematodes invade only a sharply limited range of snail hosts, these often being found within a single genus.

[44] W. W. Cort, D. B. McMullen, and S. Brackett, *J. Parasitol.*, 21: 433 (1935).

Chapter XV

THE CESTODIASES

THE CESTODE PARASITES occur both as dwellers in the intestinal lumen and as somatic tissue invaders in both man and animals. Generally, the immunological response to the lumen-dwelling forms is meager, and sometimes it is impossible to demonstrate. In contrast, powerful immune reactions usually are made to the somatic parasites. The site occupied by each cestode should therefore be kept in mind while reading the present chapter.

DIPHYLLOBOTHRIUM INFECTIONS

NATURAL RESISTANCE

HOST RESTRICTION

The most important member of the genus *Diphyllobothrium,* namely, *Diphyllobothrium latum,* has a comparatively broad choice of host in all of its developmental stages. As an adult it occurs in most fish-eating mammals, particularly in the carnivora (dog, fox, cat, mink, bear, sea lion, walrus), but also in man and pig. The procercoid stage is confined to several species of copepod of the genera *Diaptomus* and *Cyclops.* A large number of fresh-water fish serve as hosts for the plerocercoid or sparganum stage, some of the commoner forms being pike, perch, eel, white fish, salmon, and trout.

Another species of this genus, *Diphyllobothrium mansoni,* has some importance as a human parasite in the Far East. Its adult stage occurs in many carnivores, but probably never in man. The first larval stage infects copepods of the genera *Diaptomus* and *Cyclops.* The second larval stage invades snakes and frogs principally, but also man, both by transmission from the cold-blooded vertebrates and by ingestion of the copepod host.

Man is also susceptible to experimental infection with the sparganum of one other species of *Diphyllobothrium, Diphyllobothrium mansonoides,* a form living as an adult in several carnivora (for example, dog, cat, and bobcat). The first larval stage infects several species of *Cyclops,* and the second larval stage, or sparganum, invades the water snake and field mouse, as well as (probably) man and certain monkeys. The sparganum is able to reestablish itself without further development on transfer to several animals, including man, *Macacus rhesus* and ring-tail monkeys, and mice and rats.

From the foregoing it is clear that tapeworms of the genus *Diphyllobothrium* have a broad potential host range not only for their adult stage but also for the sparganum stage. The factors which determine natural resistance are not yet known. The age of the host may be significant. One species of *Diphyllobothrium* which is found naturally in gulls occurs almost exclusively in young birds. This form is regularly eliminated by the gull when an age is reached at which the host's body temperature is established at a high level and at which the host is completely feathered.[1]

ACQUIRED IMMUNITY

RESISTANCE TO REINFECTION

Little is yet known of immunity acquired through infection with the *Diphyllobothrium* tapeworms, although according to one report an immunity against reinfection is developed by man, lasting two or three years. Furthermore, dogs which already harbor *Taenia serrata* are refractory to a superimposed infection with *Diphyllobothrium.*[2] The immunity in both cases is probably lost when the worms of the original infection are expelled,[3] and the possibility remains that the apparent immunity is more truly a matter of parasite crowding in the intestine.

ANTIBODY PRODUCTION

Antibody is produced very poorly after infection with adult *Diphyllobothrium* tapeworms and is usually not detectable.[4] How-

[1] L. J. Thomas, *Anat. Rec. (Suppl.),* 78: 104 (1940).
[2] E. Brumpt, *Précis de parasitologie,* Paris, Masson et Cie (1937); V. Tarassov, *Ann. de parasitol.,* 15: 524 (1937).
[3] R. Wigand, *Zentralbl. f. Bakt.,* 135: 216 (1935).
[4] O. Sievers, *Ztschr. f. Immunitätsforsch. u. exper. Therap.,* 84: 208 (1935).

ever, complement-fixing antibody appears in the serum of monkeys after infection with the sparganum of *Diphyllobothrium manso-noides*.[5] Antibody against the adult worms can be elicited in animals by inoculating extracts of the adult worm,[6] and it has been reported also in persons with *Diphyllobothrium* anemia after the oral administration of the worm substance to the patients.[7]

PROPHYLAXIS

Only a few efforts to protect animals against experimental infection with *Diphyllobothrium* parasites by vaccination have been reported. Puppies are said to become partially immune to *Diphyllobothrium latum* after subcutaneous or oral administration of the worm substance.[8] Monkeys given repeated injections of adult *Diphyllobothrium mansonoides* substance resist subsequent exposure to the procercoids of this cestode. The resistance of the monkeys is manifested, not by a lesser number of parasites, but by their encapsulation in the vaccinated animals compared with the controls. Furthermore, the condition simulating elephantiasis noted in the control animals after infection with procercoids is not observable in vaccinated monkeys.[9] Prophylaxis of man by vaccination is perhaps inadvisable and has not as yet been attempted.

DIAGNOSIS

Since neither the antigen of *Diphyllobothrium latum* nor antibody specific for it can regularly be found in the serum of human carriers of the parasite, serological tests are generally useless for the diagnosis of this infection.[10] Occasionally skin tests with *Diphyllobothrium latum* substance are positive, although the skin test as yet has been too little used to ascertain its value as a diagnostic aid.[11] The serums of dogs which have suffered an intensive infec-

[5] J. F. Mueller and O. D. Chapman, *J. Parasitol.*, 23: 561 (1937).
[6] O. Sievers, *Ztschr. f. Immunitätsforsch. u. exper. Therap.*, 84: 208 (1935).
[7] O. Sievers, *Acta Med. Scandinav.*, 96: 289 (1938).
[8] T. Ohira, *Tr. Far East. Assoc. Trop. Med., 9th Cong.*, 1: 601 (1935).
[9] J. F. Mueller and O. D. Chapman, *J. Parasitol.*, 23: 561 (1937) ; J. F. Mueller, *Am. J. Trop. Med.*, 18: 303 (1938).
[10] O. Sievers, *Ztschr. f. Immunitätsforsch. u. exper. Therap.*, 84: 208 (1935).
[11] M. Brunner, *J. Immunol.*, 15: 83 (1928).

tion with *Diphyllobothrium mansoni* deviates complement when added to an extract of the adult parasite.[12]

The detection of complement-fixing antibodies serves to identify infection with the sparganum of *Diphyllobothrium mansonoides* in *Macacus rhesus*. The presence of as few as two spargana in the tissues suffices to elicit the fixation antibodies.[13]

TAENIA INFECTIONS

NATURAL RESISTANCE

HOST RESTRICTION

Cestodes of the genus *Taenia* are characterized by extremely limited choice of host both for the adult and for the larval (cysticercus) stage. Often the adult parasite, particularly, invades only a single vertebrate species. *Taenia saginata* and *Taenia solium*, for example, occur as adults only in man. The cysticercus of *Taenia saginata* likewise has a sharply restricted host range, this form occurring only in cattle. The range of the cysticercus of *Taenia solium* is slightly broader, including both man and pig.

The animal *Taenias* also have a restricted choice of host. *Taenia serrata* is found as an adult only in the dog and the cat and as a cysticercus only in the rabbit. Likewise, the adult *Taenia crassicollis* infects only felines including the cat and several wild cats, and its cysticercus only rats and mice.

Although few species of animals are susceptible to infection with each of the *Taenia* cestodes, the factors responsible for the natural resistance of other animals are obscure. In some cases natural resistance is correlated with the presence of certain enzymes in the digestive juice, although such a relationship is not yet established experimentally. Older rats are more resistant to cysticercosis than young rats. Female rats are more resistant to cysticercosis than are male animals. The females lose some of this resistance if castrated or if given the male sex hormone, whereas male rats treated with female sex hormone manifest an enhanced resistance.[14]

[12] M. Ravetta, *Haematologica*, 18: 69 (1937).
[13] J. F. Mueller and O. D. Chapman, *J. Parasitol.*, 23: 561 (1937).
[14] D. H. Campbell, *Science*, 89: 415 (1939); D. H. Campbell and L. R. Melcher, *J. Infect. Dis.*, 66: 184 (1940); M. R. Curtis, W. F. Dunning and F. D. Bullock, *Am. J. Cancer*, 17: 894 (1933).

ACQUIRED IMMUNITY

RESISTANCE TO REINFECTION

The fact that man usually suffers infection only with a single intestinal tapeworm is often interpreted as evidence of immunity to reinfection. However, the readiness with which tapeworms are regenerated in man from scolices not dislodged along with the proglottids by anthelminthics suggests either that any immunity against reinfection is of very brief duration or else that the initial infection must persist in order that immunity be manifested.

The question of resistance to a superimposed infection with cestodes has been studied carefully in animals infected with either the adult or the larval stage of *Taenia crassicollis*. The presence of adult worms in the intestine of the cat does not protect this animal from reinfection.[15] Rats, on the other hand, which have suffered an initial somatic infection with the cysticerci resist a second feeding of onchospheres.[16] The resistance of the rat persists for at least two months, even when those cysticerci which have developed from the initial feeding of onchospheres are surgically removed.[17] Likewise, rabbits become resistant to reinfection with onchospheres of *Taenia serrata*, and cows acquire resistance to reinfection with the onchospheres of *Taenia saginata* as a result of an initial infection with the homologous cysticerci.[18] The resistance against the cysticercus of rats is transmitted by female animals to their young.[19]

The resistance acquired against either somatic or intestinal cestodes is generally rigidly specific. An established infection with *Taenia serrata* in the dog, however, is said to inhibit an artificially superimposed infection with *Diphyllobothrium latum*,[20] although this effect may more safely be credited to crowding than to an immune response.

[15] H. M. Miller, Jr., *J. Prevent. Med.*, 6: 17 (1932).
[16] H. M. Miller, Jr., *Proc. Soc. Exper. Biol. & Med.*, 28: 467 (1931).
[17] H. M. Miller, Jr., and E. Massie, *J. Prevent. Med.*, 6: 31 (1932).
[18] K. B. Kerr, *Am. J. Hyg.*, 22: 169 (1935), and *J. Parasitol.*, 20: 328 (1934); W. J. Penfold, H. B. Penfold, and M. Phillips, *M. J. Australia*, 1: 417 (1936).
[19] H. M. Miller, Jr., *Proc. Soc. Exper. Biol. & Med.*, 29: 1124 (1932), and *Am. J. Hyg.*, 21: 456 (1935).
[20] R. Wigand, *Zentralbl. f. Bakt.*, 135: 216 (1935).

ANTIBODY PRODUCTION

Antibody is regularly demonstrable in somatic *Taenia* infections, although in the intestinal taeniases its demonstration is difficult or impossible. In *Taenia solium* cysticercosis of man and of pig, complement-fixing antibodies and precipitins are detectable.[21] Two types of functional antibody have been described in rats infected with cysticerci of *Taenia crassicollis*. The first is detectable during the first week of infection and acts directly on the larvae before their encystment and sometimes destroys them. It is an absorbable substance which can also be elicited by vaccination. The second antibody is detectable only several weeks after infection and acts on larvae after their encystment. The latter substance is not absorbable and is not elicited by vaccination.[22]

PASSIVE IMMUNITY

The serum from animals with somatic *Taenia* infections confers to normal animals resistance against the homologous parasite. This fact has been demonstrated most conclusively in the case of rats infected with the cysticerci of *Taenia crassicollis*. If the serum is given simultaneously with the feeding of onchospheres, it prevents almost completely the development of the cysticerci, although when given more than nine days after the onchospheres are fed, little or no inhibition of cysticercal development occurs.[23] Serum obtained from rats which have been heavily infected for at least ten days is best for passive protection, but that from rats artificially immunized with tapeworm substance also serves.[24] Immunity against infection with the cysticerci of *Taenia serrata* can also be passively transferred in the serum from infected or artificially immunized rabbits to normal rabbits.[25]

[21] W. P. MacArthur, *Tr. Roy. Soc. Trop. Med. & Hyg.*, 26: 525 (1933) ; J. Rothfeld, *Deutsche Ztschr. f. Nervenheilk.*, 137: 93 (1935) ; A. Trawinski, *Zentralbl. f. Bakt.*, 136: 116 (1936).
[22] D. H. Campbell, *J. Immunol.*, 35: 205 (1938).
[23] H. M. Miller, Jr., *Proc. Soc. Exper. Biol. & Med.*, 30: 82 (1932), and *Am. J. Hyg.*, 19: 270 (1934).
[24] H. M. Miller, Jr., and M. L. Gardiner, *J. Prevent. Med.*, 6: 479 (1932).
[25] K. B. Kerr, *Am. J. Hyg.*, 22: 169 (1935) ; A. B. Leonard, *Am. J. Hyg.*, 32: 117 (1940).

MECHANISM OF IMMUNITY

The mechanism of the immunity against reinfection with cysticerci undoubtedly depends primarily upon the action of humoral factors, inasmuch as serum transferred from highly immune animals will completely protect normal animals. The serum may be directly parasiticidal in function, but probably the fixed tissues of the host also play a role. The intestinal mucosa of immune rabbits, for example, seems to present a significant mechanical barrier against infection with onchospheres of *Taenia serrata*. At least, the further development of onchospheres is completely inhibited in immune animals infected by gavage, whereas, if hatched onchospheres are injected into the mesenteric vein, they experience some development. Usually, however, the developing forms are soon killed from local tissue responses initiated undoubtedly by the presence of specific antibody. In normal rabbits, for example, the slight local tissue response which generally occurs to the cysticerci of *Taenia serrata* can be markedly accelerated and intensified by the injection of a specific immune serum.[26]

PROPHYLAXIS

When rats are repeatedly injected parenterally with the substance of dried, adult *Taenia crassicollis*, they acquire resistance to infection with the cysticerci of this parasite.[27] The resistance thus acquired persists for at least several months after the last immunizing injection.[28] Partial protection is also afforded by injecting the rats with antigens from other worms of the same genus or with material from worms of the related genus *Hymenolepis*.[29] To be effective for prophylaxis an antigenic emulsion must contain the proteins of the worm.[30] At least, when the purified polysaccharide of the cysticerci of *Taenia crassicollis* is injected, little or no immunity is developed, even though antibody is formed against the polysaccharide.[31]

In similar manner immunity can be conferred upon rabbits by

[26] A. B. Leonard, *Am. J. Hyg.*, 32: 117 (1940).
[27] H. M. Miller, Jr., *Proc. Soc. Exper. Biol. & Med.*, 27: 926 (1930).
[28] H. M. Miller, Jr., *J. Prevent. Med.*, 6: 37 (1932).
[29] H. M. Miller, Jr., *Am. J. Hyg.*, 21: 27 (1935).
[30] D. H. Campbell, *Am. J. Hyg.*, 23: 104 (1936).
[31] D. H. Campbell, *J. Infect. Dis.*, 65: 12 (1939).

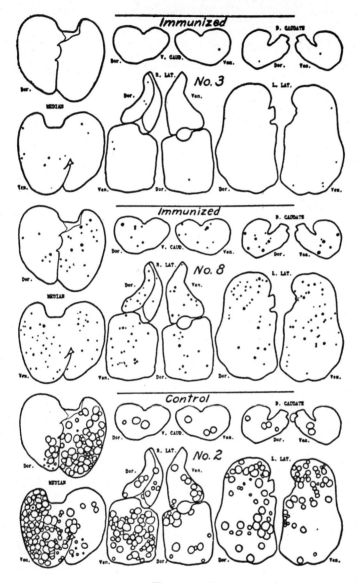

FIGURE 3

DIAGRAMS OF LIVER LOBES OF TWO IMMUNIZED AND
ONE CONTROL RAT INFECTED WITH 600 ONCHOSPHERES
OF *TAENIA CRASSICOLLIS*

Relative number and size of living cysts and of dead cysts in artificially
immunized and control animals are shown. The rats were autopsied 26 days
after infection.

vaccination with fresh or powdered adult *Taenia serrata*.[32] Resistance against infection with the adult *Taenia* cestodes is not developed by vaccination.[33]

DIAGNOSIS

Somatic *Taenia* infections can be rather easily diagnosed by immunological methods. The complement fixation test and the precipitin test have been employed successfully to identify human cysticercosis with *Taenia solium*.[34] Pig infections with the same parasite have been detected by the precipitin reaction.[35]

Skin tests also have been employed in the somatic taeniases. Human beings with cysticercosis due to *Taenia solium* and rabbits infected with the larvae of *Taenia serrata* give a positive test.[36] Since these skin reactions can be obtained with antigens from related cestodes, as well as with the specific parasite, the response must be of a group character.[37] Skin reactions have also been reported in human intestinal taeniasis,[38] although they are observed less consistently than in the somatic infections.

MULTICEPS INFECTION

NATURAL RESISTANCE

Cestodes of the genus *Multiceps* occur primarily in animals, although rarely human infections also are reported. Three species of the genus have most significance, *Multiceps multiceps*, *Multiceps glomeratus*, and *Multiceps serialis*. *Multiceps multiceps* is found almost exclusively as an adult in the dog, although the wolf also is probably susceptible. The coenurus or larval stage occurs in the brain of many animals, chiefly herbivores, such as sheep, goat, cow, horse, antelope, gazelle, and chamois. Monkey and man also harbor this coenurus. *Multiceps glomeratus* is comparatively little known,

[32] K. B. Kerr, *Am. J. Hyg.*, 22: 169 (1935).
[33] T. Ohira, *Tr. Far East. Assoc. Trop. Med., 9th Congr.*, 1: 601 (1935).
[34] W. P. MacArthur, *Tr. Roy. Soc. Trop. Med. and Hyg.*, 26: 525 (1933) ; J. Rothfeld, *Deutsche Ztschr. f. Nervenheilk.*, 137: 93 (1935) ; A. Trawinski and J. Rothfeld, *Zentralbl. f. Bakt.*, 134: 472 (1935).
[35] A. Trawinski, *Zentralbl. f. Bakt.*, 136: 116 (1936).
[36] D. R. A. Wharton, *Am. J. Hyg.*, 14: 477 (1931).
[37] L. Morenas, *Lyon Méd.*, 151: 636 (1933).
[38] M. Brunner, *J. Immunol.*, 15: 83 (1928) ; H.-L. Chung and T. T'ung, *Tr. Roy. Soc. Trop. Med. & Hyg.*, 32: 697 (1939).

but has been found as a coenurus in the gerbille and in man. The mouse and rabbit can also be experimentally infected.[39] The dog is susceptible to the adult worm. *Multiceps serialis* in its adult stage infects the dog, the wolf, and the fox. The coenurus invades intramuscular connective tissue of several rodents, including rabbit, squirrel, and coypu, and certain primates, including man, baboon, and mandrill.

ACQUIRED IMMUNITY

Little is yet known of the possible immunity acquired by man and animals after *Multiceps* infection. No resistance is acquired by dogs against the adult worm as the result of a first infection with *Multiceps glomeratus*.[40] Antibody appears in rabbits three to four weeks after infection with the coenurus of *Multiceps serialis*. One proved human case reported several years ago, however, gave neither skin nor fixation tests.[41] Rabbits infected experimentally with the coenurus of *Multiceps glomeratus* give a skin reaction to the antigens of the specific parasite, but not to antigens from larval *Multiceps serialis* or *Taenia serrata*.[42] The serum of a rabbit with the coenurus of *Multiceps multiceps* has long been known to contain antibody, since it will sensitize passively a guinea pig to the homologous worm substance. The serum of one such rabbit continued to harbor the sensitizing substance for at least eight months after the surgical removal of the coenurus.[43]

ECHINOCOCCUS INFECTION

There are several species of the genus *Echinococcus* besides *Echinococcus granulosus,* and some of these may be responsible for hydatid disease in man. As yet, however, these forms if present in man have not been satisfactorily differentiated, and practically all the reported human cases are considered due to the single species *Echinococcus granulosus.* Essentially all the immunological information on echinococcus infection as yet available is also referred to *Echinococcus granulosus,* although the designation possibly is often incorrect.

[39] P. A. Clapham, *J. Helminthol.,* 18: 45 (1940).   [40] *Ibid.*
[41] G. Bonnall, C. Joyeux, and P. Bosch, *Bull. Soc. path. exot.,* 26: 1060 (1933).
[42] P. A. Clapham, *J. Helminthol.,* 18: 45 (1940).
[43] P. Bosch, *Marseille-méd.,* 71: 291 (1934).

NATURAL RESISTANCE

HOST RESTRICTION

The adult stage of *Echinococcus granulosus* occurs only in the dog, the wolf, the jackal, and possibly the cat.[44] The larval or hydatid stage, on the other hand, invades many different kinds of animal, including sheep, cow, moose, antelope, horse, zebra, pig, camel, elephant, kangaroo, giraffe, tapir, rabbit, squirrel, cat, leopard, *Macacus* and *Cynomolgus* monkeys, and man.

FACTORS INFLUENCING NATURAL RESISTANCE

Very few of the factors which influence natural resistance to *Echinococcus granulosus* have yet been established, because of the difficulties attending the experimental study of this infection. The digestive juice probably plays a role in the resistance of most hosts to the adult stage of the parasite. At least the membranes of the hydatid are digested by the intestinal juice of many resistant animals, but not by that of the susceptible dog or cat.[45] In an effort to depress their natural resistance to this parasite, pigeons have been kept on a vitamin-free diet for a considerable period. The birds do not become susceptible, however, either to the adult or the larval parasite.[46]

ACQUIRED IMMUNITY

RESISTANCE TO REINFECTION

No adequate evidence is yet available to show whether or not infection with hydatid disease confers resistance to reinfection. The fact that many persons in whom an initial cyst is ruptured later develop many cysts hardly contra-indicates the acquisition of immunity, for severe anaphylactic shock is usually experienced by a patient as the result of cyst rupture. At this time the principal specific defense forces of the host are momentarily completely or largely incapacitated, and the patient is probably peculiarly susceptible to reinfection. Since at other times, on the contrary, antibody is present in considerable concentration, the immune response

[44] F. Lorincz, *Zentralbl. f. Bakt.*, 129: 1 (1933).
[45] D. A. Berberian, *J. Helminthol.*, 14: 21 (1936).
[46] P. Pavlov, *Bull. Soc. path. exot.*, 33: 93 (1940).

to infection must be intense and might effectively inhibit reinfection with the homologous parasite.

ANTIBODY PRODUCTION

Complement-fixing antibodies and precipitins reactive with hydatid fluid have long been known to be formed after infection with hydatid disease. Little or no information is yet available as to the period required for the serum reactions to become positive. Antibody usually persists in the serum for at least several months after surgical removal of the cysts.

PASSIVE TRANSFER

No adequate attempt has been reported to determine whether or not resistance to hydatid disease can be passively transferred with the serum, largely because of the difficulties attending investigations of experimental infections with this parasite. It is known that serum from a dog with any of various intestinal *Taenias* does not protect mice from hydatid "sand" injected intraperitoneally,[47] but serum from such an infection is certainly poor in protective antibody, if not entirely devoid of this substance. Greater success might attend an experiment in which serum from an animal with a heterologous somatic cestode infection were used, since such serums generally are comparatively rich in antibody. Undoubtedly, however, the best effect, if any, would be obtained with specific immune serum.

MECHANISM OF IMMUNITY

Humoral antibody and the cellular agencies together probably account for any resistance that is acquired against hydatid disease. The walling off of the parasite by the laying down of a fibrous capsule is the most obvious evidence of this defense. Such a response is accelerated and magnified in the case of animals which have become partially resistant at the time of infection.

PROPHYLAXIS

Sheep and probably some other susceptible animals can be partially protected from infection with the hydatid stage of *Echinococ-*

[47] F. Dévé, *Compt. rend. Soc. de biol.*, 113: 1443 (1933).

cus granulosus by previous vaccination with killed antigens prepared from the hydatid cyst fluid and membranes. The vaccinated animals wall off subsequently established parasites more successfully than do normal animals. An Arthus type of reaction generally occurs about each small cyst in the immunized animal.[48] Dogs also are said partially to resist infection with the intestinal adult stage of *Echinococcus granulosus* after vaccination with hydatid cyst material.[49]

Attempts to immunize laboratory rodents against experimental infection by subcutaneous injections of hydatid membrane have not succeeded.[50] No curative effect upon developed cysts is revealed following the administration of hydatid "anatoxin," [51] an antigenic product obtained by formolizing hydatid fluid.[52]

DIAGNOSIS

Although antibody does not usually develop in animals with the intestinal stage of *Echinococcus granulosus,* it appears quite regularly in persons and animals with somatic infections with the larval stage of this parasite. The detection of this antibody serves admirably, therefore, to identify hydatid disease in man as well as in lower animals.

The precipitin test has had comparatively little use in the diagnosis of hydatid disease, for it is positive in known cases less often than other procedures. In one survey the serums of only about 50 percent of the proved cases tested gave a precipitin test.[53] The complement fixation test as first devised for hydatid disease by Ghedini is a fairly reliable diagnostic procedure, both for human and animal infections. Success with the procedure depends largely on the skill of the technician. When proper methods are followed, the test has a high percentage of accuracy,[54] and it is especially useful in diagnosing recurrent or residual cysts in patients already

[48] E. L. Turner, E. W. Dennis, and D. A. Berberian, *J. Parasitol.,* 23: 43 (1937).
[49] E. L. Turner, E. W. Dennis, and D. A. Berberian, *J. Egyptian M. A.,* 18: 636 (1935) ; E. L. Turner, D. A. Berberian, and E. W. Dennis, *J. Parasitol.,* 22: 14 (1935).
[50] F. Dévé, *Compt. rend. Soc. de biol.,* 115: 1025 (1934).
[51] *Ibid.,* p. 954.
[52] I. L. Y. Apphatie, *Rev. sud-amér. de méd. et de chir.,* 3: 785 (1932).
[53] F. Hoder, *Fortschr. d. Med.,* 51: 959 (1933).
[54] R. H. Goodale and H. Krischner, *Am. J. Trop. Med.,* 10: 71 (1930) ; F. Hoder, *Fortschr. d. Med.,* 51: 959 (1933).

operated on.[55] Unfortunately the community in antigens among various cestodes leads to positive results as well in other cestodiases, although with reasonable interpretation of clinical signs and symptoms such confusing results can generally be recognized and ruled out.

The simplest procedure for diagnosing hydatid disease is the skin test, in which a small amount (0.5 cc.) of hydatid fluid antigen is injected intradermally. Both immediate (Magath) and delayed (Casoni) skin reactions usually occur in human cases.[56] The immediate response develops as a wheal two to four centimeters in diameter with pseudopods, the maximum size being attained in ten to twenty minutes. Gradually thereafter this immediate reaction subsides. The delayed response, which is of a true local anaphylactic or Arthus type, begins one-half hour or so after the injection of antigen, reaches its peak in two to six hours, and gradually recedes during the ensuing twenty-four to thirty-six hours. The skin test has proved useful in the hands of most investigators, up to 100 percent positive results having been reported in known cases of hydatid disease.[57] The test is positive in infected animals, as well as in man, and can also be elicited in animals which have been previously immunized by a series of injections of hydatid fluid.[58] The repetition of skin tests in man is usually discouraged, since normal persons also, if tested several times, finally become positive.[59] The skin test is consistently negative in dogs with the intestinal stage of *Echinococcus granulosus*.[60]

The skin reaction and the test for serum antibody are positive so long as cysts remain in the patient, and they may continue so for from five to seven years after the surgical removal of all cysts.[61] Positive reactions ten years or more after operation, however, in-

[55] K. D. Fairley and C. H. Kellaway, *Australian and New Zealand J. Surg.*, 2: 236 (1933).

[56] J. H. Botteri, *Klin. Wchnschr.*, 8: 836 (1929).

[57] E. and B. von Bassewitz, *Brasil-Med.*, 43: 1138 (1929); K. D. Fairley, *M. J. Australia*, 1: 472 (1929); H.-L. Chung and T. T'ung, *Tr. Roy. Soc. Trop. Med. & Hyg.*, 32: 697 (1939).

[58] E. Cubone, *Boll. d. Ist.-Sieroterap. milanese*, 8: 519 (1929).

[59] E. Sergent, M. Fourestier, and E. Jiminez-Galliano, *Bull. Acad. Med.*, 121: 180 (1939); E. Rist, *Presse Méd.* 47: 201 (1939); R. Rubegni, *Policlinico (Seg. pratica)*, 46: 1859 (1939).

[60] E. L. Turner, E. W. Dennis, and D. A. Berberian, *J. Parasitol.*, 21: 180 (1935).

[61] A. M. Bonanno, *Boll. d. Sez. Ital., Soc. Internat. di Microb.*, 3: 67 (1931).

dicate reinfection or incomplete removal of the initial cyst.[62] Negative reactions show freedom from infection in at least 95 percent of all cases.[63]

Antigen for the biologic diagnosis of hydatid disease is usually obtained as the fluid from hydatid cysts. Pure, untreated cyst fluid is commonly regarded as the best material for the purpose,[64] but the active elements sometimes occur in such dilution in the native fluid that various procedures for their concentration have been proposed.[65] The cyst membranes are generally deficient in suitable antigens.

Antigens which serve for the skin test, as well as for the in vitro tests with serum, are present also in many heterologous cestodes. In fact they often occur in these heterologous sources in greater amount than in the specific parasite. They have been derived from *Taenia saginata, Taenia serrata, Taenia crassicollis, Hymenolepis fraterna, Moniezia expansa, Raillietina cesticillus,* and *Diphyllobothrium mansonoides.* A protein-free polysaccharide from *Taenia crassicollis* also serves as antigen for the skin test (Figure 4).[66]

The fact that antigens for diagnosing hydatid disease occur in so many heterologous cestodes indicates that group reactions are rather general in the cestodiases. These are seen best in somatic infections. Cysticercosis in man, for example, can be identified by skin tests or fixation tests in which hydatid fluid is the antigen. Likewise, a positive skin test has been obtained in one human case of experimental sparganosis tested with hydatid fluid.[67] Occasionally positive tests have also been reported in the intestinal taeniases.

When the antibody-containing serum from a patient with echinococcus disease is injected locally into the skin of a normal person, the normal person will then give an immediate type of skin reaction (Prausnitz-Küstner test) if hydatid fluid antigen is injected to the same site. Usually an interval of twenty-four to forty-eight hours must elapse before the antigen can be injected, perhaps because the antibodies must first fix themselves upon the tissue cells.

[62] K. D. Fairley, *M. J. Australia,* 1: 472 (1929).
[63] C. H. Kellaway and K. D. Fairley, *M. J. Australia,* 19th Yr.: 340 (1932).
[64] F. Cantani, *Boll. d. Sez. Ital., Soc. Internat. di Microb.,* 1: 195 (1929).
[65] E. W. Dennis, *J. Parasitol.,* 23: 62 (1937).
[66] J. T. Culbertson and H. M. Rose, *J. Clin. Investigation,* 20: 249 (1941).
[67] *Ibid.*

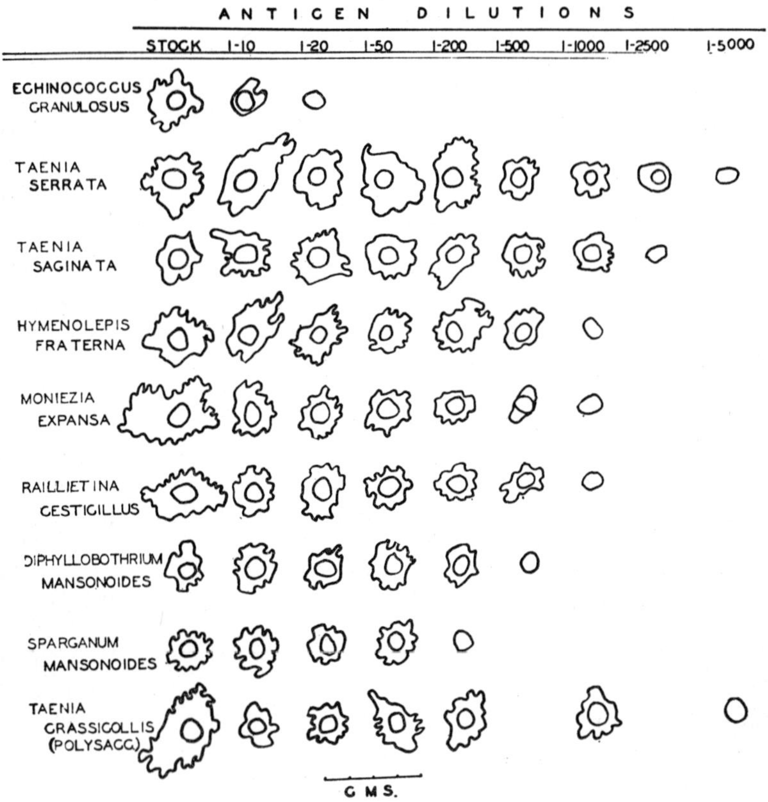

FIGURE 4

IMMEDIATE SKIN REACTIONS IN A PATIENT WITH ECHINO-
COCCUS DISEASE AFTER INJECTION WITH THE DESIG-
NATED DILUTIONS OF EQUIVALENT EXTRACTS OF
VARIOUS CESTODES

Tests with a purified polysaccharide derived from *Taenia crassicollis* also
are shown. The inner circle represents the outline of the initial bleb; the outer
irregular line shows the greatest limits attained by the wheal in fifteen minutes.

Antigens from any of the related cestodes which elicit the reaction in an infected patient will also serve for the test in the passively sensitized person.[68]

HYMENOLEPIS INFECTIONS

NATURAL RESISTANCE

HOST RESTRICTION

Two species of the genus Hymenolepis have been studied immunologically, *Hymenolepis nana* (including the rodent strain, *Hymenolepis nana*, variety *fraterna*) and *Hymenolepis diminuta*. *Hymenolepis nana* is found in human beings, certain monkeys, gerbilles, rats, and mice, and after experimental infection in guinea pigs. *Hymenolepis diminuta* is found as an adult in man, mouse, rat, monkey, and possibly the dog and as a larval form in various insects, including lepidopterans, ear-wigs, fleas, and cockroaches.

FACTORS INFLUENCING NATURAL RESISTANCE

The factors responsible for susceptibility or natural resistance to *Hymenolepis* cestodes have not been determined. Age certainly is significant. Persons of the five- to fourteen-year age group are most frequently infected with *Hymenolepis nana*,[69] and younger rats and mice are more susceptible than older animals to the rodent strain *Hymenolepis fraterna*.[70] A poor diet, such as one consisting of bread and water,[71] as well as an intercurrent infection with bacterial disease,[72] predisposes rodents to *Hymenolepis fraterna*.

ACQUIRED IMMUNITY

RESISTANCE TO REINFECTION

Mice and rats already infected with *Hymenolepis fraterna* or *Hymenolepis diminuta* resist a superimposed infection with the homologous parasite.[73] There are two points of view at present on the cause of this resistance. According to one, no true immunity is developed, and the apparent resistance to reinfection is more prop-

[68] *Ibid.*   [69] G. F. Otto, *J. Parasitol.*, 21: 443 (1935).
[70] D. A. Shorb, *Am. J. Hyg.*, 18: 74 (1933).   [71] *Ibid.*
[72] A. V. Hunninen, *J. Parasitol.*, 22: 84 (1936).
[73] A. V. Hunninen, *Am. J. Hyg.* 22: 414 (1935) ; M. Palais, *Compt. rend. Soc. de biol.*, 117: 1016 (1934) ; D. A. Shorb, *Am. J. Hyg.*, 18: 74 (1933).

erly a "pseudo-premunization," consisting simply in competition for the available space in the intestine of the host, with the result that the worms given in the reinfecting dose are crowded out. If the worms of the initial infection are dislodged by an anthelminthic prior to administering the second infecting dose of larvae of *Hymenolepis diminuta,* then no such resistance is shown against the superimposed dose.[74] No very concrete evidence has been presented to support the point of view that a true immunity is developed. However, the young of resistant mother mice likewise resist infection with *Hymenolepis fraterna* for some time after birth, their resistance apparently resulting from the passage in the mother's milk of protective substances from the mother to the young.[75] Powerful specific immune responses can generally not be expected against parasites such as these of the genus *Hymenolepis,* which are primarily or exclusively dwellers in the intestinal lumen.

PROPHYLAXIS

Efforts thus far to protect against *Hymenolepis* by vaccination with antigen from the homologous worm have failed.[76]

OTHER CESTODE INFECTIONS

RAILLIETINA

Tapeworms of the genus *Raillietina* have not been extensively studied immunologically. The form found in man, *Raillietina madagascariensis,* occurs also in rats, although its other host relationships are not yet established. An age resistance is developed by the chicken to *Raillietina cesticillus,* fowls more than two and one-half months old being more resistant than those less than one month.[77] An initial heavy infection with this parasite, however, does not protect chicks against reinfection six to twelve weeks later.[78] Birds suffer a significant retardation in growth as the result of infection.[79] On the other hand, the metabolism of the worms

[74] A. C. Chandler, *Am. J. Hyg.,* 29: 105 (1939, sec. D).
[75] D. A. Shorb, *Am. J. Hyg.,* 18: 74 (1933).
[76] A. C. Chandler, *Am. J. Hyg.,* 31: 17 (1940, sec. D).
[77] J. E. Ackert and W. M. Reid, *J. Parasitol.,* 23: 558 (1937).
[78] G. W. Luttermoser, *J. Parasitol. (Suppl.),* 24: 14 (1938).
[79] P. D. Harwood and G. W. Luttermoser, *Proc. Helminthol. Soc. Washington,* 5: 60 (1938); J. E. Ackert and A. A. Case: *J. Parasitol. (Suppl.),* 24: 14 (1938).

is severely upset if the host be starved for from twenty to forty-eight hours, and long chains of proglottids are characteristically broken off from the adult worm in the intestine.[80]

DIPYLIDIUM

The most significant member of the genus *Dipylidium* is *Dipylidium caninum*, which infects dogs and cats primarily and occasionally man. Young children are most heavily infected, although infections are never frequent in persons of any age. Nothing is established concerning the possible specific immune responses to the parasite.

MONIEZIA

Moniezia expansa is an exceedingly common parasite of sheep and is found also in goats and cattle. Apparently age is not a factor in the natural resistance to this form.[81] Experimental work on acquired immunity to this parasite has been severely handicapped until recently, when Stunkard [82] determined that orabatid mites serve as intermediate hosts of the worm.

[80] W. M. Reid, *J. Parasitol. (Suppl.)*, 26: 16 (1940).
[81] N. R. Stoll, *J. Parasitol.*, 24: 527 (1938).
[82] H. W. Stunkard, *Science*, 86: 312 (1937); and *Parasitology*, 30: 491 (1938).

Chapter XVI

THE NEMATODIASES

THE NEMATODE PARASITES of man and animals which have significance immunologically can conveniently be divided into six groups of which the type genera are, respectively, *Trichinella, Ascaris, Enterobius, Ancylostoma* (or *Necator*), *Wuchereria,* and *Strongyloides.* The immune responses to representative species of all of these type genera and to the more important related forms in each group will be discussed in this chapter.

INFECTIONS WITH *TRICHINELLA* AND RELATED FORMS

1. *TRICHINELLA* INFECTION

NATURAL RESISTANCE

HOST RESTRICTION

The only species found in the genus *Trichinella* is the very important form *Trichinella spiralis,* the cause of trichiniasis. The host range of this parasite is probably greater than that of any other nematode. It occurs naturally in wild rats, as well as in many other meat-eating animals, including dog, fox, cat, bear, marten, mongoose, wild boar, pig, and man. Such herbivorous animals as monkeys,[1] hamsters,[2] rabbits, and guinea pigs can also be infected. Chickens,[3] pigeons,[4] and crows [5] are susceptible, although the parasite does not thrive in birds and the possibility of infection successively through a series of birds is questionable. Cold-blooded animals are resistant to the parasite.[6]

---

[1] O. R. McCoy, *Proc. Soc. Exper. Biol. & Med.,* 30: 85 (1932).
[2] E. A. Mauss, *J. Parasitol. (Suppl.),* 25: 29 (1939) ; and *Am. J. Hyg.* 32: 75 (1940, sec. D)'.
[3] D. L. Augustine, *Science,* 78: 608 (1933).
[4] K. Matoff, *Tierärztl. Rundschau,* 42: 401 (1936).
[5] P. Pavlov, *Ann. de parasitol.,* 15: 434 (1937).   [6] *Ibid.,* p. 440.

FACTORS INFLUENCING NATURAL RESISTANCE

The age and the diet of the host significantly influence natural resistance to *Trichinella spiralis*.[7] Old dogs, for example, are more resistant than young ones, since a smaller percentage of the larvae fed develop to adults in the intestine of the mature animal.[8] In old pigeons the parasite fails to attain maturity, whereas in young birds it does reach the adult stage, and muscle invasion occurs.[9] As to diet, vitamin A seems most important, since rats on a vitamin-A-deficient diet are more susceptible to *Trichinella spiralis* than those on a normal diet.[10] A vitamin-E-free diet has been found by one investigator to enhance slightly the resistance of rats.[11] The administration of irradiated ergosterol is sometimes advised to enhance calcification of the encysted larvae,[12] although other authorities have found the use of this and similar substances too dangerous for general employment as a means of enhancing natural resistance after infection.[13]

ACQUIRED IMMUNITY

RESISTANCE TO REINFECTION

Animals which have recovered from the effects of an initial infection with *Trichinella spiralis* resist reinfection. This has been clearly demonstrated in rats,[14] as well as in guinea pigs,[15] hogs,[16] and, less completely, in monkeys.[17] No information is available in the case of man, although probably man also would acquire resistance to a second infection.

Immunity is transmitted from immune mother rats, rabbits, and hamsters to their young. The resistance is temporary, being lost by

[7] G. W. Bachman, *Rev. de med. trop. y parasitol., bacteriol., clin. y lab.*, 4: 121 (1938) ; E. H. Marchant, *J. Parasitol. (Suppl.)*, 25: 23 (1939).
[8] K. Matoff, *Tierärztl. Rundschau*, 43: 399 (1937).
[9] K. Matoff, *Tierärztl. Rundschau*, 42: 401 (1936).
[10] O. R. McCoy, *Am. J. Hyg.*, 20: 169 (1934).
[11] H. Zaiman, *J. Parasitol. (Suppl.)*, 26: 44 (1940).
[12] W. W. Wantland, *Proc. Soc. Exper. Biol. & Med.*, 32: 438 (1934), and *J. Parasitol.*, 24: 167 (1938).
[13] T. von Brand, G. F. Otto, and E. Abrams, *Am. J. Hyg.*, 27: 461 (1938).
[14] O. R. McCoy, *Am. J. Hyg.*, 14: 484 (1931).
[15] H. Roth, *Am. J. Hyg.*, 30: 35 (1939, sec. D).
[16] G. W. Bachman and R. Rodriguez Molina, *Am. J. Hyg.*, 18: 266 (1933).
[17] O. R. McCoy, *Proc. Soc. Exper. Biol. & Med.*, 30: 85 (1932).

the young after the third week of life. Presumably the transmission occurs through the mothers' milk.[18] One report has appeared of a positive skin test in the month-old child of an immune human mother, antibody apparently being transmitted from the mother to the child.[19]

ANTIBODY PRODUCTION

Antibody appears rather promptly in the serum of animals experimentally infected with *Trichinella spiralis*. Precipitin has been reported in the blood as early as the fifth day after infection, when only the adult worms are in the gut, and no larvae are yet in the muscles.[20] It is not regularly detected, however, until after several weeks.[21] The complement-fixing antibody has been reported by the third day, although it usually appears about the twentieth day and increases in concentration thereafter until the thirty-fifth day after infection.[22] Once present in the serum, antibody persists for at least several months, and some records in man indicate its persistence for from four to nine years.[23] It is associated chiefly with the euglobulins but also in part with the pseudoglobulin fraction of the serum.[24]

Trichinella antigen occurs in the serum of experimentally infected rabbits within twenty-four hours after feeding infective larvae and probably accounts for the antibody which is developed a few days later. It is noteworthy that this antigen occurs in the blood prior to larval invasion of the muscles.[25]

PASSIVE TRANSFER

The absence of any other method of treatment early caused physicians to employ serum from recovered or convalescent cases of trichiniasis in the treatment of this disease. Some improvement was occasionally described, and this was duplicated by some investigators in animal infections. However, resistance in passively

[18] E. A. Mauss, *Am. J. Hyg.*, 32: 75 (1940, sec. D).
[19] Z. Bercovitz, personal communication to the author (1940).
[20] G. W. Bachman, *J. Prevent. Med.*, 3: 465 (1929).
[21] J. T. Culbertson and S. S. Kaplan, *Parasitology*, 30: 156 (1938).
[22] G. W. Bachman and R. Rodriguez Molina, *Am. J. Hyg.*, 18: 266 (1932).
[23] H. Theiler, D. L. Augustine, and W. W. Spink, *Parasitology*, 27: 345 (1935).
[24] E. A. Mauss, *J. Parasitol. (Suppl.)*, 26: 43 (1940).
[25] J. Bozicevich and L. Detre, *Pub. Health Rep.*, 55: 683 (1940).

immunized persons or animals was never absolute, and the helpful effect of the serum was therefore believed to result from its possession of an antitoxic rather than an antiparasitic character.[26] Recently serum, when given prophylactically to mice, has again been shown to have some effect, acting almost exclusively on the ingested larvae developing to adults in the intestine of the infected animals. The serum appears to prevent the maturation of the larvae and usually causes their early elimination. The effect is in this case definitely upon the parasite itself. No effect, however, has been demonstrated upon larvae migrating through the blood or musculature. These very young larval forms evidently are less vulnerable to the effects of the serum than are the ingested larvae in the intestine which are approaching the adult stage.[27] Apparently the serum must be given parenterally to produce its effect, for no influence follows its administration by gavage.[28]

MECHANISM OF IMMUNITY

Acquired immunity in trichiniasis probably depends primarily on the action of the antibody developed in this disease, although as yet the direct function of the antibody in protection has not been fully demonstrated. There seems little question that the acquired resistance is directed against the intestinal phase of the parasite, for if infective larvae are fed to an immune animal they are promptly eliminated without development.[29] Such eliminated larvae are not killed by passage through an immune animal, however, for they readily infect normal animals to which they are subsequently fed. Although an increase in the intestinal secretion of mucus and of peristalsis have been suggested as the chief factors operative in expelling the larvae from the gut of immune rats,[30] it seems likely that the actual inhibition of development of the larvae is largely an effect of the serum antibody, for similar inhibition is seen in passively immunized animals.[31] To produce its ef-

[26] A. Trawinski, *Zentralbl. f. Bakt.*, 134: 145 (1935).
[27] J. T. Culbertson and S. S. Kaplan, *Parasitology*, 30: 156 (1938).
[28] G. W. Bachman and J. Oliver Gonzalez, *Proc. Soc. Exper. Biol. & Med.*, 35: 215 (1936).
[29] O. R. McCoy, *Am. J. Hyg.*, 32: 105 (1940, sec. D), and *J. Parasitol. (Suppl.)*, 24: 35 (1938); H. Roth, *Am. J. Hyg.*, 30: 35 (1939).
[30] O. R. McCoy, *Am. J. Hyg.*, 32: 105 (1940, sec. D).
[31] J. T. Culbertson and S. S. Kaplan, *Parasitology*, 30: 156 (1938).

fect, antibody may actually diffuse from the blood to the intestinal lumen, although this would hardly be required, since the parasites characteristically become so intimately associated with the tissues by penetrating the intestinal wall that exposure to the circulating antibody would be inevitable. Further evidence that serum antibody is significant in immunity to *Trichinella spiralis* is provided by the fact that infective larvae which are exposed to a powerful immune serum are found to be inhibited in development when later fed to animals, thereafter being only 30 percent as infective as larvae not so exposed.[32] Antibody is actually precipitated about the mouths of the exposed larvae, and many of them are thus immobilized and killed. Adult worms likewise are affected by the serum, and antibody precipitated about the vulvas of females in immune serum prevents the discharge of embryos.[33]

Some authorities still feel, however, that the immune response does not require that the remainder of the body besides the intestine come into play either as a source of antibody or in any other capacity. A good deal of support is given this view by the results of an ingenious experiment recently reported in which rats were infected by transplanting into the duodenum from 200 to 700 living *Trichinella* adults, all of only one sex, which had been segregated previously from the intestinal lumens of other rats. Despite the fact that no reproduction could occur, and hence no larvae could enter the somatic tissue, when these rats were fed infective larvae twenty-two days later, they were relatively resistant compared with the controls.[34] Such an experiment might easily be pointed to as proving that the immunity in trichiniasis originates in and is localized strictly to the intestine. Unfortunately, however, the experiment is not unequivocal, since antigens of the adult *Trichinella* have been shown regularly to enter the circulation of infected animals even in the absence of larval invasion. Such antigen has been detected as early as twenty-four hours after rabbits were fed infective forms, and at this time the adult parasites were not developed sufficiently for larval invasion to occur. Antibody production against these circulating antigens, nevertheless, has been shown to

[32] E. A. Mauss, *Am. J. Hyg.*, 32: 80 (1940, sec. D).
[33] J. Oliver Gonzalez, *J. Infect. Dis.*, 67: 292 (1940).
[34] C. V. Anderson and A. B. Leonard, *J. Parasitol. (Suppl.)*, 26: 42 (1940).

follow. It occurs even when blood containing such antigens is transfused to normal rabbits.[35]

The body cells also play some role in acquired immunity to *Trichinella*. Possibly this is largely through producing antibody, or through collectively immobilizing sensitized parasites. The eosinophiles, however, are known to have a further function, possibly of a more mechanical nature. They become concentrated in the intestinal mucosa, where they form a definite barrier to penetration by the adult parasites.[36] Eosinophiles also commonly are noted in the neighborhood of larvae encysted in the muscle.

PROPHYLAXIS

Rats can be protected against infection with *Trichinella spiralis* by the repeated injection of antigens prepared of heat-killed or dried larvae,[37] and even more effectively by the inoculation of living larvae parenterally.[38] None of these methods serves so well in prophylaxis as does a prior infection with the parasites.[39] Hogs are said to acquire no immunity through vaccination, although they do resist reinfection after recovery from an initial attack of trichiniasis.[40] The metabolic products of *Trichinella spiralis* in muscle are also reported to induce some degree of immunity to reinfection with the homologous parasite when fed to rats, rabbits, and guinea pigs.[41] The possibility of developing resistance in man artificially has not been investigated, since little or no general need for such a procedure is evident at this time.

DIAGNOSIS

The diagnosis of trichiniasis is possible through detecting specific serum antibody in vitro [42] and through skin tests.[43] The precipitin antibody does not usually appear in the serum before the

[35] J. Bozicevich and L. Detre, *Pub. Health Rep.*, 55: 683 (1940).
[36] V. D. van Someren, *J. Helminthol.*, 16: 83 (1938).
[37] O. R. McCoy, *Am. J. Hyg.*, 21: 200 (1935).
[38] P. Pavlov, *Ann. de parasitol.*, 15: 448 (1937).
[39] G. W. Bachman and J. Oliver Gonzalez, *Proc. Soc. Exper. Biol. & Med.*, 35: 215 (1936).
[40] G. W. Bachman and R. Rodriguez Molina, *Am. J. Hyg.*, 18: 266 (1932).
[41] L. A. Spindler, *J. Washington Acad. Sci.*, 27: 36 (1937).
[42] G. W. Bachman, *J. Prevent. Med.*, 3: 465 (1929).
[43] G. W. Bachman, *J. Prevent. Med.*, 2: 513 (1928).

second week after infection,[44] and it is best detected about the fourth or fifth week.[45] It persists up to nine years or so after recovery.[46] The precipitin test can be used also for diagnosing trichiniasis in pigs prior to slaughter.[47] The complement fixation test has had only very limited diagnostic use in trichiniasis.

The skin test has largely superseded the precipitin test as a routine diagnostic procedure because of the greater simplicity of its performance. It first becomes positive about three weeks after infection,[48] and it persists for from three to nine years after recovery.[49] In man both an immediate and a delayed reaction generally occur. Most of those who have tried the skin test have found it a most valuable diagnostic aid,[50] although some authorities still prefer older techniques.[51] The skin test serves also to diagnose trichiniasis of animals, although only the delayed reaction generally occurs. The test is recommended especially for identifying pig infections,[52] and it gives promise of attaining general adoption for that purpose.

2. *TRICHOCEPHALUS* INFECTION

Little immunological information is yet available on worms of the genus *Trichocephalus*. Several closely related species are known,

[44] W. W. Spink, *New England J. Med.*, 216: 5 (1937).

[45] H. Theiler and D. L. Augustine, *Zentralbl. f. Bakt.*, 135: 299 (1935).

[46] H. Theiler, D. L. Augustine, and W. W. Spink, *Parasitology*, 27: 345 (1935).

[47] A. Trawinski, *Berl. Tierärztl. Wchnschr.*, 50: 223 (1934), and *Ztschr. f. Fleisch-u. Milch-Hyg.*, 45: 166 (1935).

[48] H. Theiler and D. L. Augustine, *Zentralbl. f. Bakt.*, 135: 299 (1935); W. W. Spink and D. L. Augustine, *J. A. M. A.*, 104: 1801 (1935).

[49] H. Theiler, D. L. Augustine, and W. W. Spink, *Parasitology*, 27: 345 (1935); M. Warren, E. H. Drake, and R. S. Hawkes, *Ann. Int. Med.*, 13: 2141 (1940).

[50] W. W. Spink, *New England J. Med.*, 216: 5 (1937); O. R. McCoy, J. J. Miller, Jr., and R. D. Friedlander, *J. Immunol.*, 24: 1 (1933); G. W. Hunter, 3, *Am. J. Hyg.*, 13: 311 (1931); I. Maternowska, *Rozprawy Biolog.*, 11: 93 (1933); R. D. Friedlander, *Am. J. M. Sc.*, 188: 121 (1934); E. H. Drake, R. S. Hawkes, and M. Warren, *J. A. M. A.*, 105: 1340 (1935); G. F. Otto, *J. Parasitol.*, 22: 530 (1936); D. L. Augustine, *New England J. Med.*, 216: 463 (1937); J. Bozicevich, *Pub. Health Rep.*, 53: 2130 (1938); M. M. Schapiro, B. L. Crosby, and M. M. Sickler, *J. Lab. & Clin. Med.*, 23: 681 (1938); W. Sawitz, *Am. J. Pub. Health*, 27: 1023 (1937); J. E. Andes, R. A. Greene, and E. L. Breazeale, *J. A. M. A.*, 114: 2271 (1940).

[51] R. A. Kilduffe, *Am. J. M. Sc.*, 186: 802 (1933); L. S. Heathman, *Am. J. Hyg.*, 23: 397 (1936); T. R. Failmesger and J. E. Spalding, *Am. J. Dis. Child.*, 58: 129 (1939); J. B. McNaught, *Am. J. Trop. Med.*, 19: 181 (1939).

[52] D. L. Augustine and H. Theiler, *Parasitology*, 24: 60 (1932); I. Maternowska, *Zentralbl. f. Bakt.*, 129: 284 (1933); A. Trawinski, *Berl. Tierärztl. Wchnschr.*, 50: 223 (1934); A. Lichterman and I. Kleeman, *Am. J. Pub. Health*, 29: 1098 (1939).

such as *Trichocephalus trichiura* in man, *Trichocephalus vulpis* in the dog and the fox, *Trichocephalus campanulus* and *Trichocephalus serratus* in the cat, *Trichocephalus discolor* in the cow, *Trichocephalus ovis* in the sheep and the goat, *Trichocephalus suis* in the pig, *Trichocephalus leporis* in the rabbit, and *Trichocephalus muris* in the rat and the mouse. For the most part, the different worms are confined to the hosts named. The human parasite, for example, does not occur in animals. It is found in children more frequently than in adults. Infected persons give a skin reaction to *Trichinella* antigen.[53]

3. CAPILLARIA INFECTION

Capillaria hepatica is a near relative of worms of the genus *Trichocephalus*. It has been reported from several rodents (rats, mice, prairie dogs, muskrats, beavers, rabbits), a ruminant (peccary), a carnivore (dog), and certain primates (spider and capuchin monkeys, chimpanzees, and human beings).

Rats present evidence of an age resistance after experimental infection with *Capillaria hepatica,* since old animals tolerate proportionately larger infecting doses and show fewer liver lesions than do young rats. By the fourth week after an initial infection rats become refractory to a superimposed infection. The acquired immunity lasts for at least two months thereafter. Mice, on the other hand, manifest only a partial age resistance and acquire no immunity to reinfection.[54]

INFECTIONS WITH *ASCARIS* AND RELATED FORMS

1. *ASCARIS* INFECTIONS

NATURAL RESISTANCE

HOST RESTRICTION

The most important member of the genus *Ascaris*, namely, *Ascaris lumbricoides,* is found in man, certain monkeys, and pigs. The strain found in each of these hosts is specific for that host and not infective for the alternate species.[55] When embryonated eggs

[53] O. R. McCoy, J. J. Miller, Jr., and R. D. Friedlander, *J. Immunol.,* 24: 1 (1933).
[54] G. W. Luttermoser, *J. Parasitol.,* 23: 559 (1937), and *Am. J. Hyg.,* 27: 321 (1938).
[55] D. L. Augustine, *Am. J. Hyg.,* 30: 29 (1939, sec. D).

of the worm are fed to imperfect hosts, such as the laboratory rodents, they reach only the larval stage in the lung and never attain maturity as adult intestinal worms.[56]

FACTORS INFLUENCING NATURAL RESISTANCE

Individuals can be infected with *Ascaris* at any age, although young persons are more frequently and more intensely infected than older individuals. Pigs can be infected during at least their first five months of life, although some slight evidence of natural resistance is manifested by older pigs.[57] No difference in resistance between the sexes is known. The vitamin-A level of the diet may influence natural resistance,[58] although most investigators have failed to demonstrate such an effect.[59]

ACQUIRED IMMUNITY

RESISTANCE TO REINFECTION

Human beings and pigs acquire only very slight immunity to reinfection with *Ascaris*.[60] If the parasites of a first infection be eliminated by anthelminthics, reinfection can then occur.[61] Mice and guinea pigs, on the other hand, resist fatal somatic infections if previously given small doses of embryonated eggs. Very few larvae reach the liver or lungs of such animals previously infected with the somatic tissue stages.[62] The immunity acquired from prior infection is, however, of brief duration.[63]

ANTIBODY PRODUCTION

Most of the careful studies on antibody production to *Ascaris* have been performed in experimental somatic infections of rodents. In the rabbit infected with *Ascaris megalocephala* complement-

---

[56] E. Roman, *Compt. rend. Soc. de biol.*, 130: 1168 (1939).

[57] D. O. Morgan, *J. Helminthol.*, 9: 121 (1931).

[58] S. Kurisu, *Sei-I-Kai M. J.*, 50: 7 (1931).

[59] E. de Boer, *Tijdschr. v. Diergeneesk.*, 62: 965 (1935) ; P. A. Clapham, *J. Helminthol.*, 12: 165 (1934).

[60] E. Roman, *Compt. rend. Soc. de biol.*, 130: 1168 (1939) ; D. O. Morgan, *J. Helminthol.*, 9: 121 (1931).

[61] W. W. Cort, L. Schapiro, and N. R. Stoll, *Am. J. Hyg.*, 10: 614 (1929) ; G. F. Otto, *J. A. M. A.*, 95: 194 (1930) ; G. F. Otto and W. W. Cort, *J. Parasitol.*, 20: 245 (1934).

[62] O. Wagner, *Ztschr. f. Immunitätsforsch. u. exper. Therap.*, 78: 372 (1933).

[63] K. B. Kerr, *Am. J. Hyg.*, 27: 28 (1938).

fixing antibodies are found during the five weeks after infection, with their peak concentration about the fifteenth day.[64] Precipitins can be detected in serum from rabbits and guinea pigs given *Ascaris lumbricoides* sometimes for eight months.[65] These animals also respond with antibody if injected parenterally with coelomic fluid of *Ascaris* [66] or with a protein-free polysaccharide of the worm.[67] Antibodies developed by injecting rabbits with suspensions of isolated tissues of *Ascaris* react best with the homologous tissues. For example, an anticuticle serum reacts best with the cuticle antigen. Cuticle antigens of various ascarids must have much in common, however, for antibodies produced against the cuticle of one species will react indiscriminately with cuticle test antigens of many different mammalian ascarids.[68]

MECHANISM OF IMMUNITY

Humoral antibody probably influences the immunity acquired against somatic infections with *Ascaris,* although its role has not yet been demonstrated. It is possible that the antibody has in part the character of an antitoxin, for toxin-like materials from the worm are believed to cause lesions in organs which the worms themselves never invade.[69] There seems greater probability that the antibody behaves as an opsonin and acts in conjunction with the defensive body cells. The activity of the defective cells in immune animals is definitely enhanced compared with that in normal animals, since the cells increase in number as a result of a first infection and become mobilized in strategic sites in order better to repel invasion by a second group of larvae. These cells surround the migrating larvae of a superimposed infection, check their progress, and finally destroy them.[70] All of this occurs very soon after the larvae enter the somatic tissues, and few of the invaders therefore succeed in reaching the liver or the lungs of immune animals.[71]

[64] W. K. Blackie, *J. Helminthol.,* 9: 91 (1931).
[65] F. A. Coventry, *J. Prevent. Med.,* 3: 43 (1929).
[66] O. Dubelsky and E. Golubewa, *Zentralbl. f. Bakt.,* 108: 449 (1928).
[67] D. H. Campbell, *J. Infect. Dis.,* 59: 266 (1936).
[68] G. A. Canning, *Am. J. Hyg.,* 9: 207 (1929).
[69] W. K. Blackie, *J. Helminthol.,* 8: 93 (1930).
[70] K. B. Kerr, *Am. J. Hyg.,* 27: 28 (1938).
[71] O. Wagner, *Ztschr. f. Immunitätsforsch. u. exper. Therap.,* 78: 372 (1933).

PROPHYLAXIS

Vaccination of normal hosts against *Ascaris* has not been successful. Mice are said to become immune to somatic infections with *Ascaris lumbricoides*, however, after the oral administration of dried or powdered *Ascaris* substance.[72]

DIAGNOSIS

Although complement-fixing antibodies and precipitins are both developed in *Ascaris* infections, tests for antibodies are not routinely employed in the diagnosis of ascariasis. The skin test, however, has had somewhat widespread trial. A few investigators have found the skin reaction a reliable index of *Ascaris* infection,[73] but, especially in human beings, many discrepancies occur.[74] The skin of normal persons can be rendered sensitive by repeated testing.[75] Many persons, furthermore, give a skin reaction even though never infected, although some form of prior contact with *Ascaris* antigen is probably essential.[76] Many laboratory workers, for example, become sensitized by handling the parasite, even after it has been preserved.

2. TOXOCARA INFECTION

Toxocara canis and *Toxocara felis* are found, respectively, in the dog and the fox, and in the cat, the leopard, and the lion. Both have also been recorded from man. The immunology of the infection has not been thoroughly studied with either parasite. A marked age resistance is manifested by the natural hosts of each parasite. Dogs more than six months old, for example, are seldom infected with the canine species. Feeding a diet deficient in vitamin A to dogs of a resistant age leads to loss of resistance, and older animals can thus be rendered susceptible to infection. The increased sus-

---

[72] *Ibid.*

[73] F. A. Coventry, *J. Prevent. Med.*, 3: 43 (1929); F. Diehl and P. Schwoerer: *Arch. f. exper. Path. u. Pharm.*, 183: 1 (1936).

[74] W. Jadassohn, *Arch. f. Dermat. u. Syph.*, 156: 690 (1928); O. Hegglin: *Schweiz. med. Wchnschr.*, No. 1: 11 (1929); O. K. Khaw, *Arch. f. Schiffs- u. Tropen-Hyg.*, 33: 46 (1929); E. M. Konus and S. A. Gakoubovitch, *Med. Par. and Parasit. Dis.*, 6: 107 (1937).

[75] W. Schoenfeld, *Arch. f. Dermat. u. Syph.*, 175: 54 (1937).

[76] T. L. Jones and A. A. Kingscote, *Am. J. Hyg.*, 22: 406 (1935).

ceptibility may result from depression of the flow from the intestinal glands of dogs on vitamin-A-deficient diet.[77] A specific immunity is acquired by cats against reinfection with *Toxocara felis*, this resistance not requiring the persistence of the worms from the original infection.[78]

3. HETERAKIS INFECTION

The most important species of the genus *Heterakis* is *Heterakis gallinae*, a parasite of turkeys. Its importance lies in its serving as a vector for *Histomonas meleagridis*, a mastigophoran which causes blackhead in the turkey. The nematode also infects chickens. A second species, *Heterakis spumosa*, infects rats and mice.

Infections with *Heterakis gallinae* are influenced very little by the age of the host [79] or by the host's diet. At least a diet deficient in vitamin A does not lower the resistance of chickens to infection with this parasite.[80] Fowls with leukaemia generally suffer more intense infections than normal birds,[81] although those with tuberculosis harbor fewer worms than normal birds.[82] Recovery from a first infection confers to birds little or no protection against reinfection.[83]

Both a natural age resistance and an acquired immunity to reinfection have been demonstrated in rats with *Heterakis spumosa*. The acquired immunity persists even after all the worms are eliminated by carbon tetrachloride.[84]

4. ASCARIDIA INFECTION

NATURAL RESISTANCE

HOST RESTRICTION

The most important members of the genus *Ascaridia* are *Ascaridia lineata* and *Ascaridia galli*, the common roundworms of

[77] W. H. Wright, *J. Parasitol.*, 21: 433 (1935).
[78] M. P. Sarles and N. R. Stoll, *J. Parasitol.*, 21: 277 (1935).
[79] P. A. Clapham, *J. Helminthol.*, 12: 71 (1934).
[80] P. A. Clapham, *J. Helminthol.*, 11: 9 (1933).
[81] P. A. Clapham, *J. Helminthol.*, 16: 53 (1938).
[82] D. O. Morgan and J. E. Wilson, *J. Helminthol.*, 16: 165 (1938), and 17: 177 (1939).
[83] P. A. Clapham, *J. Helminthol.*, 12: 71 (1934).
[84] G. F. Winfield, *Am. J. Hyg.*, 17: 168 (1933).

both wild and domestic fowls. Turkeys also are susceptible to these parasites, although they are more resistant than chicks.[85]

FACTORS INFLUENCING NATURAL RESISTANCE

The genetic constitution of the chick is of importance in its natural resistance to *Ascaridia lineata*. Heavy breeds or heavy strains within breeds are usually more resistant than lighter ones.[86] The significance of the genetic constitution in resistance has been revealed experimentally by introducing peculiarly susceptible cockerels to a resistant flock of chickens. The level of natural resistance in the next generation is then definitely depressed.[87]

Older chickens are more resistant to *Ascaridia* than are young birds,[88] the maximum resistance being attained at about ninety-three days of age.[89] The resistance of the older birds is explained by the presence of thermostable growth-inhibiting substances in the mucus secretion of the goblet cells in the intestine of the older birds.[90] More goblet cells for the secretion of the mucus are found per unit area in the intestine of the older birds.[91]

A purely vegetable diet is less adequate than one containing animal protein for maintaining natural resistance to *Ascaridia lineata*. Vitamins also are important. In chicks on a diet deficient in vitamin A more and larger worms are found.[92] More worms develop likewise in chicks with a vitamin B deficiency.[93] The absence of vitamin D does not influence resistance to infection with *Ascaridia lineata,* although birds on a D-deficient diet grow more slowly than control birds.[94] Resistance to *Ascaridia* is also lowered by repeated hemorrhage.[95]

[85] J. E. Ackert and L. L. Eisenbrandt, *J. Parasitol.*, 21: 200 (1935).

[86] J. E. Ackert and others, *J. Agric. Res.*, 50: 607 (1935).

[87] J. E. Ackert and J. H. Wilmoth, *J. Parasitol.*, 20: 323 (1934).

[88] J. E. Ackert, *Trans. Dynamics of Develop.*, 10: 413 (1935).

[89] J. E. Ackert, D. A. Porter, and T. D. Beach, *J. Parasitol.*, 21: 205 (1935).

[90] J. E. Ackert, S. A. Edgar, and L. P. Frick, *Tr. Am. Micros. Soc.*, 58: 81 (1939), and *Proc. 3d Internat. Congr. Microbiol.*, p. 481 (1939) ; J. E. Ackert and L. P. Frick, *J. Parasitol. (Suppl.)*, 26: 14 (1940).

[91] J. E. Ackert and S. A. Edgar, *J. Parasitol. (Suppl.)*, 24: 13 (1938), and 26: 14 (1940).

[92] J. E. Ackert, M. F. McIlvaine, and N. Z. Crawford, *Am. J. Hyg.*, 13: 320 (1931) ; O. Seifried, *München. Tierärzt. Wchnschr.*, 84: 540 (1933).

[93] J. E. Ackert and L. O. Nolf, *Am. J. Hyg.*, 13: 337 (1931).

[94] J. E. Ackert and L. A. Spindler, *Am. J. Hyg.*, 9: 292 (1929).

[95] D. A. Porter and J. E. Ackert, *Am. J. Hyg.*, 17: 252 (1933).

ACQUIRED IMMUNITY

A slight measure of immunity to reinfection is acquired by chicks from an initial infection with *Ascaridia lineata*. The basis of the immunity is obscure, but it probably depends on the development of specific antibody. The young ascarids characteristically burrow into the intestinal mucosa, and those of a superimposed feeding would be at this time affected by the circulating antibody.[96] A slight immunity is also developed by chicks after vaccination with *Ascaridia lineata* antigens.[97]

INFECTIONS WITH *ENTEROBIUS* AND RELATED FORMS

NATURAL RESISTANCE

The oxyurid nematodes individually have sharply restricted host choice. For example, the most important member of the group, the human pinworm *Enterobius vermicularis,* is confined to man. Man, for his part, is infected with no other oxyurid worm. Comparatively little natural resistance is acquired with age by man against *Enterobius vermicularis*. The incidence of infection generally reflects the relative exposure. However, in one large survey in Washington, D.C., the incidence of pinworm infection was 35 percent in pre-school-age children, 51 percent in school-age children, and only 22 percent in adults.[98]

ACQUIRED IMMUNITY

Practically no specific immunity is acquired by man from an infection with pinworm. The infection is maintained in an individual only through reinfection, and reinfection can occur at any time.

Skin tests with the specific antigen have been tried for the diagnosis of the human infection, but with only limited success.[99] Antigen from the rabbit oxyurid, *Passalurus ambiguus,* also has

[96] G. L. Graham, J. E. Ackert, and R. W. Jones, *Am. J. Hyg.,* 15: 726 (1932).
[97] L. L. Eisenbrandt and J. E. Ackert, *Am. J. Hyg.,* 32: 1 (1940).
[98] E. B. Cram and L. Reardon, *Am. J. Hyg.,* 29: 17 (1939, sec. D).
[99] W. H. Wright and J. Bozicevich, *J. Parasitol.,* 23: 562 (1937).

been employed in human cases, with apparently somewhat better results than with the specific material.[100] The rabbit worm antigen has the advantage of being more easily produced.

INFECTIONS WITH HOOKWORMS AND RELATED FORMS

1. ANCYLOSTOMA AND NECATOR INFECTIONS

NATURAL RESISTANCE

HOST RESTRICTION

The hookworms of the genus *Ancylostoma* are quite limited in their choice of host. The species found in man, *Ancylostoma duodenale*, probably develops only in man, although reports occasionally appear concerning its presence in dogs, cats, lions, pigs, and certain monkeys. Animal species of *Ancylostoma* will not mature in man, although, as in the case of *Ancylostoma braziliense* and *Ancylostoma caninum* from the dog, the infective larval stage does penetrate human skin. The larvae do not experience further development in man, although they may migrate in the skin for years thereafter, causing a form of "creeping eruption." The New World hookworm of man, *Necator americanus*, has a somewhat broader host range than the species of *Ancylostoma*. It has been found in several monkeys, as well as in pangolins, pigs, dogs, rhinoceri, and certain rodents.

It is difficult to explain the fact that only partial development of the hookworms occurs in some unnatural hosts. A marked decrease in host specificity can sometimes be induced, however, by treating the hookworm larvae with an emulsion of tissues of the normal host. Following such treatment, the larvae frequently experience further development in the strange host. For example, human hookworm larvae which are treated with an emulsion of human lung tissue develop in the rabbit to the point of sexual differentiation preceding the fourth ecdysis. Biologic significance must, therefore, be ascribed to the passage through somatic tissues which these parasites experience.[101]

[100] H. Tsuchiya and T. C. Bauerlein, *J. Lab. & Clin. Med.*, 24: 627 (1939).
[101] K. Nakajima, *Jap. J. Exper. Med.*, 10: 115 (1932).

FACTORS INFLUENCING NATURAL RESISTANCE

Although such a general factor as the genetic constitution of the host influences profoundly the natural resistance of animals to hookworms,[102] other considerations also have significance. Chief among these are the character of the diet and the age of the host. From experimental studies carried out upon dogs it is clear that susceptibility to hookworm disease increases when the quality of the diet is reduced. The worms in dogs on a poor diet develop faster and produce more eggs than those in animals on an adequate diet.[103] Diets low in minerals and vitamins seem most likely to undermine resistance.[104] Essentially similar observations are made in human hookworm disease.[105] Factors which lead to anemia, such as periodic bleeding or a milk diet, also render hosts more susceptible to hookworm infection.[106] The administration of iron salts exclusively to animals that are on a deficient diet generally fails to restore their natural resistance to the normal level,[107] although in the therapy of human hookworm disease, it is true that administration of iron is frequently attended with success.[108]

Age is not a very obvious factor in the natural resistance of man to hookworm infection, for the infection of man may occur at any age. Among dogs, however, younger animals suffer much heavier infections than older animals.[109] Little or no cellular response to the migrating larvae is seen in the skin of young dogs which are infected percutaneously, but in old dogs the progress of the larvae is quickly checked, and many forms are destroyed. A smaller percentage of the larvae given to old dogs, therefore, reach maturity compared with that in young dogs.[110]

[102] A. O. Foster, *Am. J. Hyg.*, 22: 65 (1935).

[103] A. O. Foster and W. W. Cort, *Am. J. Hyg.*, 16: 241 (1932), and 21: 302 (1935).

[104] A. O. Foster and W. W. Cort, *Am. J. Hyg.*, 16: 582 (1932).

[105] W. W. Cort, *J. Parasitol.*, 19: 142 (1932); A. O. Foster and W. W. Cort, *Am. J. Hyg.*, 16: 241 (1932); C. F. Ahmann and L. M. Bristol, *South. M. J.*, 26: 959 (1933).

[106] A. O. Foster, *Am. J. Hyg.*, 24: 109 (1936).

[107] G. F. Otto and J. W. Landsberg, *Am. J. Hyg.*, 31: 37 (1940, sec. D).

[108] T. Kobayashi, *Sang*, 3: 129 (1929).

[109] C. A. Herrick, *Am. J. Hyg.*, 8: 125 (1928); M. P. Sarles, *Am. J. Hyg.*, 10: 453 (1929).

[110] M. P. Sarles, *Am. J. Hyg.*, 10: 683 and 693 (1929).

ACQUIRED IMMUNITY

RESISTANCE TO REINFECTION

Man does not acquire a very powerful immunity to reinfection with hookworms as a result of recovery from an initial infection. For example, reinfection occurs promptly after the worms of the first infection are eliminated by drugs.[111] Dogs and cats, on the other hand, offer a partial immunity to superimposed experimental infections with *Ancylostoma caninum*,[112] and this immunity can be raised to a fairly high level by repeated reinfection.[113] Mice also can be protected against a fatal somatic infection with *Ancylostoma caninum* by prior exposure to small doses of living larvae. Severe reactions of an Arthus type are seen about migrating larvae in the tissues of the immune animals.[114] Acquired resistance to skin penetration by the larvae of *Ancylostoma caninum* has also been demonstrated in guinea pigs and in man.[115]

ANTIBODY PRODUCTION

Only recently has circulating antibody been very conclusively demonstrated in hookworm infection. The serum of dogs immune to *Ancylostoma caninum* is now known to contain a specific antibody, and this antibody has been shown to act directly upon living infective larval forms exposed to it in vitro. The reaction between the serum antibody and the parasite substance goes on slowly, being first visible microscopically in about five hours. A granular precipitate develops first at the oral opening and the excretory pore of the larval worm, but later in the oesophagus and the intestine. After about five days the larvae are killed by the antibody.[116]

PASSIVE TRANSFER

The injection of serum from an immune animal does not completely protect a normal dog against the dog hookworm. Dogs which are given an immune serum suffer less from the effects of in-

[111] W. W. Cort, L. Schapiro, and N. R. Stoll, *Am. J. Hyg.*, 10: 614 (1929).
[112] O. R. McCoy, *Am. J. Hyg.*, 14: 268 (1931).
[113] G. F. Otto and K. B. Kerr, *Am. J. Hyg.*, 29: 25 (1939, sec. D).
[114] K. B. Kerr, *Am. J. Hyg.*, 24: 381 (1936).
[115] F. Fulleborn, *Scritti Med. in Onore del Sen. Prof. N. Gabbi, Gior. di clin. med.* p. 37 (1930); K. Kitamura, *Jap. J. Derm. & Urol.* 31: 866 (1931).
[116] G. F. Otto, *J. Parasitol. (Suppl.)*, 25: 29 (1939).

fection, however, and fewer mature parasites are recoverable than from control animals.[117] Serum from mice recovered from a somatic infection with *Ancylostoma caninum* also protects a small percentage of normal mice against a lethal dose of hookworm larvae.[118]

MECHANISM OF IMMUNITY

The mechanism of the specific immunity acquired against hookworm infection is dependent upon the direct antagonistic effects of both the cells and the antibody of the plasma upon the larval parasites in the somatic tissues. Practically no effect has yet been demonstrated upon the adult worms in the intestine. The defensive cells check the progress of and frequently immobilize the migrating larvae in the tissue [119] after the antibody has attacked the worm directly and interfered, perhaps, both mechanically and chemically with the normal physiological processes of the larvae.[120] The function of the defense mechanism seems peculiarly sensitive to factors which debilitate the host.[121]

PROPHYLAXIS

Dogs can be rendered resistant to *Ancylostoma caninum* by a series of twenty-five to thirty successive infections with gradually increasing numbers of the homologous larvae.[122] The use of killed larvae, however, is not effective for prophylaxis. For example, mice inoculated with killed forms are as susceptible as normal mice to somatic infection with the homologous parasite.[123] Vaccination has not yet been tried as a means of protecting man from infection with hookworm.

DIAGNOSIS

The diagnosis of hookworm disease in man does not usually require immunological methods. Nevertheless some investigators

[117] G. F. Otto, *J. Parasitol. (Suppl.)*, 24: 10 (1938).
[118] K. B. Kerr, *Am. J. Hyg.*, 27: 60 (1938).
[119] J. E. Stumberg, *Am. J. Hyg.*, 15: 186 (1932).
[120] G. F. Otto, *Am. J. Hyg.*, 31: 23 (1940, sec. D).
[121] W. W. Cort and G. F. Otto, *Rev. Gastroenterol.*, 7: 2 (1940).
[122] G. F. Otto and K. B. Kerr, *Am. J. Hyg.*, 29: 25 (1939, sec. D); G. F. Otto, K. B. Kerr, and J. W. Landsberg, *J. Parasitol.*, 23: 560 (1937).
[123] K. B. Kerr, *Am. J. Hyg.*, 27: 52 (1938).

find skin tests a fairly reliable index of hookworm disease.[124] Most authorities, however, do not favor the skin test as a diagnostic procedure in this infection, because of the group character of the reaction obtained.[125] Hookworm antigens also elicit a skin reaction in many other nematode infections, and antigens from other nematodes, such as *Ascaris lumbricoides,* elicit positive responses in hookworm patients.[126]

2. OESOPHAGOSTOMUM INFECTION

Worms of the genus *Oesophagostomum* have been but little studied immunologically. The different species are known, however, to have rather limited host range. *Oesophagostomum apiostomum,* for example, is found in several different apes and monkeys, and has been reported in man, but infests no other hosts. The administration of copper and iron in drinking water to pigs with *Oesophagostomum dentatum* benefits the host, aiding it to throw off the ill effects of the infection, but it appears to permit the worms also to thrive.[127] Some slight degree of immunity to reinfection is said to accrue to calves which have recovered from an initial infection with *Oesophagostomum radiatum.*[128]

3. SYNGAMUS INFECTION

Gapeworms are somewhat restricted in host range, although usually several different species can serve as host. The cattle gapeworm, *Syngamus laryngeus,* infects cattle, water buffaloes, goats, and possibly man. Another species, *Syngamus trachea* occurs in chickens, turkeys, partridges, and some other birds. Age is a factor in the natural resistance of fowls to *Syngamus trachea.* Chicks more than ten weeks old are generally more resistant than younger

[124] R. Arnaud, *Ann. Soc. belge de méd. trop.,* 12: 5 (1932); A. B. Vattuone, *M. J. Australia,* 20th Year: 645 (1933).

[125] J. H. H. Pirie, F. Retief, and A. L. Ferguson, *Proc. Transvaal Mine Med. Officers' Assoc.,* 9: 19 (1929); J. E. Stumberg and R. Rodriguez Molina, *Porto Rico J. Pub. Health & Trop. Med.,* 7: 37 (1931); G. W. Bachman and R. Rodriguez Molina, *Porto Rico J. Pub. Health & Trop. Med.,* 7: 287 (1932).

[126] G. W. Bachman and R. Rodriguez Molina, *Am. J. Trop. Med.,* 12: 279 (1932).

[127] L. A. Spindler, *J. Parasitol.,* 20: 325 (1934).

[128] R. L. Mayhew, *J. Parasitol. (Suppl.),* 25: 31 (1939); and *J. Parasitol.,* 26: 345 (1940).

birds,[129] although even yearling hens sometimes can be infected.[130] A diet deficient in calcium, as well as in vitamin A, is said to predispose chicks to infection.[131] Female partridges appear to be peculiarly susceptible to infection.[132] Some authorities feel that the strain of egg-laying lowers the resistance of female birds to this parasite.[133]

4. TRICHOSTRONGYLUS INFECTION

The trichostrongyle worms generally can infect several species of animals. One species, *Trichostrongylus colubriformis*, for example, is found in men, baboons, sheep, gazelles, goats, camels, antelopes, bharals, and squirrels. Another, *Trichostrongylus orientalis*, occurs in man, fat-tailed sheep, and Chinese camels.

Little is known of the factors which influence natural resistance to the trichostrongylid nematodes. Immunity is acquired, however, as a result of prior infection with these parasites. Young lambs placed on infective pasture develop a firm immunity within five months, which enables them to resist infections fatal to normal animals.[134] Immunity can also be conferred artificially to sheep and goats by repeated small doses of larvae.[135] Rabbits likewise can be immunized within six to eight weeks against *Trichostrongylus calcaratus* by giving progressively increasing doses of larvae.[136]

5. HAEMONCHUS INFECTION

The sheep wireworm, *Haemonchus contortus*, is found commonly in sheep throughout the world. It occurs also in such other ruminants as goats, cattle, moose, antelopes, chamois, bison, deer, bharals, argali, and caribou, and has been reported from man. The nutritional state of an animal is important in natural resistance to *Haemonchus*. Poorly fed lambs are more susceptible to infection

[129] P. A. Clapham, *Proc. Roy. Soc.,* London, s. B., 115: 18 (1934), and *J. Helminthol.,* 17: 192 (1939).

[130] D. O. Morgan, *J. Helminthol.,* 9: 117 (1931); ·R. H. Waite, Maryland State Coll. Agricult., Bull., No. 234: 103.

[131] P. A. Clapham, *Proc. Roy. Soc.,* London, s. B., 115: 18 (1934).

[132] S. C. Whitlock, *J. Parasitol.,* 23: 426 (1937); P. A. Clapham, *J. Helminthol.,* 17: 192 (1939).

[133] S. C. Whitlock, *J. Parasitol.,* 23: 426 (1937).

[134] E. L. Taylor, *J. Helminthol.,* 12: 143 (1934).

[135] J. S. Andrews, *J. Agric. Res.,* 58: 761 (1939).

[136] M. P. Sarles, *J. Parasitol.,* 19: 61 (1932).

than those well fed.[137] In older sheep, however, dietary deficiencies must be severe before the resistance can be affected.[138] Specific immunity to reinfection is acquired from prior infection,[139] although it is generally partial rather than absolute,[140] and sometimes it is of very low degree.[141] Proteins of the worm occur in the serum of heavily infected animals in sufficient amount to shock specifically sensitized guinea pigs.[142]

6. NIPPOSTRONGYLUS INFECTION

Worms of the genus *Nippostrongylus* are not of economic importance. One species deserves mention in some detail, however, because the results obtained with it in immunological studies serve admirably to demonstrate several principles of immunity applicable to helminths infections generally.

NATURAL RESISTANCE

Nippostrongylus muris is probably exclusively a rodent parasite, and may be restricted to rats and mice. Even some mice are relatively poor hosts for the parasite, however, for in the deer mouse the parasite fails to attain sexual maturity.[143] Old rats and mice have greater natural resistance to it than young animals.[144] The diet affects the natural resistance, for rats which are fed exclusively on a diet of whole milk [145] or on one with a deficiency in vitamin A [146] are more susceptible to the parasite.

ACQUIRED RESISTANCE

RESISTANCE TO REINFECTION

Rats, as well as mice, which have recovered from a previous infection with *Nippostrongylus muris* acquire an immunity to rein-

---

137 A. H. H. Fraser and D. Robertson, *Emp. J. Exper. Agric.*, 1: 17 (1933).

138 I. C. Ross and H. McL. Gordon, *Australian Vet. J.*, 9: 100 (1933).

139 N. R. Stoll, *Am. J. Hyg.*, 10: 384 (1929); R. L. Mayhew, *J. Parasitol. (Suppl.)*, 26: 17 (1940).

140 N. R. Stoll, *Am. J. Hyg.*, 16: 783 (1932).

141 I. C. Ross and H. McL. Gordon, *Australian Vet. J.*, 9: 100 (1933).

142 J. E. Stumberg, *Am. J. Hyg.*, 18: 247 (1933).

143 D. A. Porter, *Am. J. Hyg.*, 22: 444 (1935); *J. Parasitol.*, 21: 314 (1935).

144 C. M. Africa, *J. Parasitol.*, 18: 1 (1931); A. C. Chandler, *Am. J. Hyg.*, 16: 750 (1932); D. A. Porter, *Am. J. Hyg.*, 22: 444 (1935).

145 D. A. Porter, *Am. J. Hyg.*, 22: 467 (1935).

146 L. A. Spindler, *J. Parasitol.*, 20: 72 (1933).

fection.[147] Usually the immunity is partial rather than absolute, and it is demonstrable by the smaller number of worms in the immune animals, or the smaller number of eggs in their feces. The acquired resistance in rats reaches its peak about two weeks after infection and gradually diminishes thereafter, unless the rat is reinfected.[148] Usually a heavy infection is required before a significant immunity develops. Apparently part of the immunity is acquired by rats from the intestinal stage of the parasite independently of the development in the somatic tissues, for rats resist reinfection even when initially infected with adult worms given by duodenal tube.[149]

ANTIBODY PRODUCTION

Antibody is demonstrable in vitro in the serum from rats infected with *Nippostrongylus muris*. It is precipitated about the oral opening and the excretory pore and within the oesophagus and intestine of larval worms placed in such immune serum. The treated worms are eventually so affected by the antibody as to be disabled or killed.[150]

PASSIVE TRANSFER

Immunity to *Nippostrongylus muris* can be conferred on normal rats by injecting them with serum from immune animals.[151] The serum acts not only on the larval stages migrating through the somatic tissues of the host but also on the adult parasites, which are promptly dislodged by it.

MECHANISM OF IMMUNITY

The earlier point of view considered that the immunity to *Nippostrongylus muris* depended upon an interference with the parasite nutrition. Antienzymes were believed developed by the host to counteract the enzymes elaborated by the parasite to digest its

[147] C. M. Africa, *J. Parasitol.*, 18: 1 (1931) ; B. Schwartz, J. E. Alicata, and J. T. Lucker, *J. Washington Acad. Sc.*, 21: 259 (1931) ; D. A. Porter, *Am. J. Hyg.*, 22: 444 (1935).
[148] A. C. Chandler, *Am. J. Hyg.*, 22: 243 (1935).
[149] L. A. Spindler, *J. Parasitol.*, 20: 326 (1934), and *Am. J. Hyg.*, 23: 237 (1936).
[150] M. P. Sarles, *J. Parasitol.*, 23: 560 (1937).
[151] M. P. Sarles and W. H. Taliaferro, *J. Infect. Dis.*, 59: 207 (1936), and *J. Parasitol. (Suppl.)*, 24: 35 (1938).

food.[152] However, the recent demonstration of antibody in the serum of immune animals, the direct antagonism shown in vitro by this antibody upon the parasite, and the successful passive transfer of immunity to *Nippostrongylus muris* have demonstrated conclusively that immunity to *Nippostrongylus muris* has a true antibody basis.[153] The immunity, although resulting from a generalized immune response by the host, seems to be most effective upon the parasites in certain strategically placed organs. Larval forms are affected particularly in the skin and the lungs, and the adults in the intestinal mucosa. The worm is immobilized in these sites through the combined action of the specific antibody and the defensive cells of the host. The antibody incapacitates the parasite by directly attacking or interfering with its vital functions—including, certainly, that of nutrition—by chemically uniting with its tissues. The defensive cells meanwhile accumulate about the worm, at first loosely and later as a fibrotic nodule from which the larva cannot escape. The worm gradually becomes entirely immobilized, dies, and its debris finally is removed by the phagocytes.[154]

7. Infections with Other Related Forms

DICTYOCAULUS FILARIA

Dictyocaulus filaria occurs in sheep, goats, and some wild ruminants. Lambs in the field become comparatively resistant by the seventh month of life. This resistance is in part natural, being acquired with age, but also in part the result of a specific immune response to an early infection.[155]

METASTRONGYLUS ELONGATUS

The lungworm, *Metastrongylus elongatus*, is found in pigs, wild boars, sheep, oxen, and, rarely, in man. Among pigs, young animals suffer the most severe effects. Recovery from a severe infection results in a partial immunity to reinfection.[156]

[152] A. C. Chandler, *Am. J. Hyg.*, 22: 157 (1935), and 23: 46 (1936).
[153] M. P. Sarles and W. H. Taliaferro, *J. Infect. Dis.*, 24: 35 (1938).
[154] W. H. Taliaferro and M. P. Sarles, *J. Parasitol.*, 23: 561 (1937), and *J. Infect. Dis.*, 64: 157 (1939).
[155] G. Kauzal, *Australian Vet. J.*, 10: 100 (1934).
[156] B. Schwartz and J. T. Lucker, *J. Parasitol.*, 21: 432 (1935).

Infections with Filarioid Forms

NATURAL RESISTANCE

An extraordinarily limited host range is characteristic of all the filarial worms. Man, for example, is the only vertebrate susceptible to *Wuchereria bancrofti*, *Loa loa*, and *Onchocerca volvulus*. Likewise, the dog is the only vertebrate host of *Dirofilaria immitis*. On the other hand, a member of the group somewhat remotely related to those species just named, *Dracunculus medinensis*, the guinea worm or fiery serpent, is infective for many hosts including man, fox, raccoon, mink, dog, horse, cow, skunk, and monkey.

ACQUIRED IMMUNITY

Very little experimental data is available upon acquired immunity to filarid worms, because experimental infections of animals and man with these forms are either difficult or as yet impossible. It is known, however, that rabbits which have been first immunized with *Dirofilaria immitis* antigen and subsequently transfused with blood from a dog with *Dirofilaria immitis* infection eliminate the introduced microfilariae more readily than normal rabbits similarly transfused.[157] A homologous antiserum from such immune rabbits manifests a marked lethal action in vitro upon the microfilariae.[158]

Most of the immunological studies upon these worms have been concerned with the diagnosis of the infections. Both skin tests and complement fixation tests have been used for the diagnosis of *Wuchereria* infections.[159] Antigens for these tests are generally prepared from an adult filarid from dogs, *Dirofilaria immitis*, since this species is comparatively easily obtained in quantity and contains antigens effective for the tests in man. *Contortospiculum rheae* from the South American ostrich has also been shown to supply the necessary antigens and to serve for skin tests.[160] Saline extracts of the worms are generally used in skin tests, but an alcoholic extract is preferred for the fixation test. The reactions are definitely of a

[157] H. Murata, *Fukuoka Acta Med.*, 32: 54 (1939)
[158] J. G. Arnold, Jr., and T. L. Duggan, *J. Parasitol.*, 23: 561 (1937).
[159] W. H. Taliaferro and W. A. Hoffman, *J. Prevent. Med.*, 4: 261 (1930); N. H. Fairley, *Tr. Roy. Soc. Trop. Med. & Hyg.*, 24: 635 (1931), and 25: 220 (1932).
[160] W. Mohr and H. Lippelt, *Klin. Wchnschr.*, 19: 157 (1940).

group character.[161] Skin tests and fixation reactions can also be elicited with the same antigens in loaiasis,[162] onchocerciasis,[163] and dracontiasis.[164] A specific antigen prepared from the guinea worm also serves for skin tests in dracontiasis.[165] An adhesion reaction can also be obtained in vitro with the blood of persons with filariasis. In positive reactions leucocytes begin to adhere to the microfilariae in about one hour after the blood is drawn.[166] The reaction depends on the presence of specific antibody in the serum acting in much the same manner as an opsonin.

INFECTIONS WITH *STRONGYLOIDES*

NATURAL RESISTANCE

Nematodes of the genus *Strongyloides* have a comparatively limited host range. *Strongyloides stercoralis* of man, for example, infects man, as well as dogs, cats, and foxes, although the infections in the carnivores are poor and transient. *Strongyloides papillosus* infects sheep, goats, cattle, wild ruminants, rabbits, and minks. *Strongyloides ratti* infects only rats and guinea pigs.[167] An age resistance has been described in rats for *Strongyloides ratti*.[168] The age resistance seems to be explained largely by the better capacity of the old rats to make a specific immune response.[169]

ACQUIRED IMMUNITY

Experimental studies on *Strongyloides ratti* infection of rats show that an initial infection confers resistance to reinfection.[170]

---

[161] J. Rodhain and A. Dubois, *Rev. belge de sc. méd.*, 3: 613 (1931), and *Tr. Roy. Soc. Trop. Med. & Hyg.*, 25: 377 (1932) ; W. Mohr and H. Lippelt, *Klin. Wchnschr.*, 19: 157 (1940).

[162] A. Connal, *West African M. J.*, 7: 113 (1934) ; G. C. Low, *J. Trop. Med.*, 37: 359 (1934).

[163] A. C. Chandler, G. Milliken, and V. T. Schuhardt, *Am. J. Trop. Med.*, 10: 345 (1930) ; F. Fülleborn, *Arch. f. Dermat. u. Syph.*, 164: 216 (1931) ; V. L. Gutiérrez, *Rev. Mexic. de Biol.*, 11: 1 (1931) ; J. Rodhain and A. Dubois, *Tr. Roy. Soc. Trop. Med. & Hyg.*, 25: 377 (1932) ; L. Van Hoof, *Tr. Roy. Soc. Trop. Med. & Hyg.*, 27: 609 (1934).

[164] G. J. Stefanopoulo and J. Daniaud, *Bull. Soc. path. exot.*, 33: 149 (1940).

[165] G. W. St. C. Ramsay, *Tr. Roy. Soc. Trop. Med. & Hyg.*, 28: 399 (1935).

[166] C. G. Pandit, S. R. Pandit, and P. V. S. Iyer, *Indian J. M. Research*, 16: 946 (1929).

[167] A. J. Sheldon and G. F. Otto, *Am. J. Hyg.*, 27: 298 (1938).

[168] A. J. Sheldon, *J. Parasitol.*, 22: 533 (1936).

[169] H. J. Lawlor, *J. Parasitol. (Suppl.)*, 25: 30 (1939).

[170] A. J. Sheldon, *Am. J. Hyg.*, 25: 53 (1937).

Usually the resistance becomes demonstrable in about one month, worms of the initial infection being expelled at that time.[171] The filariform larvae are strongly agglutinated by an immune serum in vitro, and as they penetrate the skin of an immune animal they elicit a severe local reaction.[172] The resistance to *Strongyloides ratti* is passively transferred with the serum to normal rats. The immunity can also be induced artificially by vaccination with heat-killed larvae of the homologous parasite.[173]

[171] A. J. Sheldon, *Am. J. Hyg.*, 26: 352 (1937).

[172] S. Sato, *Fukuoka-Ikwadaigaku-Zasshi*, 26: 88 (1933).

[173] A. J. Sheldon, *Am. J. Hyg.*, 29: 47 (1939, sec. D); H. J. Lawlor, *Am. J. Hyg.*, 31: 28 (1940, sec. D).

Chapter XVII

RESPONSE TO ARTHROPODS

SOME PERSONS suffer severely from contact with insects or other arthropods, whereas other individuals are but little affected. Often a tolerance of these pests is acquired by persons after prolonged residence in an infested community. For example, newcomers to the Adirondack Mountains in New York State generally are attacked by the black flies which are found there, whereas older residents are annoyed but little.[1] Likewise, in the San Francisco area of California, where fleas and mosquitoes abound, new residents suffer from these pests chiefly during their first several months.[2] After this time, they seem to become less attractive to the insects. These differences or changes probably result from the development by the individuals of a true immunity by reason of continued contact with the offending arthropod.

Immune responses of persons or of animals to arthropods generally follow bites, stings, or infections by these creatures. In every case in which an immune response is made, antigens of the parasite must get into the tissue of the host, and the reaction in all involves a specific response (perhaps with antibody formation) by the host to these antigens. In the case of bites the antigens are contained in the saliva which the arthropod injects. In stings the antigens occur in the inoculated venom. In actual infections the antigens are secreted or excreted by the parasite itself while resident in or migrating through the host's tissue.

Before the effect of an arthropod bite or sting can correctly be interpreted as an immune response, it is first necessary to prove that the substance which the arthropod injects is without effect in a

---

[1] R. Matheson, *Medical Entomology*, Thomas (Springfield) (1932).
[2] L. S. Cherney, C. M. Wheeler, and A. C. Reed, *Am. J. Trop. Med.*, 19: 327 (1939).

normal person. This control has seldom been employed, and many reported cases of "sensitization" to arthropod bites or stings are not truly immune responses. They are rather evidence of the susceptibility of local tissue to the native toxic effects of the injected arthropod substance. In the same way man exhibits a marked susceptibility to the toxins of the diphtheria bacillus or the streptococcus when these are injected into the skin. After an individual has been bitten or stung many times by an arthropod, however, he acquires a true sensitivity to the arthropod substances, often manifested merely by his capacity to neutralize the toxic effect of the substance which the arthropod introduces. This capacity is quite analogous with that of man for neutralizing the diphtheria and the streptococcus toxins after he has been immunized with these antigens.

RESPONSE TO BITES

Immune responses to arthropod bites generally involve the blood-sucking forms, which include, among insects, mosquitoes, flies, fleas, lice, and such hemipterans as bedbugs, and, among arachnids, ticks and mites. In the case of all these forms, saliva containing the antigens of the parasite is inoculated beneath the skin of the host through the inserted proboscis in a manner analogous to that of injecting any antigenic solution by means of a hypodermic syringe. The arthropod inoculates the saliva in order to prevent coagulation of the blood which it ingests, the saliva mixing with this blood before it is withdrawn from the host.

THE BITES OF INSECTS

Any of the biting insects potentially can lead to an immune response, although only the blood sucking forms are of practical significance in this respect. Mosquitoes [3] are the worst offenders, although certain midges,[4] and flies,[5] fleas,[6] and lice [7] are also of

[3] A. Brown and others, *South. M. J.*, 31: 590 (1938); O. Hecht, *Zool. anzeiger*, 87: 94 (1930); E. N. Pawlowsky, A. K. Stein, and P. P. Perfiljew, *Ztschr. f. Parasitenk.*, 1: 484 (1928).
[4] A. Hase, *Ztschr. f. Parasitenk.*, 6: 119 (1933).
[5] E. N. Pawlowsky, A. K. Stein, and P. P. Perfiljew, *Ztschr. f. Parasitenk.*, 5: 1 (1932); S. Szentkiralyi and F. Lorincz, *Dermat. Wchnschr.*, 96: 289 (1933).
[6] A. A. Boycott, *Nature*, 118: 591 (1926).
[7] E. Grübel, *Dermat. Wchnschr.*, 79: 1182 (1924).

importance. A succession of bites is probably required before an individual becomes sensitive to the bite, although sometimes no possibility of prior contact seems obvious.[8] Usually the reactions which develop in sensitive persons to the bites are mild, resembling the immediate type of skin reaction seen in tests for hay fever allergies. Sometimes, however, where a greater immune response has been made, either because of unusually severe exposure or because of an unexpectedly great reactivity of the patient, a typical Arthus reaction can occur. One interesting case of acquired sensitivity to the bite of a mosquito (*Aëdes aegypti*) has been reported concerning a child living in an area with a large mosquito population (near Jacksonville, Florida). When two and one-half years old, the child had comparatively mild reactions to mosquito bites. The severity of the reaction increased as the child grew, however, until, when nine years of age, the child experienced with each bite a severe Arthus response with necrosis. Injections of extracts of mosquito substance failed to desensitize the patient significantly. The sensitivity to *Aëdes aegypti* could be passively transferred to a normal person by inoculating locally serum from the child, and a local reaction occurred when the mosquito bit the inoculated area of the normal person.[9]

Vaccination.—Persons sometimes can be immunized against the effects of insect bites by vaccination with the substance of the offending agent. This has been reported in persons sensitive to flea bite, the vaccine being prepared from the adult flea bodies. The vaccine has been tried experimentally in flea-infested areas near San Francisco with some success, although the routine use of such flea vaccine has not yet replaced other control measures directed against the fleas themselves.[10]

Homologous vaccines, perhaps containing the "toxins" of the insect, have been used to desensitize persons who give a severe reaction to mosquito bites.[11] In the case referred to in the previous paragraph, which was hypersensitive to *Aëdes aegypti,* no signifi-

[8] E. N. Pawlowsky, A. K. Stein, and P. P. Perfiljew, *Ztschr. f. Parasitenk.,* 5: 1 (1932).

[9] A. Brown and others, *South. M. J.,* 31: 590 (1938).

[10] L. S. Cherney, C. M. Wheeler, and A. C. Reed, *Am. J. Trop. Med.,* 19: 327 (1939).

[11] E. B. McKinley, *Proc. Soc. Exper. Biol. & Med.,* 26: 806 (1929).

cant improvement resulted from the administration of such a vaccine.[12]

THE BITES OF ARACHNIDS

Ticks,[13] mites,[14] and probably spiders, on biting individuals either defensively or for obtaining blood as food, elicit an immune response. In some cases a true venom is inoculated during the bite, which in the host body probably acts as does a true toxin by inducing the production of specific antitoxin. Such an antitoxin has, however, as yet not been experimentally demonstrated.[15] The acquisition of immunity by repeated exposure to these toxins likewise has not been shown. For example, sheep may suffer repeatedly the typical paralysis which follows the bite of certain ticks. The acquisition of immunity to spider venom by man also has not been proved, although animals do acquire such an immunity to the same species of poisonous spider.

The most thoroughgoing studies on the immune response to tick bite are those of Trager, who finds that guinea pigs after repeated infestation with larvae of *Dermacentor variabilis* manifest a typical Arthus reaction to the bite, which prevents the larvae from feeding successfully upon the immune host.[16] The sensitization can also be induced in the animal artificially by vaccination with tick substance. A true antibody is evidently produced, for specific complement fixation reactions can be obtained with the serum of rabbits vaccinated with the tick antigen.[17]

Apparently an immune response by a host can be effective only upon ticks such as *Dermacentor variabilis,* which feed slowly. Adult argasid ticks (for example, *Argas persicus*), which engorge in five to ten minutes, experience no difficulty in feeding upon specifically immune chickens. The immune response of the chicken, however,

---

[12] A. Brown and others, *South. M. J.*, 31: 590 (1938).

[13] W. Trager, *J. Parasitol. (Suppl.)*, 24: 20 (1938).

[14] C. M. Africa, *Philippine J. Sc.*, 50: 205 (1933); L. H. Dunn, *Am. J. Trop. Med.*, 13: 475 (1933).

[15] I. C. Ross, *Parasitology*, 18: 410 (1926); P. Regendanz and E. Reichenow, *Arch. f. Schiffs- u. Tropen-Hyg.*, 35: 255 (1931); A. W. Blair, *Arch. Int. Med.*, 54: 831 (1934).

[16] W. Trager, *J. Parasitol.*, 25: 57 (1939).

[17] W. Trager, *J. Parasitol.*, 25: 137 (1939).

does act against the larval argasid ticks which require at least four days for engorgement.[18]

An immunity to the bites of mites also occurs. A severe local reaction—dermatitis—has been reported to many species, such as *Trombicula irritans* and *Pediculoides ventricosus*. Presumably such reactions can develop only after sensitization, since natives long resident in an infested area develop an immunity to the dermatitis and even to attack by the mites. Antibody has been detected in the host's serum during one mite infestation—namely, that of the ear lobe mite, *Psoroptes communis cuniculi* in rabbits.[19]

RESPONSE TO STINGS

It is a long-established fact that bee keepers, stung repeatedly by bees, gradually react less and less to the bee venom and finally not at all. The inference is that the keeper has become "immune" to the venom. A definite immunity is developed rather quickly against bee sting, sometimes in three weeks or so, although several years usually are required for the immunity to reach its peak. Often a more-or-less absolute or perfect immunity is finally acquired to the chemical effects of the sting, and the individual becomes accustomed to the mechanical injury as well. Some animals, such as frogs, birds, and skunks, have a natural immunity to bee venom.[20]

Sensitivity to bee sting can be reduced by repeatedly injecting an extract of the bee.[21] Apparently the immune response has a group character, as would be expected, for the injection of an extract of the honey bee (*Apis mellifica*) is effective also for immunizing individuals to the stings of yellow jackets and other wasps, as well as to the stings of ants.[22] The issue is still not clear, however, whether such injections lead to desensitization or to an elevation of the immunity to a threshold level which prevents injury to the body by the venom. The evidence seems to favor the second point of view.

Very little experimental work has yet been done to determine

---

[18] W. Trager, *J. Parasitol.*, 26: 71 (1940).

[19] J. T. Culbertson, *Proc. Soc. Exper. Biol. & Med.*, 32: 1239 (1935).

[20] B. F. Beck, *Bee Venom Therapy*, New York, Appleton-Century (1935).

[21] D. C. Fisher and C. Center, *J. Allergy*, 5: 519 (1934); R. L. Benson and H. Semenov, *J. Allergy*, 1: 105 (1930); L. I. B. Braun, *South African Med. Record*, 23: 408 (1925).

[22] H. E. Prince and P. G. Secrest, *J. Allergy*, 10: 379 (1939).

whether an immunity is developed by man to scorpion stings, although desert animals which come in frequent contact with scorpions are said to acquire such an immunity.[23] Fatal stings in man usually occur in those five years old or less, although death of persons as much as twenty years of age has been reported.[24] Several stings simultaneously are fatal to adults.[25] An antiserum against scorpion venom is effective both prophylactically and therapeutically in animals and greatly reduces the symptoms in human cases. Apparently to be effective the antiserum must be specific for the precise species of scorpion supplying the venom.[26]

RESPONSE TO INFECTIONS

Arthropods which themselves penetrate the tissue of man sometimes call forth powerful immune responses. The larvae of flies are of especial importance in this respect. The experimental infection with one species, *Cordylobia anthropophaga*, has been most carefully studied and guinea pigs, monkeys, dogs, and man have all been shown to acquire a specific immunity from an initial infection with this form.[27] In immune guinea pigs the larvae of the second infection are usually dead within six days. The acquired immunity is first confined locally in the skin, but later it spreads to other areas. It lasts for at least several months. The immunity can be induced by vaccinating an animal with an emulsion of the larvae.[28] Antibody specific for the body fluids of the larva appear in the animal's serum after either infection or vaccination.[29]

An essentially similar immunity appears in guinea pigs after an initial cutaneous infection with the larvae of *Cochliomyia americana*. The acquired immunity is presumably localized in the skin, and animals remain susceptible to reinfection on the side of the body opposite that which harbored the initial infection. In this case the acquired immunity persists about forty days. A local skin im-

---

[23] W. H. Wilson, *Records Egypt. Gov. School Med.*, Cairo, 2: 7 (1904).

[24] R. M. Linnell, *Lancet*, 177: 11 (1914).

[25] C. C. Hoffman, *Anales Inst. Biol. Univ. Mexico*, 2: 291 (1931), and 3: 243 (1932).

[26] Todd, cited by W. A. Riley and O. A. Johannsen, *Medical Entomology*, New York, McGraw-Hill (1938).

[27] D. B. Blacklock and M. G. Thompson, *Ann. Trop. Med.*, 17: 443 (1923).

[28] D. B. Blacklock and R. M. Gordon, *Ann. Trop. Med.*, 21: 181 (1927).

[29] D. B. Blacklock, R. M. Gordon, and J. Fine, *Ann. Trop. Med.*, 24: 5 (1930).

munity can be developed to a slight degree by injecting a suspension of dried larval tissue.[30]

From the results described above it would seem probable that cattle could be successfully immunized against warbles by vaccination. The attempts made thus far to do so, however, have failed.[31] Nevertheless, cattle which are infected with warbles definitely respond immunologically to the parasite. For example, if a warble is accidentally crushed when in the tissue, the infected cow sometimes manifests a severe local inflammation or even symptoms of generalized anaphylactic shock.

Immune responses are also noted to mites. For example, following the ingestion of the tyroglyphid mites which are added to impart the characteristic flavor to a famous cheese, the Altenburger Milbenkäse, sensitive persons sometimes experience a definite digestive upset. No immune response to scabies, which is caused by the burrowing mite *Sarcoptes scabeii,* has yet been demonstrated.

[30] F. A. Borgstrom, *Am. J. Trop. Med.,* 18: 395 (1938).
[31] C. W. McIntosh, *Rep. Vet. Direct. Gen. Canada,* 51–52 (1932–33).

Part Three

APPLIED IMMUNOLOGY

Chapter XVIII

CLASSIFICATION OF PARASITES

PARASITES are generally classified according to morphological criteria. Different species are included in a single genus and different genera grouped in a single family because they are similar structurally. Relative nearness in relationship, therefore, depends on relative identity in structure. In a few cases, however, two species with identical morphology are considered distinct if they characteristically infect different hosts. Each of these parasites may have become rather perfectly adjusted physiologically to its own host, and neither can survive in the host of the alternate parasite. Thus natural susceptibility and resistance of the host is likewise useful for the purpose of classification.

In comparatively recent years immunological tests have also been invoked to classify the parasites, the relationships being based upon the relative identity of the antigenic constitution of the parasites. The serum from an animal immune to one parasite will react best in vitro with the substance of that parasite; it may also react with the substance of the related forms, usually less intensely. The nearness of relationship to the homologous parasite is usually shown by the relative intensity of the heterologous reactions. For the most part the findings from these immunological studies have corroborated the relationships already established from structural considerations. In a few cases, however, new and unexpected taxonomic points of view have resulted from the application of the immunological procedures.

GROUP RELATIONSHIPS

Immunological procedures have been employed both to establish the large taxonomic groups of parasites and to determine relationships within single groups. The results are as yet incomplete in all cases, however, and much of the data which is available requires corroboration before acceptance. The field is an especially favorable one for future experimentation.

REACTIONS BETWEEN GROUPS

Immunological reactions are of value in classifying only those parasites which have some antigens in common. Since no antigens are common to some large groups, immunological reactions cannot be employed to establish taxonomic relationships between these forms. For example, no antigens have been described as common to the different classes of protozoans or to any group of protozoans and the helminths. However, some antigens are common to two or more of the helminth classes. For example, reactions occur when antigens of such tapeworms as *Taenia pisiformis* and *Moniezia expansa* are tested with antiserums against such nematodes as *Ascaris suum*, *Ascaridia lineata*, and *Toxocara canis*, although, of course, they are weaker than those between each antiserum and the antigens of the homologous parasite. The group of spiny-headed worms (Acanthocephala) also has been shown to be more closely related antigenically to the flatworms than to the round worms. This observation holds considerable interest for systematists, since the acanthocephalids are usually classified with the round worms, from purely morphological considerations.[1]

The precise chemical nature of the antigens occurring simultaneously in different parasite groups is as yet not clear. Certain polysaccharides have been derived from various worms, however, which are absolutely specific. Even those from two such closely related nematode species as *Ascaris lumbricoides* and *Ascaris suum* are antigenically distinct.[2] Generally lipoids are thought to have very much broader specificity.

RELATIONSHIPS WITHIN GROUPS

In some groups of parasites the taxonomic relationships (including the differentiation of species) have been worked out almost exclusively by immunological procedures. In others, little, if any, use of these procedures has been made.

---

[1] L. L. Eisenbrandt, *Proc. Soc. Exper. Biol. & Med.*, 35: 322 (1936), and *Am. J. Hyg.*, 27: 117 (1938).

[2] D. H. Campbell, *J. Parasitol.*, 23: 348 (1937).

Amoebae.—The most thoroughgoing study of the classification of amoebae by immunological procedures has endorsed the earlier classification based on morphology and biochemical reactions. A considerable antigenic similarity is indicated in the pathogen *Endamoeba histolytica* and the free-living forms *Flabellula citata, Flabellula myra, Mayorella conipes, Mayorella bigemma,* and *Chaos diffluens,* although an extract of these free-living forms fails to fix complement when mixed with the serum of a patient infected with *Endamoeba histolytica.*[3] In contrast, an extract of any strain of *Endamoeba histolytica* will serve as antigen for the fixation test in amoebiasis.[4]

Some authorities consider *Endamoeba dispar* a separate pathogenic species from *Endamoeba histolytica.* They point out that the dog is immune to the specific parasite after recovery from *Endamoeba dispar* infection, but remains susceptible to *Endamoeba histolytica.*[5] Others believe the two forms identical.

Leishmania.—The leishmanias of kala azar, oriental sore, and espundia cannot be differentiated morphologically or by biochemical reactions, and the usual classification of the organisms rests upon the pathology of the infections they produce. Some doubt prevails, however, that the differences in pathology are properly related to distinct organisms, since the relative susceptibility of the host may about as well explain some of the observed differences. For example, oriental sore and espundia may be merely local manifestations of the generalized kala azar. However, some immunological evidence for differences among the parasites causing these diseases has also come to light. The serums from rabbits inoculated severally with cultures of *Leishmania donovani, Leishmania tropica,* and *Leishmania braziliensis* generally agglutinate the homologous organisms best,[6] although occasionally strong cross-reactions are reported.[7] If the rabbit antiserum against the various species is added to cultures of homologous and heterologous leishmanias, lysis occurs only in the tubes of homologous culture and growth

---

[3] L. Heathman, *Am. J. Hyg.,* 16: 97 (1932).
[4] P. E. Menendez, *Am. J. Hyg.,* 15: 785 (1932).
[5] T. Simĭc, *Ann. de parasitol.,* 13: 345 (1935).
[6] A. Laurinsich, *Pediatria,* 39: 345 (1931) ; G. Franchini and E. Pirami, *Arch. ital. di sc. med. colon.,* 11: 666 (1930).
[7] J. C. Ray, *Arch. f. Schiffs- u. Tropen-Hyg.,* 33: 598 (1929).

continues in the other tubes.[8] Less conclusive results to support the separate etiologies of these different clinical pictures have been obtained by the adhesin test, using the serum of mice which have been injected with cultures of the various leishmanias. In these tests essential identity is indicated for *Leishmania donovani* and *Leishmania tropica,* as well as for the canine strains of each.[9]

Trypanosomes.—The trypanosomes are easily differentiated into several large groups by morphology alone. Thus the so-called pathogenic forms, the *lewisi* group, *Trypanosoma cruzi,* and the trypanosomes of birds and of cold-blooded animals can all be identified. Within each group, however, some species bear close resemblance structurally. Various members of the *lewisi* group, for example, are identical in morphology. These can often be differentiated by their infectivity. The type species *Trypanosoma lewisi* infects rats, but not mice, whereas another species of the group, *Trypanosoma duttoni,* infects mice, but not rats.

The pathogenic trypanosomes also can to some extent be differentiated by host susceptibility. Those which naturally infect animals characteristically do not infect man, and those of the *vivax* group are distinct in that they do not infect the laboratory rodents. They can best be differentiated, however, through immunological tests. This has been done by the French workers chiefly in goats and sheep, which typically recover from infections with these forms and thereafter resist reinfection with the homologous species. Since their immunity is rigidly and narrowly specific, however, and heterologous species readily produce infections in recovered animals, strains of trypanosomes can somewhat easily be identified and differentiated by appropriate immunological tests in these animals. A similar test can also be performed in mice. If an initial infection with a given pathogenic trypanosome is cured by the administration of a suitable drug, the mouse will resist reinfection with the homologous parasite while remaining susceptible to heterologous species. Unfortunately the results from these tests in mice have led to confusion because of the extraordinarily narrow specificity of the immunity. Even relapse strains within a given species behave in these tests as distinct species.

[8] F. da Fonseca, *Am. J. Trop. Med.,* 12: 453 (1932), and 13: 113 (1933).
[9] N. I. Chodukin and M. S. Sofieff, *Arch. f. Schiffs- u. Tropen-Hyg.,* 34: 369 (1930).

Other immunological procedures, such as anaphylactic tests in guinea pigs, have also been employed for classifying the trypanosomes. *Trypanosoma lewisi* can thus be differentiated from the pathogenic species, but the pathogens cannot by this means be distinguished one from another.[10]

Malarias.—The malarias of man, monkeys, and birds can be differentiated by immunological procedures. The four human malaria parasites are all distinct morphologically and are just as definitely so by immunological procedures, since recovery from an infection with one will not protect against the others.[11] Indeed immunity in malaria is specific for a given strain, and reinjection with a heterologous strain, even of the same species, will result in infection.[12] By immunity tests strains within species can be identified.

Immunological tests have indicated that at least seven distinct species of bird malarial parasites exist which are infective for canaries, these being *Plasmodium cathemerium, Plasmodium praecox, Plasmodium circumflexum, Plasmodium elongatum, Plasmodium nucleophilum, Plasmodium rouxi,* and *Plasmodium vaughani.*[13] Immunity against only the homologous parasite follows recovery from one of these species, and infection with others can usually be expected. The species also are distinct in morphology, however, and both morphologic and immunologic facts must be considered in the differentiation of species. Distinct immunological strains are recognized within several species, although these strains usually appear to have many antigens in common.[14]

Coccidia.—Immunological tests can be used to differentiate various coccidia when these infect the same host. A rabbit which is immune to *Eimeria perforans,* for example, is still susceptible to *Eimeria stiedae,*[15] and a chicken which has acquired an immunity to *Eimeria tenella* remains susceptible to *Eimeria necatrix.*[16] All the

---

[10] H. Furukawa, *Japan M. World,* 8: 136 (1928).

[11] S. P. James, W. D. Nicol, and P. G. Shute, *Am. J. Trop. Med.,* 15: 187 (1935).

[12] M. F. Boyd, W. K. Stratman-Thomas, and H. Muench, *Am. J. Hyg.,* 20: 482 (1934) ; M. F. Boyd, W. K. Stratman-Thomas, and S. F. Kitchen, *Am. J. Trop. Med.,* 16: 139 (1936) ; M. F. Boyd and W. K. Stratman-Thomas, *Am. J. Hyg.,* 17: 55 (1933).

[13] R. D. Manwell, *Am. J. Trop. Med.,* 15: 265 (1935).

[14] R. D. Manwell and F. Goldstein, *Am. J. Hyg.,* 30: 115 (1939, sec. C) ; R. D. Manwell, *Am. J. Hyg.,* 27: 196 (1938).

[15] G. W. Bachman, *Am. J. Hyg.,* 12: 641 (1930).

[16] E. E. Tyzzer, H. Theiler, and E. E. Jones, *Am. J. Hyg.,* 15: 319 (1932).

coccidia have a comparatively restricted host range, many forms being infective only for one or two species.

Trematodes.—Immune reactions have not been extensively used for classifying or differentiating the trematodes. Yet the inter-relationships of certain trematode families have been studied by the precipitin test.[17] Furthermore, it is known that the schistosomes of mammals all have some antigens in common, since any mammalian schistosome will provide antigens useful for the fixation test in human schistosomiasis.[18] The liver fluke, *Fasciola gigantica*, evidently also possesses some antigens like those of schistosomes, since extracts of these forms are also useful in the skin test for schistosomiasis.[19]

Cestodes.—Immunological procedures have not been much tried for classifying the cestodes, although their use is strongly indicated for this purpose. Species whose adults are structurally similar, yet which are evidently distinct because of differences in infectivity (such as *Taenia serrata* and *Taenia crassicollis*), could possibly be shown to have distinct antigenic constitution by appropriate immunological procedures. Two species, *Moniezia expansa* and *Dipylidium caninum*, have been indicated by precipitin tests to be more closely related to each other than either is to *Taenia crassicollis*.[20] Such a result was expected, however, from a study of the morphologies of the several worms. The various cestodes are known to have many antigens in common. For example, an antiserum prepared by injecting an animal with either *Taenia* or *Diphyllobothrium* substance reacts in the test tube with both the specific and the alternate antigen.[21] Furthermore, antigenic extracts from practically any cestode serve to elicit skin tests in hydatid disease.[22]

Nematodes.—Certain recognized relationships among nematodes and especially among the ascarids have been confirmed by immune

[17] R. W. Wilhelmi, *J. Parasitol. (Suppl.)*, 25: 31 (1939), and *Biol. Bull.*, 79: 64 (1940).

[18] N. H. Fairley, *J. Helminthol.*, 11: 181 (1933).

[19] A. Hassan and M. Betashe, *J. Egyptian M. A.*, 17: 991 (1934).

[20] R. W. Wilhelmi, *J. Parasitol. (Suppl.)*, 25: 31 (1939), and *Biol. Bull.*, 79: 64 (1940).

[21] L. L. Eisenbrandt, *Am. J. Hyg.*, 27: 117 (1938); O. Sievers, *Ztschr. f. Immunitätsforsch. u. exper. Therap.*, 84: 208 (1935).

[22] L. Morenas, *Compt. rend. Soc. de biol.*, 110: 321 (1932); J. T. Culbertson and H. M. Rose, *J. Clin. Investigation*, 20: 249 (1941).

reactions.[23] *Ascaridia lineata* of the chicken, for example, has been found through precipitin tests to be more closely related to the *Ascaris* of pigs or the *Toxocara* of dogs than to *Heterakis papillosa* of chickens.[24] Among the filarid nematodes, also, many are known to have common antigens. An extract of *Dirofilaria immitis* from the dog, for example, will serve for skin tests or for fixation tests in all the human filariases.[25] Antigens suitable for skin testing in human filariasis also have been derived from *Ascaris lumbricoides* [26] and from *Contortospiculum rheae*.[27]

The various stages of a parasite species have, so far as is known, the same antigenic constitution.[28] Antigens from two forms which are suspected to represent different stages of the same parasite should, then, react equally with an antiserum prepared against either. Use has been made of this fact in completing the life cycles of certain parasites. Since, for example, by agglutination tests *Leishmania tropica* from man and *Herpetomonas papatasii* from an invertebrate are the same in antigenic structure, these forms are considered successive stages of one species of parasite by some authorities.[29] Probably the method will eventually have somewhat greater use for the purpose among helminths, although, until the present, it has had but little application.[30]

[23] B. Schwartz, *J. Parasitol.*, 6: 115 (1920).
[24] L. L. Eisenbrandt, *Am. J. Hyg.*, 27: 117 (1938).
[25] W. H. Taliaferro and W. A. Hoffman, *J. Prevent. Med.*, 4: 261 (1930); J. Rodhain and A. Dubois, *Rev. belge de sc. méd.*, 3: 613 (1931); N. H. Fairley, *Tr. Roy. Soc. Trop. Med. & Hyg.*, 25: 220 (1932).
[26] J. Rodhain and A. Dubois, *Tr. Roy. Soc. Trop. Med. & Hyg.*, 25: 377 (1932).
[27] W. Mohr and H. Lippelt, *Klin. Wchnschr.*, 19: 157 (1940).
[28] R. W. Wilhelmi, *J. Parasitol. (Suppl.)*, 25: 31 (1939), and *Biol. Bull.*, 79: 64 (1940).
[29] S. Adler and O. Theodor, *Ann. Trop. Med.*, 20: 355 (1926).
[30] H. W. Stunkard, *J. Parasitol.*, 26: 1 (1940).

Chapter XIX

VACCINATION AGAINST PARASITES

PROPHYLAXIS through vaccination is possible in animal infections with representatives of nearly all groups of parasites. Only in rare cases, however, have the fundamentals of such protection been worked out adequately so as to permit the application of the methods to corresponding human infections.

Vaccination may be carried out by (1) infection with small numbers of living virulent parasites, (2) administration of living but avirulent strains of homologous parasites, and (3) inoculation of killed homologous organisms. The essential requisite, whatever the method employed, is the intensive stimulation of the host with the antigens of the parasite. The immune response thus engendered is generally characterized by the development of antibodies, although sometimes the demonstration of these antibodies is difficult or impossible.

EXAMPLES OF VACCINATION IN DIFFERENT DISEASES

AMOEBIASIS

Vaccination against *Endamoeba histolytica* has as yet not been investigated. Such studies have until now been prevented because of the difficulty experienced in obtaining the amoebae in sufficient concentration and purity to prepare a vaccine.

LEISHMANIASIS

Oriental sore is one of the few parasitic infections against which man is known to acquire protection through vaccination. Vaccination against the disease is rather widely resorted to, apparently with considerable success, in those parts of the world where a large percentage of the general population suffers from oriental sore.[1] To secure protection, fully virulent *Leishmania tropica* apparently must be inoculated into the skin and a typical lesion must be experienced. On recovery from this initial infection the individual is immune to reinfection. Even when the first lesion occurs in some hidden area of the skin, the recovered individual is nevertheless protected against the danger of disfiguration from lesions in an exposed site, such as the face. Experimental work in animals, even when living organisms are used as the vaccine, however, does not support vaccination as a protective method. Monkeys, for example, can be reinfected readily after recovery from an initial experimental lesion.[2] The injection of killed cultures either to man or to animals confers no protection. The vaccination of man against kala azar has not been tried, and efforts to protect animals by this procedure have thus far been unsuccessful.[3]

TRYPANOSOMIASIS

Attempts to protect man against trypanosome infections by vaccination have not yet been reported. In Africa the vaccination of domesticated animals with very small doses of virulent organisms has been tried and some favorable results have been reported.[4] However, perfect protection is so seldom obtained even by those who have devised the methods that the routine use of such vaccination for protection is not advised. The chief stumbling blocks appear to be the multiplicity of biologic strains of trypanosomes which are potentially pathogenic for domesticated animals in the endemic areas and the capacity of each of these to vary even further as its need arises. The chance seems remote, if not nonexistent, for the preparation of a vaccine of sufficient biologic breadth to protect against all these infective strains. Experimentally, however, animals can be protected against any specific immunologic strain by vaccination with killed homologous organisms.

The small laboratory rodents can be protected often perfectly

[1] A. P. Lawrow and P. A. Dubowskoj, *Arch. f. Schiffs- u. Tropen-Hyg.*, 41: 374 (1937); E. I. Marzinowsky, *Bull. Soc. path. exot.*, 21: 638 (1928).

[2] L. Parrot, *Compt. rend. Soc. de biol.*, 100: 411 (1929).

[3] B. Malamos, *Arch. f. Schiffs- u. Tropen-Hyg.*, 41: 416 (1937); T. J. Kurotchkin, *Nat. M. J. China*, 17: 458 (1931).

[4] C. Schilling and others, *Ztschr. f. Immunitätsforsch. u. exper. Therap.*, 89: 112 (1936).

against trypanosomes of the *lewisi* group by the injection of killed suspensions of homologous trypanosomes.[5] The problem in this case, however, is a comparatively simple one, since only a single biologic strain of each species exists. Indeed, there is even a group reaction, the same antigens occurring in different species of parasites, and mice can be immunized against *Trypanosoma duttoni* by vaccination with killed *Trypanosoma lewisi*.[6]

MALARIAS

Experimental attempts to protect man and monkey against malaria through vaccination have failed except when an individual has suffered a typical infection of comparative severity. The inoculation of vaccines consisting of killed organisms is without protective effect.[7] In bird malaria, however, some protection is said to follow vaccination with organisms which have been killed with formaldehyde or rendered avirulent by prolonged exposure to low temperature.[8]

COCCIDIOSES

Chicks, as well as pigs, cattle, and some other animals, can be specifically protected against coccidiosis by feeding very small doses of fully virulent coccidia.[9] Symptoms often become rather acute, but the infections are generally self-limiting, and resistance for short periods after recovery is the rule. Larger doses of coccidial cysts can be used in chicks, and a somewhat higher level of immunity can be developed, if the cysts are heated prior to their administration.[10] The parenteral injection of dead coccidial substance does not lead to protection.[11]

[5] W. H. Taliaferro, *Am. J. Hyg.*, 16: 32 (1932) ; J. T. Culbertson and W. R. Kessler, *Am. J. Hyg.*, 29: 33 (1939, sec. C).

[6] W. R. Kessler, unpublished experiments.

[7] M. D. Eaton and L. T. Coggeshall, *J. Exper. Med.*, 70: 141 (1939).

[8] E. Sergent, E. Sergent, and A. Catanei, *Arch. Inst. Pasteur d'Algerie*, 12: 10 (1934) ; W. B. Redmond, *J. Parasitol. (Suppl.)*, 25: 28 (1939) ; W. D. Gingrich, *J. Infect. Dis.*, 68: 46 (1941).

[9] E. E. Tyzzer, *Am. J. Hyg.*, 10: 269 (1929) ; H. E. Biester and L. H. Schwarte, *J. Am. Vet. M. A.*, 81: 358 (1932) ; W. T. Johnson, Oreg. Agric. Exp. Stat., *Director's Report*, 230 (1927), and *J. Parasitol.*, 19: 160 (1932).

[10] H. A. Jankiewicz and R. H. Scofield, *J. Am. Vet. M. A.*, 84: 507 (1934).

[11] E. E. Tyzzer, *Am. J. Hyg.*, 10: 269 (1929) ; E. R. Becker, *Am. J. Hyg.*, 21: 389 (1935) ; G. W. Bachman, *Am. J. Hyg.*, 12: 641 (1930).

TREMATODIASES

Little experimentation on vaccination against trematodes has yet been done. Rabbits can be protected against *Fasciola hepatica* by the injection of the homologous substance,[12] but the use of such vaccination in sheep and cattle—species which so frequently suffer from fascioliasis—has not yet been tried. The infection in these animals is probably of sufficient economic importance to warrant the development of methods for vaccination.

Vaccination of man against schistosomiasis also has not yet been attempted, despite the fact that specific means of protection against the disease might have application in endemic areas. The fact that man responds immunologically rather powerfully following infection suggests that an effective immunity might follow vaccination.

CESTODIASES

Animals can be protected against subsequent infection with larval cestodes both by recovery from a prior mild infection and by vaccination with the killed homologous cestode substance. The best evidence of such protection is seen in experimental cysticercosis of rats and rabbits.[13] Oxen also are protected against subsequent heavy infections if they first experience a mild attack of cysticercosis.[14] Probably man likewise could be protected by vaccination against infection with cysticerci, although because cysticercosis is quite rare in man, need hardly exists for such prophylactic measures.

Vaccination against hydatid or echinococcus disease with killed antigens is sometimes partially successful in sheep,[15] and its use in man is not contraindicated. An individual who already is infected with echinococcus disease might benefit by vaccination with the antigens of the parasite. Such a vaccinated person might thereafter resist reinfection from a ruptured cyst and might even destroy those cysts which are already present. There is need for experimental

---

[12] K. B. Kerr and O. L. Petkovich, *J. Parasitol.*, 21: 319 (1935).

[13] H. M. Miller, Jr., *Proc. Soc. Exper. Biol. & Med.*, 27: 926 (1930) and 28: 467 (1931); K. B. Kerr, *Am. J. Hyg.*, 22: 169 (1935).

[14] W. J. Penfold and H. B. Penfold, *J. Helminthol.*, 15: 37 (1937).

[15] E. L. Turner, E. W. Dennis, and D. A. Berberian, *J. Parasitol.*, 23: 43 (1937); H. B. Penfold, *M. J. Australia*, 1: 375 (1938).

work on this problem, for it would have considerable practical application.

NEMATODIASES

Experimental animals can be protected through vaccination against many nematodes, including ascarids,[16] hookworms,[17] and some of their relatives, as well as *Strongyloides* [18] and *Trichinella*.[19] Protection is sometimes conferred by inoculating killed antigens, although actual infection with small numbers of parasites must often be resorted to. No effort has been made thus far to duplicate any of these results in man, probably in part because most of these infections are of limited severity in man or can be controlled easily through treatment with chemotherapeutic agents. Trichiniasis is one exception. This disease is sometimes fatal to man, and no method of specific treatment is available. For the most part, however, human infections with *Trichinella* are very mild. Furthermore, the disease does not occur in man with sufficient frequency to require the vaccination of the general population.

Whether or not mild infections with *Trichinella* confer to man a specific immunity against contracting a subsequent severe infection has not been proved, although certainly such an effect would be expected from the results obtained with *Trichinella* infections in experimental animals.

THE PREPARATION OF VACCINES

The vaccines employed for protecting animals from parasitic infection in many cases represent merely the living, fully virulent homologous parasites obtained either in culture or else directly or indirectly from an animal harboring them. In other cases these forms before administration are exposed to various physical or chemical agents to reduce their virulence without killing them. Often they are killed outright, either by desiccation or gentle heating or by treatment with formaldehyde, phenol, or other disinfec-

---

[16] O. Wagner, *Ztschr. f. Immunitätsforsch. u. exper. Therap.*, 78: 372 (1933); K. B. Kerr, *Am. J. Hyg.*, 27: 28 (1938).

[17] G. F. Otto and K. B. Kerr, *Am. J. Hyg.*, 29: 25 (1939, sec. D).

[18] A. J. Sheldon, *Am. J. Hyg.*, 25: 53 (1937).

[19] O. R. McCoy, *Am. J. Hyg.*, 14: 484 (1931), and 21: 200 (1935); H. Roth, *Am. J. Hyg.*, 30: 35 (1939, sec. D).

tant. Usually these killed vaccines are prepared as suspensions or extracts of the isolated parasites.

VACCINES OF VIRULENT ORGANISMS

Virulent *Leishmania tropica* serve as vaccine in oriental sore. A culture of these parasites is generally employed,[20] although the essential initial lesion can also be established by direct transfer of material from a primary lesion in a patient to the skin of a normal person. Likewise, the injection of a few fully virulent pathogenic trypanosomes [21] or the feeding of small numbers of fully virulent coccidia [22] protects domestic animals against subsequent infection with the homologous forms. The administration of small numbers of malaria organisms has been reported to lead to the protection of man.[23] Cattle also are protected against Texas fever if first inoculated with the virulent causal piroplasm when young, or if the infection in older animals is controlled by the administration of trypan blue after parasites have appeared in the peripheral blood.[24] Likewise, the administration of small numbers of virulent onchospheres of the taeniid cestodes [25] or of the infective larvae of ascarids,[26] hookworms,[27] *Strongyloides*,[28] and trichinae [29] serves for vaccinating against subsequent infection with the corresponding parasites.

VACCINES OF ORGANISMS OF REDUCED VIRULENCE

It is extraordinarily difficult to reduce the virulence of an animal parasite while preserving its other natural qualities. In very few

[20] A. P. Lawrow and P. A. Dubowskoj, *Arch. f. Schiffs- u. Tropen-Hyg.*, 41: 374 (1937) ; E. I. Marzinowsky, *Bull. Soc. path. exot.*, 21: 638 (1928).
[21] C. Schilling and others, *Ztschr. f. Immunitätsforsch u. exper. Therap.*, 89: 112 (1936).
[22] E. E. Tyzzer, *Am. J. Hyg.*, 10: 269 (1929) ; H. E. Biester and L. H. Schwarte, *J. Am. Vet. M. A.*, 81: 358 (1932) ; W. T. Johnson, *J. Parasitol.*, 19: 160 (1932).
[23] C. Schilling, *Deutsche med. Wchnschr.*, 65: 1264 (1939).
[24] E. Sergent and others, *Ann. Inst. Pasteur*, 41: 721, 1175 (1927).
[25] H. M. Miller, Jr., *Proc. Soc. Exper. Biol. & Med.*, 27: 926 (1930), and 28: 467 (1931) ; K. B. Kerr, *Am. J. Hyg.*, 22: 169 (1935).
[26] O. Wagner, *Ztschr. f. Immunitätsforsch. u. exper. Therap.*, 78: 372 (1933) ; K. B. Kerr, *Am. J. Hyg.*, 27: 28 (1938).
[27] G. F. Otto and K. B. Kerr, *Am. J. Hyg.*, 29: 25 (1939, sec. D).
[28] A. J. Sheldon, *J. Parasitol.*, 22: 533 (1936), and *Am. J. Hyg.*, 25: 53 (1937).
[29] O. R. McCoy, *Am. J. Hyg.*, 14: 484 (1931), and 21: 200 (1935) ; H. Roth, *Am. J. Hyg.*, 30: 35 (1939, sec. D).

cases has this been done so that thereafter the organisms can be used for vaccination. Success has been reported with the plasmodia of bird malaria by subjecting these organisms to prolonged exposure to low temperature.[30] It has also been reported with the coccidia of chickens by gentle heating.[31]

KILLED VACCINES

Vaccines consisting of isolated homologous organisms killed by desiccation or heat or else by treatment with chemicals have been prepared for several parasitic infections. A good vaccine against *Trypanosoma lewisi* of the rat, for example, can be made by formolizing the parasites after separation from the blood of an intensely infected young rat.[32] A formolized homologous vaccine has been used in bird malaria.[33] With the helminths the isolated parasites are usually killed by desiccation, then (after trituration, in the case of the large forms) resuspended and extracted in such sterilizing solutions as 0.5 percent phenol or formalin. Effective vaccines for inoculating animals have been prepared in this or an essentially similar manner for such helminths as *Fasciola hepatica*,[34] *Taenia serrata, Taenia crassicollis*,[35] *Nippostrongylus muris*,[36] *Strongyloides ratti*,[37] and *Trichinella spiralis*.[38]

[30] W. B. Redmond, *J. Parasitol. (Suppl.)*, 25: 28 (1939).
[31] H. A. Jankiewicz and R. H. Scofield, *J. Am. Vet. M. A.*, 84: 507 (1934).
[32] J. T. Culbertson and W. R. Kessler, *Am. J. Hyg.*, 29: 33 (1939, sec. C).
[33] W. D. Gingrich, *J. Infect. Dis.*, 68: 46 (1941).
[34] K. B. Kerr and O. L. Petkovich, *J. Parasitol.*, 21: 319 (1935).
[35] H. M. Miller, Jr., *Proc. Soc. Exper. Biol. & Med.*, 27: 926 (1939), and 28: 467 (1931); K. B. Kerr, *Am. J. Hyg.*, 27: 28 (1938).
[36] A. C. Chandler, *Am. J. Hyg.*, 16: 750 (1932), and 24: 129 (1936).
[37] A. J. Sheldon, *Am. J. Hyg.*, 29: 47 (1939, sec. D).
[38] O. R. McCoy, *Am. J. Hyg.*, 21: 200 (1935).

Chapter XX

DIAGNOSIS OF PARASITIC
INFECTION

PARASITIC INFECTIONS can be diagnosed by detecting in the blood serum or tissues of the host either the antigens of the parasite or the antibody which the host has formed against these antigens. The test for antigen, which is rarely employed in diagnosis, is useful chiefly in very acute infections, and among these during only the early stages. The tests for antibody, on the other hand, are widely used and serve in both acute and chronic infections. Antibody tests often do not become positive before the second or third week after infection, since time must elapse to permit the host to react with antibody formation after invasion by the parasite.

In order that the host can form antibody it must be significantly affected by the parasite, either through the invasion of its tissues by the parasite or through the absorption of parasite antigens from the intestine. In general, parasites which dwell in the lumen of the intestine stimulate only traces of antibody at best, and immunological tests can be applied in the diagnosis of these infections with only limited success. In contrast, parasites which reach the somatic tissues or which experience a blood stream passage stimulate larger amounts of antibody, and infections by them can be identified through tests for antibody with greater facility.

In the diagnosis of infection by immunological methods one must keep clearly in mind the specific and invariable quality that homologous antigens and antibodies have of uniting with each other. If one has available a known antibody he can test a patient's specimen for the presence of the homologous antigen; if one has at hand a known antigen he can detect the corresponding antibody. Usually the detection of either the antigen of a parasite or the antibody specific for it suffices to establish that the host is infected with that parasite. Since parasites are constituted of many antigens, however, and since certain of these antigens usually occur also in related parasites, confusing group reactions—often inaccurately explained as of nonspecific character—are frequently encountered, just as in the diagnosis of bacterial diseases. Furthermore, since tests for antibody often remain positive for years after clinical recovery, positive tests, although perhaps correctly identifying the presence of a given parasite in the patient's tissues, do not prove that the parasite in question accounts for the symptoms which the patient exhibits at the time the test is made. Therefore positive immunological tests must be carefully studied and cautiously interpreted before a given parasite is declared responsible for the symptoms which a patient presents.

TESTS FOR ANTIGEN

As yet relatively little use has been made of the test for antigen in diagnosis, although, especially in intense infections, there is much to recommend it. It has been employed in leishmaniasis, trypanosomiasis, and malaria, among protozoan diseases. Leishmania antigen can be detected by the fixation test in the serum of patients or animals with kala azar, the specific antibody for the test coming from a rabbit artificially immunized with cultures of leishmania.[1] Nonspecific results, however, occasionally are obtained.[2] A similar fixation test will detect the antigens of *Plasmodium knowlesi* in the serum of intensely infected *Macacus rhesus*.[3] The serum antibody for this test can be obtained from an immune *Macacus rhesus*. A thermoprecipitinogen test has been described for experimental trypanosomiasis. When heated extracts of the tissue of a rabbit or guinea pig infected with *Trypanosoma equiperdum* are mixed with the serum of a recovered animal, a precipitation reaction promptly occurs.[4]

Among the helminthiases, both trichiniasis of rabbit and *Hae-*

---

[1] L. Nattan-Larrier and L. Grimard-Richard, *Compt. rend. Soc. de biol.*, 113: 1489 (1933); L. Nattan-Larrier and L. Grimard, *Bull. Soc. path. exot.*, 28: 658 (1935).

[2] C. Anderson and C. Disdier, *Arch. Inst. Pasteur de Tunis*, 27: 203 (1938).

[3] M. D. Eaton, *J. Exper. Med.*, 69: 517 (1939).

[4] H. A. Poindexter, *J. Exper. Med.*, 60: 575 (1934)

monchus infection of sheep can be diagnosed by testing the serum for antigen during the early days of infection. A precipitin reaction occurs when serum from an animal infected with *Trichinella* larvae a day or so earlier is mixed with a specific antiserum.[5] A more delicate test is required in the *Haemonchus* infection. If blood from a sheep with haemonchiasis is injected to a guinea pig which has previously been sensitized with *Haemonchus* substance, a rise in the absolute number of eosinophiles in the guinea pig occurs because of the presence of *Haemonchus* antigens in the sheep blood.[6]

The tests for antigen have the distinct advantage of diagnosing the infection in its early stages. This is important to the clinician, since it permits treatment to begin earlier. Indeed by the time antibody has appeared and positive tests for antibody are possible, the patient is often well along toward recovery and beyond the need of treatment. At this time the diagnosis is relatively unimportant except in a confirmatory capacity.

TESTS FOR ANTIBODY

All the different tests for antibody have been invoked for diagnosing parasitic infection. Complement fixation, precipitation, and skin tests have been most extensively employed, although agglutination and adhesin tests also have had some use.

AGGLUTINATION TESTS

Agglutination tests have been little used in the diagnosis of parasitic infections chiefly because only a few parasites can be prepared in the form of an agglutinable suspension. Nevertheless several protozoans are obtainable in this form, and the agglutination test can be used to diagnose the corresponding infections. Malaria, leishmaniasis, and trypanosomiasis have all been diagnosed by the agglutination test. *Plasmodium knowlesi* malaria of monkeys has been especially studied.[7] In this infection agglutinin appears between the fifteenth and forty-fifth day after infection, the agglutinin titer often rising thereafter to about 1:1000. Peculiarly, only the mature malaria parasites are clumped by the antibody, pre-

[5] J. Bozicevich and L. Detre, *Pub. Health Rep.*, 55: 683 (1940).
[6] J. E. Stumberg, *Am. J. Hyg.*, 18: 247 (1933).
[7] B. Malamos, *Riv. di malariol.*, 16: 91 (1937); M. D. Eaton, *J. Exper. Med.*, 67: 857 (1938).

sumably because immature stages occur so deeply within the red cell that the antibody in the immune serum cannot reach them. *Plasmodium circumflexum* of the canary is likewise agglutinated by an immune serum.[8] A similar clumping of *Plasmodium falciparum* in human serum has also been reported.[9] A number of investigators have reported finding agglutinins for *Leishmania donovani* in the serum of patients with kala azar, although the titers have generally been too weak for use in diagnosis.[10]

Agglutinins are developed by animals after experimental infection with many pathogenic trypanosomes, including *Trypanosoma gambiense, Trypanosoma brucei,* and *Trypanosoma equiperdum,*[11] as well as with trypanosomes of the *lewisi* group.[12] The test for agglutinins has been used in dourine of the horse. It has not attained general use in the African form of human trypanosomiasis.[13] Its use has been suggested in *Trypanosoma cruzi* infections.[14]

The agglutination test has not been used for diagnosing helminth infections. Serum from an animal infected with *Strongyloides* will, nevertheless, clump a suspension of the homologous infective larvae.[15] Probably the agglutination of finely divided particles of other helminths would also occur if a specific immune serum were added to a suspension of them.

PRECIPITATION TEST

The test for precipitins has been employed only rarely for diagnosing any of the protozoan infections and in none has it attained general use. The difficulty in procuring a suitable antigen has prevented its wider trial. Positive precipitin tests have been reported, nevertheless, in amoebiasis, trypanosomiasis, and malaria. The positive tests in amoebiasis have been obtained thus far only in experimental infections of cats, the antigen for such tests being procured

[8] R. D. Manwell and F. Goldstein, *J. Exper. Med.,* 71: 409 (1940).
[9] J. G. Thomson, *Proc. Roy. Soc. Med.,* 12: 39 (1919).
[10] G. di Cristina, *Pediatria,* 19: 774 (1911) ; G. Caronia, *Pathologica,* 4: 724 (1912).
[11] Lange, *Centralbl. f. Bakt., Ref.,* 50: Beiheft 171 (1911).
[12] J. T. Culbertson and W. R. Kessler, *Am. J. Hyg.,* 29: 33 (1939, sec. C).
[13] Winkler and S. Wyschelessky, *Berl. tierärztl. Wchnschr.,* 27: 933 (1911).
[14] A. Packchanian, *J. Immunol.,* 29: 84 (1935), and *Pub. Health Rep.,* 55: 2116 (1940).
[15] S. Sato, *Fukuoka Ikwadaigaku-Zasshi,* 26: 88 (1933).

by extracting scrapings of gut lesions.[16] The precipitin test in trypanosomiasis has been obtained in human infections, the antigen
being extracted from the organs of an experimentally infected animal.[17] In the tests in malaria the antigen is obtained from infected
placentas [18] or from cultures of the parasites.[19] A strong group
reaction occurs, however, for an antigen from any one species of
human malaria serves to detect antibodies against other species of
the parasite.

The Henry flocculation test, which has been used particularly in
malaria but also in leishmaniasis and trypanosomiasis, is not an
antigen-antibody reaction, and hence will not be discussed here in
detail. A positive test depends on the increased precipitability of
the serum globulin during these diseases. The reaction is entirely
nonspecific and is elicited by adding distilled water to the patient's
serum under controlled conditions. Various pigments are often
added to the water in order to render the globulin floccules more
easily visible after they have been formed.[20]

Precipitin tests have been used in the diagnosis of such helminth
infections as fascioliasis of cattle,[21] schistosomiasis,[22] cysticercosis,[23] echinococcus disease,[24] somatic ascariasis of rodents,[25] *Ascaridia* infection of chicks,[26] and trichiniasis.[27] The precipitin anti-

[16] E. H. Wagener, Univ. California, *Publ., Zoology*, 36: 15 (1924).

[17] A. Sicé, *Bull. Soc. path. exot.*, 22: 912 (1929), and 23: 459 (1930).

[18] W. H. Taliaferro and L. G. Taliaferro, *J. Prevent. Med.*, 2: 147 (1928).

[19] R. Row, *Tr. Roy. Soc. Trop. Med. & Hyg.*, 24: 623 (1931).

[20] A. F. X. Henry, *Compt. rend. Soc. de biol.*, 101: 1026 (1929); F. Trensz,
Arch. Inst. Pasteur d'Algerie, 10: 443 (1932); F. Trensz, *Bull. Soc. path. exot.*, 25:
230 (1932); F. Trensz, *Compt. rend. Soc. de biol.*, 117: 1106 (1934); V. Chorine
and R. Gillier, *Compt. rend. Acad. d. sc.* 197: 950 (1933); V. Chorine, *Riv. di
malariol.*, 13: 807 (1934); V. Chorine and D. Koechlin, *Bull. Soc. path. exot.*, 28:
375 (1935).

[21] W. A. Hoffman and T. Rivero, *Porto Rico Rev. Pub. Health & Trop. Med.*,
4: 589 (1929).

[22] W. H. Taliaferro, W. A. Hoffman, and D. H. Cook, *J. Prevent. Med.*, 2: 395
(1928), and *Porto Rico Rev. Pub. Health & Trop. Med.*, 4: 117 (1928); B. Imai,
Japan M. World, 8: 273 (1928); S. Miyaji and B. Imai, *Zentralbl. f. Bakt.*, 106:
237 (1928).

[23] J. Rothfeld, *Deutsche Ztschr. f. Nervenheilk.*, 137: 93 (1935); A. Trawinski
and J. Rothfeld, *Zentralbl. f. Bakt.*, 134: 472 (1935); A. Trawinski, *Zentralbl. f.
Bakt.*, 136: 116 (1936).

[24] F. Hoder, *Fortschr. d. Med.*, 51: 959 (1933).

[25] F. A. Coventry, *J. Prevent. Med.*, 3: 43 (1929).

[26] L. L. Eisenbrandt and J. E. Ackert, *Am. J. Hyg.*, 32: 1 (1940, sec. D).

[27] G. W. Bachman, *J. Prevent. Med.*, 3: 465 (1929); D. L. Augustine, *New*

body has also been detected in serum of dogs with hookworm disease.[28] A salt solution extract of the homologous worm is generally employed for these tests. Often the tests remain positive for years after infection, in trichiniasis, for example, sometimes being obtained after from four to nine years.[29]

A positive precipitin test requires that the serum possess a considerable amount of antibody. The precipitate formed in the reaction consists often of about 90 percent antibody and 10 percent antigen, and enough of the combination must be formed to be visible. Relatively smaller amounts of antibody are required for positive agglutination and complement fixation tests, and these tests are therefore sometimes positive when the precipitin test is negative.

COMPLEMENT FIXATION TEST

The complement fixation test is the most delicate in vitro means of detecting antibody. It has been used in nearly all the important parasitic infections of man and domesticated animals. The test is especially valuable in such protozoan infections as amoebiasis [30] and trypanosomiases, and has also been used in leishmaniasis, malaria, and coccidiosis.

The antigen for the fixation test in amoebiasis can be made either from cultures [31] or by extracting the scrapings from intestinal lesions of experimentally infected animals. The reaction becomes positive in experimental animals in from the third to the fourteenth day after infection.[32] After the infection is cured, either spontaneously or by treatment with specific drugs, the test is negative, although in relapsed cases it again becomes positive.[33]

The fixation test is useful in kala azar, as well as in cutaneous

England J. Med., 216: 463 (1937); W. W. Spink and D. L. Augustine, J. A. M. A., 104: 1801 (1935); H. Theiler and D. L. Augustine, Zentralbl. f. Bakt., 135: 299 (1935); A. Trawínski, Zentralbl. f. Bakt., 136: 238 (1936).

[28] G. F. Otto, Am. J. Hyg., 31: 23 (1940, sec. D).

[29] H. Theiler, D. L. Augustine, and W. W. Spink, Parasitology, 27: 345 (1935).

[30] C. F. Craig, Am. J. Pub. Health, 27: 689 (1937); T. B. Magath and H. E. Meleney, Am. J. Trop. Med., 20: 211 (1940).

[31] H. Tsuchiya, J. Lab. & Clin. Med., 19: 495 (1934).

[32] C. F. Craig, Proc. Soc. Exper. Biol. & Med., 30: 270 (1932).

[33] C. F. Craig, J. Lab. & Clin. Med., 18: 873 (1933).

leishmaniasis of both man and dog.[34] The antigen can be made from cultures of leishmania [35] or from the liver of infected animals.[36] As previously stated, a reversed complement fixation test has also been described in leishmaniasis, by which, early in the infection, leishmania antigens are detected in the serum of patients by mixing their serum with an antiserum from rabbits immunized with *Leishmania* cultures.[37] As yet the reversed fixation test has not had widespread adoption because of frequent nonspecific reactions.[38]

The complement fixation test is positive in infections with both pathogenic and nonpathogenic trypanosomes. It is reported in horses, as well as in dogs, with *Trypanosoma equiperdum*,[39] in cattle with *Trypanosoma hippicum*,[40] in camels with *Trypanosoma marocanum*,[41] in both humans and animals with *Trypanosoma cruzi*,[42] and in rats with *Trypanosoma lewisi*.[43] Antigens for the pathogenic species (for example, *Trypanosoma equiperdum*) can be made by extracting trypanosomes isolated from the blood of heavily infected rats.[44] Antigens for diagnosing *Trypanosoma cruzi* infections are best obtained from cultures of this parasite,[45] although they can also be prepared from the heavily infected spleens of young puppies.[46] The antigen for *Trypanosoma lewisi* can be made from cultures of the organism.[47]

Complement fixation tests are of especial importance in the diag-

---

[34] A. M. da Cunha and E. Dias, *Brasil-med.*, 53: 89 (1939) ; *Compt. rend. Soc. de biol.*, 129: 991 (1938).

[35] P. Zdrodowski and B. Woskressenski, *Bull. Soc. path. exot.*, 23: 1028 (1930); A. M. da Cunha and E. Dias, *Brasil-med.*, 53: 89 (1939).

[36] A. Georgiewsky, *Pensée Méd. d'Usbékistane et de Turquemenistane*, No. 3: 80 (1927).

[37] L. Nattan-Larrier and L. Grimard, *Bull. Soc. path. exot.*, 28: 658 (1935).

[38] C. Anderson and C. Disdier, *Arch. Inst. Pasteur de Tunis*, 27: 203 (1938).

[39] A. C. Woods and H. H. Morris, *J. Infect. Dis.*, 22: 43 (1918).

[40] H. C. Clark and J. Benavides, *Am. J. Trop. Med.*, 15: 285 (1935).

[41] H. W. Schoening, *J. Infect. Dis.*, 34: 608 (1924).

[42] C. M. Johnson and R. A. Kelser, *Am. J. Trop. Med.*, 17: 385 (1935); J. G. Lacorte, *Acta Med., Rio de Janeiro*, 1: 264 (1938).

[43] J. Marmorston-Gottesman, D. Perla, and J. Vorzimer, *J. Exper. Med.*, 52: 587 (1930).

[44] G. Zottner, *Compt. rend. Soc. de biol.*, 115: 19 (1934).

[45] R. A. Kelser, *Am. J. Trop. Med.*, 16: 405 (1936).

[46] W. Minning, *Arch. f. Schiffs- u. Tropen-Hyg.*, 39: 315 (1935).

[47] J. Marmorston-Gottesman, D. Perla, and J. Vorzimer, *J. Exper. Med.*, 52: 587 (1930).

nosis of such helminth infections as schistosomiasis of man and of animals,[48] echinococcus disease of man and of animals,[49] and human filariasis.[50] Experimentally favorable results have also been obtained in diagnosing fascioliasis of sheep,[51] sparganosis of monkeys,[52] cysticercosis of man,[53] somatic ascariasis,[54] and trichiniasis.[55] The complement fixation test is usually positive somewhat earlier than other antibody reactions because less antibody is required for the reaction to occur.

ADHESIN TESTS

The adhesin reaction has been used in diagnosing leishmaniasis of man and dog,[56] trypanosomiasis,[57] and human filariasis.[58] In the protozoan diseases red cells adhere to the parasite if the adhesin antibody is present; in filariasis the leucocytes adhere to the parasite body. The test is performed in vitro. Serum from the patient or the animal is added to a suspension containing the suspected parasite and the appropriate blood cells. The reaction is as specific as other antigen-antibody reactions.

[48] N. H. Fairley, *Arch. f. Schiffs- u. Tropen-Hyg.*, 30: 372 (1926), and *J. Helminthol.*, 11: 181 (1933); K. D. Fairley and N. H. Fairley, *M. J. Australia*, 2: 597 (1929); S. Miyaji and B. Imai, *Zentralbl. f. Bakt.*, 106: 237 (1928); M. N. Andrews, *J. Helminthol.*, 13: 25 (1935).

[49] K. D. Fairley and C. H. Kellaway, *Australian and New Zealand J. Surg.*, 2: 236 (1933); R. H. Goodale and H. Krischner, *Am. J. Trop. Med.*, 10: 71 (1930).

[50] N. H. Fairley, *Tr. Roy. Soc. Trop. Med. & Hyg.*, 24: 635 (1931), and 25: 220 (1932); R. B. Lloyd and S. N. Chandra, *Indian J. M. Research*, 20: 1197 (1933); L. van Hoof, *Tr. Roy. Soc. Trop. Med. & Hyg.*, 27: 609 (1934); A. Connal, *West African M. J.*, 7: 113 (1934); G. J. Stefanopoulo and J. Daniaud, *Bull. Soc. path. exot.*, 33: 149 (1940).

[51] O. Wagner, *Ztschr. f. Immunitätsforsch. u. exper. Therap.*, 84: 225 (1935).

[52] J. F. Mueller and O. D. Chapman, *J. Parasitol.*, 23: 561 (1937).

[53] W. P. MacArthur, *Tr. Roy. Soc. Trop. Med. & Hyg.*, 26: 525 (1933).

[54] W. K. Blackie, *J. Helminthol.*, 9: 91 (1931); F. Fulleborn and W. Kikuth, *Beih. z. Arch. f. Schiffs- u. Tropen-Hyg.*, 33: 168 (1929).

[55] G. W. Bachman and P. E. Menendez, *J. Prevent. Med.*, 3: 471 (1929).

[56] E. A. Mills and C. Machattie, *Tr. Roy. Soc. Trop. Med. & Hyg.*, 25: 205 (1931); M. T. Balachewa, *Pensée Méd. d'Usbéquistane et de Turquemenistane*, 5: 48 (1930); L. Burowa, *Pensée Méd. d'Usbékistane et de Turquemenistane*, No. 1: 20 (1928).

[57] H. L. Duke and J. M. Wallace, *Parasitology*, 22: 414 (1930); S. Raffel, *Am. J. Hyg.*, 19: 416 (1934); A. F. Brown, *Tr. Roy. Soc. Trop. Med. & Hyg.*, 26: 471 (1933); H. C. Brown and J. C. Broom, *Tr. Roy. Soc. Trop. Med. & Hyg.*, 32: 209 (1938); G. F. T. Saunders, *West African M. J.*, 5: 28 (1931); J. M. Wallace and A. Wormall, *Parasitology*, 23: 346 (1931).

[58] C. G. Pandit, S. R. Pandit, and P. V. S. Iyer, *Indian J. M. Research*, 16: 946 (1929).

SKIN TESTS

Skin tests are especially valuable diagnostic aids because of the simplicity of their performance. A small amount of a suitable antigen injected intracutaneously generally will elicit a local response if the individual is infected with the parasite. Positive skin tests usually are possible by the second or third week after infection. Skin tests have not been generally used with the protozoan infections, but among the helminthiases they have enjoyed widespread success and in some cases general adoption as the diagnostic method of choice.

Skin tests have been tried in experimental amoebiasis of dogs,[59] the leishmaniases of man and dogs,[60] malaria of man and monkeys,[61] and coccidiosis of rodents,[62] among the protozoan diseases, although in no case have particularly favorable results been obtained. The same difficulty is encountered in preparing the antigen from protozoans for the skin test as for other immunological tests. Usually saline extracts of the parasites are preferred to alcoholic extracts.

Among the helminth infections, schistosomiasis,[63] echinococcus disease,[64] trichiniasis,[65] and filariasis [66] are most satisfactorily di-

[59] R. Bieling, *Arch. f. Schiffs- u. Tropen-Hyg.*, 39: 49 (1935).

[60] G. Buss, *Arch. f. Schiffs- u. Tropen-Hyg.*, 33: 65 (1929); A. M. da Cunha, *Rev. med.-cir. do Brasil*, 39: 37 (1930); A. Dostrovsky, *Ann. Trop. Med.*, 29: 123 (1935); G. C. Gasperini, *Arch. ital. di sc. med. colon.*, 18: 430 (1937); B. Malamos, *Arch. f. Schiffs- u. Tropen-Hyg.*, 41: 240 (1937).

[61] O. Herrmann and M. Lifschitz, *Ztschr. f. Immunitätsforsch. u. exper. Therap.*, 65: 240 (1930); M. M. Tschnowitzer and W. D. Moldawskaya-Kritschewskaya, *Trop. Med. and Veterinary*, 9: 261 (1931); J. A. Sinton and H. W. Mulligan, *Indian J. M. Research*, 20: 581, 1932, and *Records Malaria Survey of India*, 3: 323 (1932).

[62] J. Chapman, *Am. J. Hyg.*, 9: 389 (1929); D. P. Henry, *Proc. Soc. Exper. Biol. & Med.*, 28: 831 (1931), and Univ. California, *Publ., Zoology*, 37: 211 (1932).

[63] N. H. Fairley and F. E. Williams, *M. J. Australia*, 2: 811 (1927); W. H. and L. G. Taliaferro, *Porto Rico J. Pub. Health & Trop. Med.*, 7: 23 (1931); H. C. Kan, *China M. J.* (*Suppl. No. 1*), 387 (1936); M. Khalil and A. Hassan, *J. Egyptian M. A.*, 15: 129 (1932).

[64] K. D. Fairley, *M. J. Australia*, 1: 472 (1929); K. D. Fairley and C. H. Kellaway, *Australian and New Zealand J. Surg.*, 2: 236 (1933); R. H. Goodale and H. Krischner, *Am. J. Trop. Med.*, 10: 71 (1930); H. M. Rose and J. T. Culbertson, *J. A. M. A.*, 115: 594 (1940).

[65] G. W. Bachman, *J. Prevent. Med.*, 2: 513 (1928); D. L. Augustine, *New England J. Med.*, 216: 463 (1937); O. R. McCoy, J. J. Miller, Jr., and R. D. Friedlander, *J. Immunol.*, 24: 1 (1933); W. W. Spink, *New England J. Med.*, 216: 5 (1937); A. Trawinski, *Berl. tierärztl. Wchnschr.*, 50: 223 (1934).

[66] W. H. Taliaferro and W. A. Hoffman, *J. Prevent. Med.*, 4: 261 (1930); N. H.

agnosed by the skin test. Experimentally, fascioliasis,[67] cysticercosis of rabbits,[68] ascariasis,[69] hookworm disease,[70] oxyuriasis,[71] and
dracontiasis [72] also can sometimes be identified through skin tests.

Group reactions occur very commonly in these skin tests with
helminth antigens. Often the antigens appear to occur more or less
universally throughout a given class of parasite. For example, practically any species of cestode will serve as the source of antigen for
the skin test in echinococcus disease,[73] and *Ascaris lumbricoides*
supplies antigens which elicit a reaction in many of the nematodiases.[74] Furthermore, an extract of any schistosome [75] or even of the
cattle liver fluke, *Fasciola gigantica*,[76] will serve in the skin test for
human schistosomiasis, and an extract of the dog filarid, *Dirofilaria
immitis*,[77] or of *Contortospiculum rheae*,[78] is suitable for identifying any of the human filariases. However, the best antigen for skin
tests in any infection generally is obtained from the homologous
parasite, for although strong cross reactions may occur with antigens from heterologous forms they are usually less intense than
those to antigens from the homologous parasite. Either larval or
adult parasites can be used, however, for preparing the skin-testing
antigen, since the antigenic constitution of larval and adult parasites is the same. The antigen for schistosomiasis in man, for example, is usually obtained from the liver of a snail heavily infected

---

Fairley, *Tr. Roy. Soc. Trop. Med. & Hyg.*, 25: 220 (1932); J. Rodhain and A.
Dubois, *Tr. Roy. Soc. Trop. Med. & Hyg.*, 25: 377 (1932).
   [67] H. K. Sievers and R. Oyarzun, *Compt. rend. Soc. de biol.*, 110: 630 (1932);
O. Wagner, *Ztschr. f. Immunitätsforsch. u. exper. Therap.*, 84: 225 (1935).
   [68] D. R. A. Wharton, *Am. J. Hyg.*, 14: 477 (1931).
   [69] E. M. Konus and S. A. Gakoubovitch, *Med. Par. and Parasit. Diseases*, 6:
107 (1937); W. Schoenfeld, *Arch. f. Dermat. u. Syph.*, 175: 54 (1937).
   [70] G. W. Bachman and R. Rodriguez Molina, *Am. J. Trop. Med.*, 12: 279 (1932),
and *Porto Rico J. Pub. Health & Trop. Med.*, 7: 287 (1932).
   [71] W. H. Wright and J. Bozicevich, *J. Parasitol.*, 23: 562 (1937); H. Tsuchiya
and T. C. Bauerlein, *J. Lab. & Clin. Med.*, 24: 627 (1939).
   [72] G. W. St. C. Ramsay, *Tr. Roy. Soc. Trop. Med. & Hyg.*, 28: 399 (1935).
   [73] J. T. Culbertson and H. M. Rose, *J. Clin. Investigation*, 20: 249 (1941).
   [74] M. Brunner, *J. Immunol.*, 15: 83 (1928); J. Rodhain and A. Dubois, *Rev.
belge de sc. méd.*, 3: 613 (1931).
   [75] N. H. Fairley, *J. Helminthol.*, 11: 181 (1933); N. H. Fairley and F. Jasudasan,
Indian Med. Research Mem., Suppl. to Indian J. M. Research (1930); M. Khalil
and A. Hassan, *J. Egyptian M. A.*, 15: 129 (1932).
   [76] A. Hassan and M. Betashe, *J. Egyptian M. A.*, 17: 991 (1934).
   [77] W. H. Taliaferro and W. A. Hoffman, *J. Prevent. Med.*, 4: 261 (1930); N. H.
Fairley, *Tr. Roy. Soc. Trop. Med. & Hyg.*, 24: 635 (1931).
   [78] W. Mohr and H. Lippelt, *Klin. Wchnschr.*, 19: 157 (1940).

with the sporocysts and cercariae of a mammalian schistosome. Likewise, antigen for diagnosing hydatid disease in man can be obtained from either larval or adult related taenias.

Two types of skin reaction frequently occur in man: an immediate response and a delayed reaction. The immediate response is of the type seen in hay fever allergies, with a distinct wheal and erythema developing about the inoculated site. It reaches its greatest intensity within ten to fifteen minutes and fades quickly thereafter. The delayed reaction is an Arthus type of response. It begins in half-an-hour or so and may not reach its peak for three or four hours or even longer. Often it persists for from twenty-four to forty-eight hours. The delayed reaction alone is generally seen in positive skin tests in animals.

Skin tests often remain positive for many years after infection with the helminths, even after apparent cure of the disease by drugs, as in schistosomiasis,[79] or after the surgical removal of the parasite, as in hydatid disease.[80] As already mentioned, skin tests have been reported in trichiniasis as long as nine years after infection.[81]

[79] N. H. Fairley and F. E. Williams, *M. J. Australia,* 2: 811 (1927) ; P. Manson-Bahr, *J. Helminthol.,* 7: 99 (1929) ; M. Khalil and A. Hassan, *J. Egyptian M. A.,* 15: 129 (1932).

[80] C. H. Kellaway and K. D. Fairley, *M. J. Australia,* 19th year: 340 (1932) ; E. von Bassewitz and B. von Bassewitz, *Brasil-med.,* 43: 1138 (1929).

[81] H. Theiler, D. L. Augustine, and W. W. Spink, *Parasitology,* 27: 345 (1935).

ABBREVIATIONS OF NAMES
OF PERIODICALS

This list has been compiled largely from Morris Fishbein, *Medical Writing*, Chicago, Press of American Medical Association, 1938.

Acta leidensia scholae med. trop.—Acta leidensia scholae medicinae tropicase. Leiden, Netherlands.

Acta med. Rio de Janeiro.—Acta medica. Rio de Janeiro.

Acta med. Scandinav.—Acta medica Scandinavica. Stockholm.

Am. J. Cancer.—American Journal of Cancer. New York.

Am. J. Clin. Path.—American Journal of Clinical Pathology. Baltimore.

Am. J. Hyg.—American Journal of Hygiene. Baltimore.

Am. J. M. Sc.—American Journal of the Medical Sciences. Philadelphia.

Am. J. Pub. Health.—American Journal of Public Health and the Nation's Health. New York.

Am. J. Trop. Med.—American Journal of Tropical Medicine. Baltimore.

Anales Inst. biol. Univ. México.—Anales del Instituto de biología. Universidade de México. Mexico.

Anat. Rec.—Anatomical Record. Philadelphia.

Ann. de méd.—Annales de médicine. Paris.

Ann. de parasitol.—Annales de parasitologie humaine et comparée. Paris.

Ann. Inst. Past.—Annales de l'Institut Pasteur. Paris.

Ann. Soc. belge de méd. trop.—Annales de la Société belge de médicine tropicae. Brussels.

Ann. Trop. Med.—Annals of Tropical Medicine and Parasitology. Liverpool.

Arb. a. d. Staatsinst. f. exper. Therap.—Arbeiten aus dem Staatsinstitut für experimentelle Therapie und dem Georg Speyer-Hause zu Frankfort a M. Jena.

Arch. de med. inf.—Archivos de medicina infantil. Habana.

Arch. Dermat. & Syph.—Archives of Dermatology and Syphilology. Chicago.

Arch. f. Dermat. u. Syph.—Archiv für Dermatologie und Syphilis. Berlin.

Arch. f. exper. Path. u. Pharmakol.—Naunyn-Schmiedebergs Archiv für experimentelle Pathologie und Pharmakologie. Berlin.

Arch. f. Schiffs- u. Tropen-Hyg.—Archiv für Schiffs- und Tropen-Hygiene. Leipzig.

Arch. Inst. Pasteur d'Algerie.—Archives de l'Institut Pasteur d'Algerie. Algiers.

Arch. Inst. Pasteur de Tunis.—Archives de l'Institut de Tunis. Tunis.

Arch. internat. de méd. expér.—Archives internationales de médicine expérimentale. Liége.

Arch. Int. Med.—Archives of Internal Medicine. Chicago.

Arch. ital. di sc. med. colon.—Archivio italiano di scienze mediche coloniae. Modena.

Arch. Path.—Archives of Pathology and Laboratory Medicine. Chicago.

Arch. roumaines de path. expér. et de microbiol.—Archives roumaines de pathologie expérimentale et de microbiologie. Paris.

Australian and New Zealand J. Surg.—Australian and New Zealand Journal of Surgery. Sydney.

Australian Vet. J.—Australian Veterinary Journal. Sydney.

Berl. tierärztl. Wchnschr.—Berliner tierärztliche Wochenschrift. Berlin.

Biol. Bull.—The Biological Bulletin. Lancaster, Pa.

Boll. d. Ist. sieroterap. milanese.—Bolletino dell'Istituto sieroterapica milanese. Milan.

Brasil-med.—Brasil-medico. Rio de Janeiro.

Bull. Acad. de méd., Paris.—Bulletin de l'Académie de médicine. Paris.

Bull. agric. Congo belge.—Bulletin agricole de Congo belge. Brussels.

Bull. de l'Acad. vet. de France.—Bulletin de l'Académie veterinaire de France. Paris.

Bull. et mém. Soc. méd. hôp. de Paris.—Bulletins et mémoires de la Société médicale des hôpitaux de Paris.

Bull. Neur. Inst. New York.—Bulletin of the Neurological Institute of New York. New York.

Bull. Soc. méd.-chir. de l'Indochine.—Bulletin de la Société médico-chirurgicale de l'Indochine. Hanoi.

Bull. Soc. path. exot.—Bulletin de la Société de pathologie exotique. Paris.

Canad. J. Research.—Canadian Journal of Research. Ottawa.

Canad. M. A. J.—Canadian Medical Association Journal. Montreal.

Centralbl. f. Bakt.—Centralblatt für Bakteriologie, Parasitenkunde, und Infektionskrankheiten. Jena.

Centralbl. f. Bakt., Ref.—Centralblatt für Bakteriologie, Parasitenkunde, und Infektionskrankheiten, Referate. Jena.

China M. J.—China Medical Journal. Shanghai.

Chinese M. J.—Chinese Medical Journal. Peiping.

Compt. rend. Acad. de sc.—Comptes rendus hebdomodaires des seances de l'Académie des sciences. Paris.

Compt. rend. Soc. de biol.—Comptes rendus de la Société de biologie. Paris.

Dermat. Wchnschr.—Dermatologische Wochenschrift. Leipzig.

Deutsche med. Wchnschr.—Deutsche medizinische Wochenschrift. Leipzig.

Deutsche Ztschr. f. Nervenh.—Deutsche Zeitschrift für Nervenheilkunde. Berlin.

Emp. J. Exp. Agric.—Empire Journal of Experimental Agriculture. Oxford.

Ergebn. d. Hyg., Bakt., Immunitätsforsch., u. exper. Therap.—Ergebnisse der Hygiene, Bakteriologie, Immunitätsforschung und experimentellen Therapie. Berlin.

Folia clin., chim., et micr.—Folia clinica, chimica, et microscopica. Bologna.

Fortschr. d. Med.—Fortschritte der Medizin. Berlin.

Fukuoka acta med.—Fukuoka acta medica. Fukuoka.

Fukuoka-Ikwadaigaku-Zasshi., see Fukuoka acta med.

Gazz. d. osp.—Gazzetta degli ospedali e delle cliniche. Milan.

Geneesk. tijdschr. v. Nederl.-Indië.—Geneeskundig tijdschrift voor Nederlandsch-Indië. Batavia.

Gior. di batteriol. e immunol.—Giornale di batteriologia e immunologia. Turin.

Gior. di clin. med.—Giornale di clinica medica. Parma.

Haematologica.—Haematologica Archivo. Catania.

Indian J. M. Research.—Indian Journal of Medical Research. Calcutta.

Indian J. Pediat.—Indian Journal of Pediatrics. Calcutta.

Indian M. Gaz.—Indian Medical Gazette. Calcutta.

Iowa State Coll. J. Sci.—Iowa State College Journal of Science. Ames.

J. A. M. A.—Journal of the American Medical Association. Chicago.

J. Agric. Res.—Journal of Agricultural Research. Washington, D.C.

J. Allergy.—The Journal of Allergy. St. Louis.

J. Am. Vet. M. A.—Journal of the American Veterinary Medical Association. Chicago.

Japan M. World.—Japan Medical World. Tokyo.

Jap. J. Derm. & Urol.—Japanese Journal of Dermatology and Urology. Tokyo.

Jap. J. Exper. Med.—Japanese Journal of Experimental Medicine. Tokyo.

J. Clin. Investigation.—Journal of Clinical Investigation. New York.

J. Egyptian M. A.—Journal of the Egyptian Medical Association. Cairo.

J. Exper. Med.—Journal of Experimental Medicine. New York.

J. Helminthol.—Journal of Helminthology. St. Albans.

J. Hyg.—Journal of Hygiene. London.

J. Immunol.—Journal of Immunology. Baltimore.

J. Infect. Dis.—Journal of Infectious Diseases. Chicago.

J. Lab. & Clin. Med.—Journal of Laboratory and Clinical Medicine. St. Louis.

J. M. A. Formosa.—Journal of the Medical Association of Formosa.

J. Malaria Institute of India.—Journal of the Malaria Institute of India. Calcutta.

J. Orient. Med.—The Journal of Oriental Medicine. Mukden.

J. Parasitol.—Journal of Parasitology. Baltimore.

J. Path. & Bact.—Journal of Pathology and Bacteriology. Edinburgh.

J. Pediat.—The Journal of Pediatrics. St. Louis.

J. Prevent. Med.—Journal of Preventive Medicine. Baltimore.

J. Trop. Med.—Journal of Tropical Medicine and Hygiene. London.

J. Washington Acad. Sci.—Journal of the Washington Academy of Sciences. Washington, D.C.

Kenya & East African M. J.—Kenya and East African Medical Journal. Kenya.

Klin. Wchnschr.—Klinische Wochenschrift. Berlin.

Lancet.—Lancet. London.

Marseille-méd.—Marseille-médical. Marseille.

Maryland State Coll. Agric., Bull.—Bulletin of the Maryland State College of Agriculture. College Park.

M. Clin. North America.—The Medical Clinics of North America. Philadelphia.

Med. paises cálidos.—Medicina de los paises cálidos. Madrid.

Med. Par. and Parasit. Dis.—Medical Parasitology and Parasitic Diseases. Moscow.

Mem. Inst. Oswaldo Cruz.—Memorias do Instituto Oswaldo Cruz. Rio de Janeiro.

M. J. Australia.—Medical Journal of Australia. Sydney.

München. med. Wchnschr.—Münchener medizinische Wochenschrift. Munich.

München. tierärzt. Wchnschr.—Münchener tierärztliche Wochenschrift. Munich.

Nachr. d. trop. Med.—Nachrichten der tropischen Medizin. Tiflis.

Nat. M. J. China.—National Medical Journal of China. Shanghai.

Nature. London.—Nature. London.

Nederl. tijdschr. v. geneesk.—Nederlandsch tijdschrift voor geneeskunde. Amsterdam.

New England J. Med.—New England Journal of Medicine. Boston.

Parasitology.—Parasitology. London.

Pathologica.—Pathologica; rivista mensile. Genoa.

Pediatria.—La pediatria; rivista mensile di medicina e di chirurgia dell'-infanzia. Naples.

Pensée méd. d'Usbéquistane et de Turquemenistane.—Pensée médicale d'Usbéquistane et de Turquemenistane. Tashkent.

Philippine J. Sc.—Philippine Journal of Science. Manila.

Policlinico.—Il policlinico. Rome.

Porto Rico Rev. Pub. Health and Trop. Med.—Porto Rico Review of Public Health and Tropical Medicine. San Juan.

Poult. Sci.—Poultry Science. Ithaca, N.Y.

Presse méd.—La Presse médicale. Paris.

Proc. Helminthol. Soc. Washington.—Proceedings of the Helminthological Society of Washington. Washington, D.C.

Proc. Int. Vet. Congr., N.Y.—Proceedings of the Twelfth International Veterinary Congress. New York.

Proc. Nat. Acad. Sc.—Proceedings of the National Academy of Sciences. Washington, D.C.

Proc. Roy. Soc., London. s.B.—Proceedings of the Royal Society, series B (Biological Sciences). London.

Proc. Roy. Soc. Med.—Proceedings of the Royal Society of Medicine. London.

Proc. Soc. Exper. Biol. & Med.—Proceedings of the Society for Experimental Biology and Medicine. Utica.

Proc. Third Internat. Congr. Microbiol.—Proceedings of the Third International Congress for Microbiology. New York.

Proc. Transvaal Mine Med. Officers' Assoc.—Proceedings Transvaal Mine Medical Officers' Association. Johannesburg.

Pub. Health Rep.—Public Health Reports. Washington, D.C.

Puerto Rico J. Pub. Health & Trop. Med.—Puerto Rico Journal of Public Health and Tropical Medicine. San Juan.

Records Egypt. Gov. School Med., Cairo.—Records of the Egyptian Government School of Medicine. Cairo.

Records Malaria Survey of India.—Records of the Malaria Survey of India. Calcutta.

Rev. belge sc. méd.—Revue belge des sciences médicales. Louvain.

Rev. de med. trop. y parasitol., bacteriol., clín. y lab.—Revista de medicina tropical y parasitologia, bacteriologia, clínica y laboratorio. Habana.

Rev. Gastroenterol.—The Review of Gastroenterology. New York.

Rev. med.-cir. do Brasil.—Revista medico-cirurgica do Brasil. Rio de Janeiro.

Rev. mexic. de biol.—Revista mexicana de biologia. Mexico.

Rev. sud.-am. de méd. et de chir.—Revue sud-americaine de médecine et de chirurgie. Paris.

Riforma med.—La riforma medica. Naples.

Riv. di malariol.—Rivisita di malariologia. Rome.

Riv. di parassitol.—Rivista di parassitologia. Rome.

Riv. di patol. e clin. d. tuberc.—Rivista di patologia e clinica della tuberculosi. Bologna.

Rozprawy biolog.—Rozprawy biologiczne. Lemberg.

Sang.—Le Sang. Paris.

Schweiz. med. Wchnschr.—Schweizerische medizinische Wochenschrift. Basel.

Science.—Science. New York.

Scientific Agric.—Scientific Agriculture. Gardenvale, P.Q.

Sei-I-Kai M. J.—Sei-I-Kai Medical Journal. Tokyo.

Soc. internaz. di microbiol., Boll. d. sez. ital.—Societa internazionale di microbiologia. Bolletina della sezione italiana. Milan.

South African Med. Record.—South African Medical Record. Cape Town.

South. M. J.—Southern Medical Journal. Birmingham, Ala.

Tierärztl. Rundschau.—Tierärztliche Rundschau. Berlin.

Tijdschr. v. Diergeneesk.—Tijdschrift voor diergeneeskunde. Utrecht, Amsterdam.

Tr. Am. Micr. Soc.—Transactions of the American Microscopical Society. Manhattan, Kan.

Tr. Dynamics of Develop.—Transactions on the Dynamics of Development. Moscow.

Tr. Far Eastern Assoc. Trop. Med.—Transactions of Congresses of the Far Eastern Association of Tropical Medicine. Singapore.

Trop. Med. and Veterinary.—Tropical Medicine and Veterinary. Moscow.

Tr. Roy. Soc. Trop. Med. & Hyg.—Transactions of the Royal Society of Tropical Medicine and Hygiene. London.

Tr. Third Internat. Congr. Trop. Med. & Malaria.—Transactions of the Third International Congress of Tropical Medicine and Malaria. Amsterdam.

Univ. California Publ., Zool.—University of California Publications in Zoology. Berkeley.

Vet. Med.—Veterinary Medicine. Chicago.

Virginia Agric. Exper. Sta., Tech. Bull.—Virginia Agricultural Experiment Station, Technical Bulletin. Blacksburg.

Vol. Jubil. pro Prof. S. Yoshida.—Volumen Jubilare pro Professor Sadao Yoshida. Osaka.

West African M. J.—West African Medical Journal. Lagos.

Wisconsin Agric. Exp. Sta., Bull.—Bulletin of the Wisconsin Agricultural Experiment Station. Madison.

Yale J. Biol. & Med.—Yale Journal of Biology and Medicine. New Haven.

Zentralbl. f. Bakt.—Zentralblatt für Bakteriologie, Parasitenkunde und Infektionskrankheiten. Jena.

Zool. anzeiger.—Zoologischer anzeiger. Leipzig.

Zoologica.—Zoologica. New York.

Ztschr. f. Fleisch- u. Milch-Hyg.—Zeitschrift für Fleisch- und Milch-Hygiene. Berlin.

Ztschr. f. Hyg. u. Infektionskr.—Zeitschrift für Hygiene und Infektionskrankheiten. Berlin.

Ztschr. f. Immunitätsforsch. u. exper. Therap.—Zeitschrift für Immunitätsforschung und experimentelle Therapie. Jena.

Ztschr. f. Infektionskr.—Zeitschrift für Infektionskrankheiten, parasitare Krankheiten und Hygiene der Haustiere. Berlin.

Ztschr. f. Parasitenk.—Zeitschrift für Parasitenkunde. Berlin.

INDEX